ADVANCES IN NEUROLOGY

Volume 41

Advances in Neurology

Advances in Neurology
Volume 41

The Olivopontocerebellar Atrophies

Editors

Roger C. Duvoisin, M.D.
Professor and Chairman
Department of Neurology
University of Medicine and
Dentistry of New Jersey
Rutgers Medical School
Academic Health Science Center
New Brunswick, New Jersey

Andreas Plaitakis, M.D.
Associate Professor
of Neurology
Department of Neurology
Mount Sinai School of Medicine
City University of New York
New York, New York

Raven Press ■ New York

Raven Press, 1140 Avenue of the Americas, New York, New York 10036

Made in the United States of America

Library of Congress Cataloging in Publication Data

Main entry under title:

The Olivopontocerebellar atrophies.

(Advances in neurology ; v. 41)
Includes bibliographical references and index.
1. Olivopontocerebellar atrophies. I. Duvoisin,
Roger C., 1927– . II. Plaitakis, Andreas.
III. Series. [DNLM: 1. Atrophy. 2. Cerebellum—pathology.
3. Olivary Nucleus—pathology. 4. Pons—pathology.
W1 AD684H v.41 / WL 310 049]
RC321.A276 vol. 41 616.8s [616.8′3] 84-9861
[RC394.045]
ISBN 0-89004-958-0

The material contained in this volume was submitted as previously unpublished material, except in the instances in which credit has been given to the source from which some of the illustrative material was derived.

Great care has been taken to maintain the accuracy of the information contained in the volume. However, Raven Press cannot be held responsible for errors or for any consequences arising from the use of the information contained herein.

Advances in Neurology Series

Vol. 41: The Olivopontocerebellar Atrophies
R. C. Duvoisin and A. Plaitakis, editors. 304 pp., 1984.

Vol. 40: Parkinson-Specific Motor and Mental Disorders, Role of the Pallidum: Pathophysiological, Biochemical, and Therapeutic Aspects
R. G. Hassler and J. F. Christ, editors. 601 pp., 1984.

Vol. 39: Motor Control Mechanisms in Health and Disease
J. E. Desmedt, editor. 1,224 pp., 1983.

Vol. 38: The Dementias
R. Mayeux and W. G. Rosen, editors. 288 pp., 1983.

Vol. 37: Experimental Therapeutics of Movement Disorders
S. Fahn, D. B. Calne, and I. Shoulson, editors. 339 pp., 1983.

Vol. 36: Human Motor Neuron Diseases
L. P. Rowland, editor. 592 pp., 1982.

Vol. 35: Gilles de la Tourette Syndrome
A. J. Friedhoff and T. N. Chase, editors. 476 pp., 1982.

Vol. 34: Status Epilepticus: Mechanisms of Brain Damage and Treatment
A. V. Delgado-Escueta, C. G. Wasterlain, D. M. Treiman, and R. J. Porter, editors. 579 pp., 1983.

Vol. 33: Headache: Physiopathological and Clinical Concepts
M. Critchley, A. Friedman, S. Gorini, and F. Sicuteri, editors. 417 pp., 1982.

Vol. 32: Clinical Applications of Evoked Potentials in Neurology
J. Courjon, F. Mauguiere, and M. Revol, editors. 592 pp., 1982.

Vol. 31: Demyelinating Diseases: Basic and Clinical Electrophysiology
S. Waxman and J. Murdoch Ritchie, editors. 544 pp., 1981.

Vol. 30: Diagnosis and Treatment of Brain Ischemia
A. L. Carney and E. M. Anderson, editors. 424 pp., 1981.

Vol. 29: Neurofibromatosis
V. M. Riccardi and J. J. Mulvihill, editors. 288 pp., 1981.

Vol. 28: Brain Edema
J. Cervós-Navarro and R. Ferszt, editors. 539 pp., 1980.

Vol. 27: Antiepileptic Drugs: Mechanisms of Action
G.H. Glaser, J.K. Penry, and D.M. Woodbury, editors. 728 pp., 1980.

Vol. 26: Cerebral Hypoxia and Its Consequences
S. Fahn, J.N. Davis, and L.P. Rowland, editors. 454 pp., 1979.

Vol. 25: Cerebrovascular Disorders and Stroke
M. Goldstein, L. Bolis, C. Fieschi, S. Gorini, and C.H. Millikan, editors. 412 pp., 1979.

Vol. 24: The Extrapyramidal System and Its Disorders
L.J. Poirier, T.L. Sourkes, and P. Bédard, editors. 552 pp., 1979.

Vol. 23: Huntington's Chorea
T.N. Chase, N.S. Wexler, and A. Barbeau, editors. 864 pp., 1979.

Vol. 22: Complications of Nervous System Trauma
R.A. Thompson and J.R. Green, editors. 454 pp., 1979.

Vol. 21: The Inherited Ataxias: Biochemical, Viral, and Pathological Studies
R.A. Kark, R. Rosenberg, and L. Schut, editors. 450 pp., 1978.

Vol. 20: Pathology of Cerebrospinal Microcirculation
J. Cervós-Navarro, E. Betz, G. Ebhardt, R. Ferszt, and R. Wüllenweber, editors. 636 pp., 1978.

Vol. 19: Neurological Epidemiology: Principles and Clinical Applications
Bruce S. Schoenberg, editor. 672 pp., 1978.

Vol. 18: Hemi-Inattention and Hemisphere Specialization
E.A. Weinstein and R.P. Friedland, editors. 176 pp., 1977.

Vol. 17: Treatment of Neuromuscular Diseases
R.C. Griggs and R.T. Moxley, editors. 370 pp., 1977.

Vol. 16: Stroke
R.A. Thompson and J.R. Green, editors. 250 pp., 1977.

Vol. 15: Neoplasia in the Central Nervous System
R.A. Thompson and J.R. Green, editors. 393 pp., 1976.

Vol. 14: Dystonia
R. Eldridge and S. Fahn, editors. 509 pp., 1976.

Vol. 13: Current Reviews
W.J. Friedlander, editor. 400 pp., 1975.

Vol. 12: Physiology and Pathology of Dendrites
G.W. Kreutzberg, editor. 524 pp., 1975.

Vol. 11: Complex Partial Seizures and Their Treatment
J.K. Penry and D.D. Daly, editors. 486 pp., 1975.

Vol. 10: Primate Models of Neurological Disorders
B.S. Meldrum and C.D. Marsden, editors. 270 pp., 1975.

Vol. 9: Dopaminergic Mechanisms
D.B. Calne, T.N. Chase, and A. Barbeau, editors. 452 pp., 1975.

Vol. 8: Neurosurgical Management of the Epilepsies
D.P. Purpura, J.K. Penry, and R.D. Walter, editors. 369 pp., 1975.

Vol. 7: Current Reviews of Higher Nervous System Dysfunction
W.J. Friedlander, editor. 202 pp., 1975.

Vol. 6: Infectious Diseases of the Central Nervous System
R.A. Thompson and J.R. Green, editors. 401 pp., 1974.

Vol. 5: Second Canadian-American Conference on Parkinson's Disease
F. McDowell and A. Barbeau, editors. 525 pp., 1974.

Vol. 4: International Symposium on Pain
J.J. Bonica, editor. 858 pp., 1974.

Vol. 3: Progress in the Treatment of Parkinsonism
D.B. Calne, editor. 402 pp., 1973.

Vol. 2: The Treatment of Parkinsonism—The Role of DOPA Decarboxylase Inhibitors
M.D. Yahr, editor. 303 pp., 1973.

Vol. 1: Huntington's Chorea, 1872–1972
A. Barbeau, T.N. Chase, and G.W. Paulson, editors. 901 pp., 1973.

In Memoriam

RICHARD A. BERENBERG, M.D.

The Editors note with regret the untimely death of our colleague and fellow contributor on March 26, 1984, prior to the publication of this volume.

Preface

Formerly a rare and obscure condition rarely diagnosed in living patients and chiefly the concern of the pathologist and the nosologist, olivopontocerebellar atrophy (OPCA) has become in recent years a familiar clinical syndrome comprising a large heterogenous group of morbid entities sharing common clinical and pathological features. The "splitters" have won over the "lumpers," and we must now speak of the olivopontocerebellar *atrophies*.

Neurologists, as well as their radiological colleagues, are increasingly recognizing the OPCAs on clinical grounds by the characteristic pattern of brain stem and cerebellar atrophy on computed tomography scans. New forms of OPCA have been identified, and manifestations that were previously unrecognized have been described; for example, disturbances in ocular motility and peripheral neuropathy. Others, such as parkinsonism, that were poorly appreciated, have been given new emphasis.

Less than a decade ago, P. J. Vinken and G. W. Bruy noted in their foreword to Volumes 21 and 22 of the *Handbook of Clinical Neurology* (Elsevier/North Holland, Amsterdam, 1975) that "the study of system degenerations has not progressed much beyond the description level." Within a few years, the situation has changed. Recent biochemical investigations have identified additional new entities and provided fresh and previously unsuspected insights into pathogenesis; they have also raised the possibility of developing appropriate therapies and means of prevention.

In short, a long-neglected subject is stirring with the ferment of new discoveries and changing concepts. In this volume, the OPCAs are critically assessed with regard to their clinical, pathological, radiological, and physiological characteristics in the light of the new knowledge. The traditional problem of the classification of these disorders is reconsidered. Several chapters are devoted to specific biochemical defects which have recently been identified in some of these afflictions—a central issue in the evolving OPCA story.

We are grateful to the various investigatiors in the field who consented to join us in the endeavor to bring these new developments to more general attention. The fruit of their labor is the collection of papers comprising this volume. We hope it will prove helpful to our colleagues in clinical neurology and related fields who diagnose and provide care to the patients afflicted with this important group of neurodegenerative disorders.

ROGER C. DUVOISIN
ANDREAS PLAITAKIS

Contents

Contributors

Kevin D. Barron, M.D., *Department of Neurology, Albany Medical College of Union University, Albany, New York 12208*

Richard A. Berenberg, M.D., *Department of Neurology, Northwestern University Medical School, 303 East Chicago Avenue, Chicago, Illinois 60611*

Louis R. Caplan, M.D., *Department of Neurology, Michael Reese Hospital and Medical Center, Lake Shore Drive at 31st Street, Chicago, Illinois 60616*

Sudhansu Chokroverty, M.B.B.S, F.R.C.P., F.A.C.P., *Department of Neurology, University of Medicine and Dentistry of New Jersey, Rutgers Medical School, Academic Health Science Center, CN 19, New Brunswick, New Jersey 08903*

Robert D. Currier, M.D., *Department of Neurology, The University of Mississippi Medical Center, 2500 North State Street, Jackson, Mississippi 39216*

Roger C. Duvoisin, M.D., *Department of Neurology, University of Medicine and Dentistry of New Jersey, Rutgers Medical School, Academic Health Science Center, CN 19, New Brunswick, New Jersey 08903*

Christopher G. Goetz, M.D., *Department of Neurological Sciences, Rush Presbyterian St. Luke's Medical Center, 1753 West Congress Parkway, Chicago, Illinois 60612*

Donald H. Harter, M.D., *Department of Neurology, Northwestern University Medical School, 303 East Chicago Avenue, Chicago, Illinois 60611*

George F. Howard III, M.D., *Department of Neurology, Boston University Medical School, 80 East Concord Street, Boston, Massachusetts 02118*

Yun Peng Huang, M.D., *Department of Radiology, Neuroradiology Section, Mount Sinai School of Medicine, City University of New York, One Gustave L. Levy Place, New York, New York 10029*

Harold L. Klawans, M.D., *Department of Neurological Sciences, Rush Presbyterian St. Luke's Medical Center, 1753 West Congress Parkway, Chicago, Illinois 60612*

Arnulf H. Koeppen, M.D., *Department of Neurology, Albany Medical College of Union University, and Neurology Service, Veterans Administration Medical Center, Albany, New York 12208*

Frederick E. Lepore, M.D., *Department of Neurology, University of Medicine and Dentistry of New Jersey, Rutgers Medical School, Academic Health Science Center, CN 19, New Brunswick, New Jersey 08903*

Shoichi Maruyama, M.D., *Department of Neurology, Neurological Institute, Tokyo Women's Medical College, 10 Kawada-cho, Shinjuku-ku, Tokyo, Japan*

Onur Melen, M.D., *Department of Ophthalmology, Northwestern University Medical School, 303 East Chicago Avenue, Chicago, Illinois 60611*

Hirotaro Narabayashi, M.D., *Department of Neurology, Juntendo University School of Medicine, Hongo, Bunkyo-ku, Tokyo 113, Japan*

William J. Nicklas, Ph.D., *Department of Neurology, University of Medicine and Dentistry of New Jersey, Rutgers Medical School, P.O. Box 101, Piscataway, New Jersey 08854*

Thomas L. Perry, M.D., *Department of Pharmacology, Faculty of Medicine, University of British Columbia, 2176 Health Sciences Mall, Vancouver, British Columbia, Canada V6T 1W5*

Andreas Plaitakis, M.D., *Department of Neurology, Mount Sinai School of Medicine, City University of New York, One Gustave L. Levy Place, New York, New York 10029*

Roger N. Rosenberg, M.D., *Department of Neurology, University of Texas Health Science Center at Dallas, Southwestern Medical School, 535 Harry Hines Blvd., Dallas, Texas 75235*

Caroline M. Tanner, M.D., *Department of Neurological Sciences, Rush Presbyterian St. Luke's Medical Center, 1753 West Congress Parkway, Chicago, Illinois 60612*

N. H. Wadia, M.D., F.R.C.P., F.N.A.M.S., F.A.Sc., *Ben Nevis, B. Desai Road, Bombay 400 036, India*

Tomoko Yamaguchi, M.D., *Department of Biochemistry, Tokyo Women's Medical College, 10-Kawada-cho, Shinjuku-ku, Tokyo, Japan*

The Olivopontocerebellar Atrophies

The Olivopontocerebellar Atrophies, edited by
R. C. Duvoisin and A. Plaitakis. Raven Press,
New York © 1984.

A Classification for Ataxia

R. D. Currier

*Department of Neurology, The University of Mississippi Medical Center,
Jackson, Mississippi 39216*

This chapter is presented with apologies to Barbeau, Bell and Carmichael, Brouwer and Biemond, Eadie, Greenfield, Harding, Holmes, Konigsmark and Weiner, Netsky, Plaitakis, Schut, Sjögren, Sobue, Zülch, and others who previously have attempted the clarification of chaos.

The Editors of this volume have kindly requested a summary of our investigative efforts in the dominant forms of ataxia, a work that is not yet ready for definitive publication. A tentative classification of the ataxias is presented with the thought that it should be truly tentative and subject to alteration in line with subsequent comments and criticisms.

Twenty years ago, we innocently hoped it would be possible to carry on research in the area without either a thorough reading of the literature or the existence of an acceptable classification. These hopes were worksaving at the time but were delusions which are now no longer tenable. An expansion of research recently has forced a consideration of the continuing necessity of a useful, modern classification of the ataxias. Scientific discoveries are being related to types of ataxia which may or may not be consistent with the reader's understanding of that particular type, and a common frame of reference is needed.

The decision was made to review the world literature on ataxia and to attempt a new classification based on that and our own clinical experience. Although only one-third of the review task is completed, an outline has begun to form. It is presented not as a solution but as an evolving entity which will be published again in one or two years. Meanwhile, we hope that comments for improvement will be made. A review of the variables used to construct previous classifications is summarized in Table 1.

Ultimately, of course, the definition of a chemical abnormality for each subtype of ataxia will enable a correct and final classification. A temporary and generally agreed upon structure is necessary, however; thus the physician encountering a new case, after evaluating the family history and examining the patient, can tentatively assign the patient to a position in which he can be compared with other reported cases.

Previous classifications have used clinical signs, pathologic examination, signs of involvement of other systems, and the hereditary type nearly exclusively in forming reference frames.

TABLE 1. *Variables used in previous classifications*

Heredity
Dominant
Recessive
X-linked
Unknown (sporadic)
Pathology
OPCA
Spinopontine
Cerebelloolivary
Joseph disease (basal ganglia)
Spinocerebellar
Many others
Pathology related to other systems
Gonadal
Skeletal
Others
Clinical signs and symptoms
Signs and symptoms
Reflexes
Extrapyramidal
Sensory
Anterior horn cell
Peripheral nerve
Retina (optic nerve)
Auditory
Dementia
Others
Age of onset
Infantile or congenital
Young
Middle age
Old age
Progression rate
Fast
Usual or normal
Slow, indolent
Nonprogressive
Intermittent
Race (geography)
White, Black, Indian, etc.
Scandinavian, Azorean, French, German, Japanese, etc.
Chemistry (Genetic)
Chemical
GDH abnormality
Malic enzyme
Other chemical abnormalities (aspartate, etc.)
Genetic
Linked versus not linked on 6th chromosome
Other linkage (X-linked)

The clinical symptom-sign complex in a kindred, although fairly consistent, usually shows some variation from patient to patient, a variation that may allow errors if it has first priority in the classification scheme. The pathoanatomic substrate was long hoped to be, and may eventually be, a useful classification tool; but some attempts have been misleading, sometimes due to inadequate sampling of

TABLE 2. *A tentative classification of ataxia*

I. Stationary or nonprogressive ataxias
Congenital: cerebral palsy
Injury: anoxia, stroke, heat, nutrition, toxic
II. Intermittent subtypes (very rare)
III. Progressive ataxias
A. Secondary: cancer, MS, thyroid, seizures, others
B. Sporadic: idiopathic (exist?)
C. Hereditary: primary
1. Common types
a. Dominant heredity
(1) Usual age (20–50 yr) of onset (OPCA)
(a) Usual symptoms (Marie, Nonne, Menzel, Schut) increased reflexes with cerebellar signs, dysarthria, and dysphagia
(b) Common variants
1. Decreased reflexes
2. Extrapyramidal signs (Azorean)
3. Spastic ataxia
4. Others
(2) Old age (>50 yr) onset (Richter)
(3) Childhood onset: (exist?)
b. Recessive heredity
(1) Adult onset
(a) Increased reflexes
(b) Decreased reflexes
(2) Old age onset
GDH deficiency (Plaitakis)
(3) Childhood
(a) Increased DTRs: Charlevoix (Barbeau, Hogan)
(b) Decreased DTRs: Friedreich (malic vs. taurine)
2. Rare types: dominant, X-linked, or recessive
a. Neurologic: pathologic variations
(1) Spinopontine
(2) Posterior column
(3) Cerebelloolivary
(4) Anterior horn cell: peripheral nerve
(5) With cerebral cortex changes: dementia
(6) Infantile types: with broad CNS pathology
(7) Others
b. With sense organ abnormality
(1) Ocular: retina, optic nerve, EOM weakness
(2) Ear: deafness
(3) Others
c. Body abnormality in addition to ataxia
(1) Gonadal
(2) Skeletal
(3) Others

a kindred. Thus the clinical- and/or pathologic-based classifications are not ideal as the chief differential tool in an outline. Abnormalities of other tissues, such as the gonads, although reliable for subtypes, are usually related to small or rare kindreds and thus are not useful in the broad classification of the usual ataxia patient.

A classification is proposed based first on a relatively unmistakable clinical criterion, which relates to a basic abnormality and allows broad placement of a patient or family: the inheritance pattern. The age of onset, although subject to definite variation, is usually typical and consistent, based probably on genetic-chemical differences, and enables a patient and/or kindred to be further classified. The next variable used is that of usual or unusual clinical symptomatology. In the dominant forms, the usual symptoms are imbalance, dysarthria, dysphagia, and limb ataxia. The common variations of this symptom pattern, in the dominant forms, are reflex changes, extrapyramidal rigidity and/or resting tremor, marked spasticity, and amyotrophy. An increase or decrease in tendon reflexes at an early or middle stage is also a reliable classifying characteristic for the recessive types. Finally, known chemicals or enzyme abnormalities are listed. The rare varieties—with cranial nerve abnormalities, dementia, marked distal atrophy, or changes in other organ systems and the infantile degenerative diseases—are set aside (perhaps temporarily) from the classification scheme of the common ataxias and their variations.

The proposed classification thus uses the following scheme: stationary versus progressive, hereditary versus nonhereditary, common versus rare, inheritance type, age of onset, clinical variation, and chemical-genetic subtypes.

Barbeau's thinking[1] and construction of a classification for the recessive ataxias is helpful, and several of his ideas are included in the outline presented in Table 2.

The eventual determination of the particular chemical error for each type will enable this classification to be enlarged, changed, and adorned. It is possible that some subtypes, such as the old age dominant progressive hereditary ataxia, will possess a similar or identical chemical abnormality to the common variety but at a different chromosomal locus or, if at the same locus, as an allele. It is also predictable that all the inherited ataxias will be eventually chromosomally placed either by classic linkage studies or by cloning techniques.

The uncommon varieties are not in the main section of the classification because they are many and rare. Inclusion in the main classification at this time might present a deceptively long and discouraging differential diagnosis to the clinician who then might choose to reject rather than use the classification.

---

[1]A. Barbeau, A tentative classification of recessively inherited ataxias. *Can. J. Neurol. Sci.*, Vol. 9, pp. 95–98 (1982).

The Olivopontocerebellar Atrophies, edited by R.C. Duvoisin and A. Plaitakis. Raven Press, New York © 1984.

An Apology and an Introduction to the Olivopontocerebellar Atrophies

Roger C. Duvoisin

Department of Neurology, University of Medicine and Dentistry of New Jersey, Rutgers Medical School, Academic Health Science Center, New Brunswick, New Jersey 08903

As a nosologic label, the cumbersome name "olivopontocerebellar" atrophy (OPCA) would seem neither useful nor convenient. It makes no reference to pathogenesis or clinical features; in fact, it does not fully describe the morbid anatomy. Yet it has survived the test of time and enjoys widespread recognition in either the form of the full expression or its acronym OPCA. It is now the key word to a large and growing body of literature bearing on an admittedly heterogenous but nevertheless distinctive clinicopathologic entity. The nosologic concept of OPCA is alive and thriving, and the term no doubt will continue in favor for some time until a more satisfactory terminology can be evolved to identify the group of the OPCAs as a whole, or its component entities are dispersed among other nosologies based on different principles.

THE PROTOTYPIC CASES

The term was introduced by Dejerine and Thomas (6) in an article published in 1900 in which they described two patients with a distinctive type of chronic progressive cerebellar degeneration appearing in middle age. Unsteadiness in walking and standing, fatigue, and a marked slowness and hesitation in all bodily movements were the salient clinical manifestations. The patients walked on a broad base with short, hesitant steps in constant fear of falling but without the swaying and staggering typical of the inebriated state or of other cerebellar disorders. Additional features included hypomimia, a fixed facial expression, awkwardness of the hands, minimal action tremor, and a slow, scanning speech. There was also some disturbance of ocular motility. Upward gaze was accomplished in several brief nystagmoid jerks or steps, and rapid movements, presumably pursuit movements, were "uncertain." One patient experienced diplopia. The tendon reflexes were exaggerated. The plantar reflexes were tested only in the second patient and were normally flexor. Among the important negative findings on examination were normal vision, normal fundi on ophthalmoscopy, normal sensation, and preservation of the intellect. The patients denied the occurrence of a similar or indeed of any nervous affliction in their families.

Postmortem examination was obtained in the first patient and showed a particular pattern of atrophy. To summarize the findings briefly, there was symmetric atrophy of the cerebellar cortex more marked in the hemispheres than in the vermis but preservation of the dentate nuclei, "total" atrophy of the middle cerebellar peduncle and basis pontis, and marked atrophy of the inferior olive and partial atrophy of the restiform body; finally, the pyramids and cerebral peduncles appeared smaller than normal, although no degenerating fibers were seen. These features were summarized in the descriptive term "olivopontocerebellar atrophy," which served as the title of the published report.

Dejerine and Thomas (6) sought to establish a nosologic position for the disorder that afflicted their patients. They distinguished it from the disorder described 40 years earlier by Friedreich (11) and from the heterogenous group of cases of cerebellar degeneration of adult onset collected by Marie (19) under the rubric of "hereditary cerebellar ataxia." They noted the similarity of their two patients to those described earlier by Menzel (20), although these differed in several aspects: a strong familial concentration, a younger age of onset, and the presence of choreiform movements in the initial stages of the illness. Despite these clinical and genetic differences, the two groups of patients have since been considered sufficiently similar as to warrant their inclusion under the same heading. Indeed, in the following chapter, Koeppen and Barron argue that they are the same disorder.

A moderate number of cases, some apparently sporadic and others occurring in familial concentration consistent with autosomal dominant inheritance, have been reported over the more than 80 years since Dejerine and Thomas (6) published their two cases. Berciano (5) in his recent review of the literature, collected a total of 117 cases. (It may be argued that not all these cases are properly labeled OPCA.) The dichotomous subdivision of OPCA into a sporadic type and a dominantly inherited type was firmly established by Greenfield (13) in his classic review of the cerebellar degenerations and was continued by Eadie (7,8) in his comprehensive review and more recently by Berciano (5). Eadie (9), however, found it necessary to recognize a third group of atypical or variant cases of OPCA. A number of published cases have varied considerably from the prototypic cases of Menzel (20) and of Dejerine and Thomas (6). Involvement of the striatum, for example, and the association of the morphologic features of OPCA and striatonigral degeneration (SND) has repeatedly been noted since Adams et al. (1,2) drew attention to the latter entity. Thus it has been clear for some time, even from a purely morphologic perspective, that we are considering not a mere dichotomy but a heterogenous group of disorders.

CLASSIFICATION OF KONIGSMARK AND WEINER

Kongismark and Weiner (16) recognized the heterogeneity of OPCA in their paper published in 1970 in which they proposed a classification based on clinical and genetic as well as anatomic features. They placed the previously autopsied cases into seven major groups, as follows:

I. Menzel type
II. Autosomal recessive type
III. Dominant with retinal degeneration
IV. The Schut family; dominant
V. Dominant with dementia, extrapyramidal signs, and ophthalmoplegia
VI. Other types of familial OPCA
VII. Sporadic OPCA (Dejerine–Thomas type)

Several problems have limited the usefulness of this classification. It is difficult to apply clinically. In fact, its authors unwittingly placed members of different branches of the well-known Schut family (25) in two separate groups, an error that illustrates the limitations of a classification based on clinical and morphologic grounds. Some critics have disagreed with the inclusion of the Fickler (10) and Winkler (28) families, for example, as cases of OPCA and with the family reported by Aring (3) with cavitation of the basal ganglia and diencephalon and have questioned the validity of the autosomal recessive group (see, for example, Koeppen and Barron, *this volume*). Konigsmark and Weiner (16) were uncertain about the inclusion of the Schut family, a well-studied kindred of dominantly inherited ataxia, because of the considerable variation in both the clinical manifestations and the pathologic findings. They decided to include it because the major pathology involved the inferior olive, cerebellum, and pons.

The authors were also uncertain how to categorize the sporadic cases with parkinsonian features and suggested that these might form yet another group, leaving the classification open-ended to permit the addition of new entities. Apparently, they did not consider the two cases of Dejerine and Thomas (6) to have parkinsonian features. However, Dejerine and Thomas had described immobility, facial hypomimia, slowness of movement, and hesitation on initiating movement as the more striking features of their cases. They drew no parallels with the bradykinesia of Parkinson's disease, perhaps because the "negative" manifestations of parkinsonism were not well appreciated in their time.

PARKINSONISM AND OPCA

The occurrence of parkinsonian features, including rigidity and occasionally a resting tremor of the limbs, was well documented in a number of the cases reported in the 1920s and 1930s (14,18,24). Rosenhagen (23) emphasized the frequent presence of extrapyramidal rigidity and, in his review of 45 cases, correlated the presence of parkinsonism with neuronal degeneration of the substantia nigra. Eadie (7), in his comprehensive review of 35 autopsied cases collected from the literature, again noted the common occurrence of parkinsonian features. Parkinsonism had been noted in 55% of the sporadic cases reviewed by Berciano (5). Such patients today are commonly seen in the Parkinson clinics of teaching hospitals and major centers and are often erroneously diagnosed as cases of Parkinson's disease.

In the years since Konigsmark and Weiner (16) published their review, the nosology of the OPCAs has become still more confused because of the recognition of new entities and especially the increasing frequency with which OPCA is diagnosed on clinical grounds. Until mid-century, the diagnosis of OPCA was primarily a pathologist's diagnosis made only postmortem, although Dejerine and Thomas (6) had diagnosed their second case on clinical grounds alone, relying on the similarity of the signs and symptoms. Pneumoencephalography made possible the demonstration of the cerebellar and brainstem atrophy in the living patient, greatly facilitating the clinical diagnosis. The computerized tomographic (CT) scan of the brain has proved even more helpful and enables the neuroradiologist to demonstrate the specific pattern of cerebellar hemisphere and brainstem atrophy on CT scanning (12), as Huang and Plaitakis show elsewhere in this volume. Many cases are now recognized that would formerly have been classified, for example, as instances of Parkinson's disease or idiopathic parkinsonism. As a result, the nosologic concept of OPCA has in practice become a syndrome of diverse etiology defined by its clinical manifestations and the gross pathology as demonstrated by CT scanning.

One practical consequence of this development is a broadening of the spectrum of disorders included under this diagnostic category. The OPCAs had been viewed mainly as one of the ataxias and were often placed by nosologists among the cerebellar degenerations. More recently, their affinity with the extrapyramidal disorders, especially parkinsonism, has received growing and somewhat belated recognition. No modern classification of parkinsonism can be complete which does not mention OPCA. The nosologic concept of OPCA has provided a useful diagnostic category in which the clinician may place those patients presenting with manifestations of combined involvement of the cerebellar and extrapyramidal systems. Moreover, recognition of OPCA on clinical grounds is a matter of practical importance, because the prognosis and response to therapy are not the same as in Parkinson's disease. An inverse relationship of the cerebellar and extrapyramidal features has been noted, the latter masking the former, and can be demonstrated in physiologic studies, as shown by Narabayashi *(this volume)*.

In this context, it is appropriate to consider what proportion of patients referred to the neurologist for "parkinsonism" in clinical practice in fact should be classified as cases of OPCA. The survey of 802 patients attending the Parkinson Clinic at the Columbia Presbyterian Medical Center in New York City from 1947 to 1964 reported by Hoehn and Yahr (15) included 22 "atypical" cases, five of which had cerebellar system abnormalities. Several personal cases included in that series were identified as OPCA some years later, and one ultimately was found to have glutamate dehydrogenase deficiency. The recent epidemiologic survey of parkinsonism in Rochester, Minnesota, carried out by Rajput et al. (22) found 128 cases of parkinsonism; of these, one was classified as OPCA, one as "multiple-system atrophy," and one was unclassified. Personal experience suggests that at least one or two of the patients classified as having parkinsonism or Parkinson's disease will be reclassified as OPCA within several years as the clinical picture unfolds. Goetz et al. *(this volume)* collected no less than 24 cases of OPCA from their movement disorder clinic at Rush-Presbyterian-St. Luke's Medical Center in Chicago. In my own personal consulting practice, OPCA accounts for 5 to 6% of all parkinsonism.

These considerations indicate that OPCA is more common than has previously been thought. Its prevalence must be at least as great as the estimate of 5/100,000 for all hereditary ataxias offered by Kurtzke and Kurland (17) and greater than the rate of 3/100,000 estimated by Sobue et al. (26) from a survey of ataxia in Japan.

NEW TYPES OF OPCA

In recent years, new morbid entities have been identified among the OPCAs on clinical grounds, such as the cases with slow eye movements and peripheral neuropathy reported by Wadia and Swami (27; see also Wadia, *this volume*), the cases associated with progressive autonomic failure studied by Bannister and Oppenheimer (4), and Joseph disease, another dominant disorder which resembles in its genetic and clinical features the disorder found in the Schut family (Rosenberg, *this volume*). Additional entities have been discovered on biochemical grounds: an apparently recessive disorder associated with deficiency of glutamate dehydrogenase (Plaitakis, Maruyama and Yamaguchi, and Duvoisin, *this volume*) and a dominant form associated with urinary excretion of an as yet unidentified glycolipid (Berenberg et al., *this volume*). Perry *(this volume)* has developed evidence of several different etiologic types of dominant OPCA in the postmortem material at his disposal. Although the significance of these new observations remains to be clarified by future research, they clearly portend a new era in our understanding of the OPCAs and an increase in the number of discrete morbid entities to be included under this term.

The plethora of OPCAs now confronting us calls for a new classification to contain them all, to help us think about them, to clarify their relationships, and to facilitate the recognition of new entities. One must recognize at the outset the limitations inherent in a scheme for grouping logically a variety of disorders of largely unknown etiology, some of which do not always, or only occasionally, produce OPCA. This is particularly a problem with the dominant disorders, in which phenotypic expression can be variable, and the OPCA phenotype may occur in various genotypes. In the Schut and Joseph diseases, for example, many individuals present typical OPCA features clinically and pathologically, but some instead may present a spastic paraplegia or a primarily spinocerebellar syndrome.

A similar problem is the overlapping relationship of OPCA and SND. Both may coexist in the same individual or occur separately. Oppenheimer (21) has persuasively argued that these two are but varying expressions of a common condition, for which he has proposed the inclusive term multiple system atrophy. Where are we to place the SND cases without cerebellar involvement? Still another problem awaiting future resolution is the relationship of OPCA associated with progressive autonomic failure to the Shy-Drager syndrome. Finally, the classification cannot be based on a single principle; some entities are identified on clinical grounds, others on biochemical grounds. Ultimately, when a classification based entirely on etiology can be possible, it will cut across the lines of any classification based on present knowledge.

A NEW CLASSIFICATION

The classification scheme presented in Table 1 may prove useful as a guide to a complex and rapidly changing clinical scene; it is provisional and subject to revision as new knowledge emerges. In developing this scheme, the dichotomy between dominantly inherited and sporadic OPCA was preserved. There is reason to suspect recessive inheritance in some if not all of the sporadic cases. Recessive inheritance of glutamate dehydrogenase deficiency has been noted both by Plaitakis and in my own observations summarized elsewhere in this volume. Nevertheless, since recessive inheritance has not been documented in other forms of apparently sporadic disease, it seemed prudent to combine the sporadic and recessive cases under one large heading. Within the two major headings, various forms may be grouped together. It is recognized that each type (for example, the Menzel type) may itself be etiologically diverse. It is possible, however, that with future advances in knowledge, some types presently separated in this scheme may prove to be one entity.

SUMMARY

The OPCAs are not, as Dejerine and Thomas (6) and subsequent writers have suggested, a unitary morbid entity. They comprise a heterogenous group of disorders sharing certain major clinical and morphologic features with the hereditary and acquired ataxias and with the extrapyramidal system disorders, such as Parkinson's disease and the hereditary and acquired choreas, yet distinct from both these general groups of neurodegenerative diseases. Some of the OPCAs are sharply defined morbid entities of known etiology identified on combined genetic and clinical grounds or by a unique biochemical defect; most are of uncertain provenance and may themselves represent a collection of multiple, as yet undetermined entities. The nosologic concept of OPCA survives today in part because of its

TABLE 1. *A brief classification of the OPCAs*

Dominantly inherited
Menzel type
Schut and Joseph diseases
With slow saccades and peripheral neuropathy
With retinal degeneration
With dementia and extrapyramidal features
With glycolipiduria
Sporadic and/or recessively inherited
Dejerine-Thomas type
With glutamate dehydrogenase deficiency
With striatal degeneration (multiple system atrophy)
With progressive autonomic failure

clinical usefulness in categorizing patients with mixed cerebellar and extrapyramidal syndromes and its importance in the differential diagnosis of both extrapyramidal and cerebellar disorders.

REFERENCES

1. Adams, R., Van Bogaert, L., and Van Der Ecken, H. (1961): Dégénérescences nigro-striées et cérébello-nigro-striées. *Psychiatr. Neurol. (Basel)*, 142:219–259.
2. Adams, R., Van Bogaert, L., and Van Der Ecken, H. (1964): Striatonigral degeneration. *J. Neuropathol. Exp. Neurol.*, 23:584–608.
3. Aring, C. D. (1940): Degeneration of the basal ganglia associated with olivopontocerebellar atrophy. *J. Nerv. Ment. Dis.*, 92:448.
4. Bannister, R., and Oppenheimer, D. R. (1972): Degenerative disease of the nervous system associated with autonomic failure. *Brain*, 95:457–474.
5. Berciano, J. (1982): Olivopontocerebellar atrophy. *J. Neurol. Sci.*, 53:253–272.
6. Dejerine, J., and Thomas, A. (1900): L'atrophie olivo-ponto-cérébèlleuse. *Nouv. Iconogr. Salpêt.*, 13:330–370.
7. Eadie, M. J. (1975): Olivonpontocerebellar atrophy (Dejerine-Thomas type). In: *Handbook of Clinical Neurology, Vol. 21*, edited by P. J. Vinken and G. W. Bruyn, pp. 415–443. North Holland, Amsterdam.
8. Eadie, M. J. (1975): Olivopontocerebellar atrophy (Menzel Type). In: *Handbook of Clinical Neurology, Vol. 21*, edited by P. J. Vinken and G. W. Bruyn, pp. 443–449. North Holland, Amsterdam.
9. Eadie, M. J. (1975): Olivopontocerebellar atrophy (variants). In: *Handbook of Clinical Neurology, Vol. 21*, edited by P. J. Vinken and G. W. Bruyn, pp. 451–457. North Holland, Amsterdam.
10. Fickler, A. (1911): Klinishe und pathologisch anatomische Beiträge zu den Erkrankungen des kleinhirns. *Dtsch. Z. Nervenheilk.*, 41:306–375.
11. Friedreich, N. (1876): Ueber Ataxia mit besonderer Berücksichtigung der hereditären Formen. *Virchows Arch. Pathol. Anat.*, 68:145.
12. Gilroy, J., and Lynn, G. E. (1978): Computerized tomography and auditory-evoked potentials. Use in the diagnosis of olivo-ponto-cerebellar degeneration. *Arch. Neurol.*, 35:143–147.
13. Greenfield, J. G. (1954): *The Spino-Cerebellar Degenerations*. Charles C Thomas, Springfield, Illinois.
14. Guillain, G., Mathieu, P., and Bertrand, I. (1926): Etude anatomoclinique sur deux cas d'atrophies olivo-ponto-cérébèlleuse avec rigidite. *Ann Med.*, 20:417.
15. Hoehn, M., and Yahr, M. D. (1967): Parkinsonism: Onset, progression and mortality. *Neurology*, 17:427–442.
16. Konigsmark, B. W., and Weiner, L. P. (1970): The olivopontocerebellar atrophies: A review. *Medicine*, 49:227–241.
17. Kurtzke, J. F., and Kurland, L. T. (1973): Other specific neurologic disorders. In: *Neurologic and Sense Organ Disorders*, edited by L. T. Kurland, J. F. Kurtzke, and I. D. Goldberg, pp. 210–231. Harvard University Press, Cambridge.
18. Ley, R. A. (1925): Forme atypique d'atrophie cérébèlleuse ayant evolve en syndrome rigide. *J. Belge Neurol. Psychiatr.*, 25:92.
19. Marie, P. (1893): Sur l'hérédo-ataxie cérébèlleuse. *Sem. Med.*, 13:444–447.
20. Menzel, P. (1891): Beitrag zur Kenntniss der hereditären Ataxie und Kleinhirnatrophie. *Arch. Psychiatr. Nervenkr.*, 22:160–190.
21. Oppenheimer, D. R. (1980): Multiple system atrophy and the Shy-Drager syndrome. In: *Spinocerebellar Degeneration*, edited by I. Sobue, pp. 165–170. University Park Press, Baltimore.
22. Rajput, A. H., Elveback, L. R., Beard, C. M., and Kurland, L. T. (1981): Epidemiology of Parkinson's disease in Rochester, Minnesota. In: *12th World Congress of Neurology, Kyoto, Japan, Sept. 20–25, 1981,* International Congress Series 548. Excerpta Medica, Amsterdam.
23. Rosenhagen, H. (1943): Die Primäre atrophie des Brückenfuss und der unteren oliven. *Arch. Psychiatr. Nervenkr.*, 116:163–228.
24. Scherer, H. J. (1933): Extrapyramidale storungen bei der olivo-ponto-cerebellaren atrophie. *Ztschr. Neurol.*, 145:406.

25. Schut, J. W. (1954): Hereditary ataxia. Clinical study through six generations. *Arch. Neurol. Psychiatry*, 63:535–567.
26. Sobue, I., Takayanagi, T., and Yamamoto, H. (1980): Clinical features of spinocerebellar degenerations in Japan. In: *Spinocerebellar Degenerations*, edited by I. Sobue, pp. 3–16. University of Tokyo Press, Tokyo.
27. Wadia, N. H., and Swami, R. K. (1971): A new form of heredo-familial spinocerebellar degeneration with slow eye movements. *Brain*, 94:359–374.
28. Winkler, C. (1923): A case of olivo-pontine cerebellar atrophy and our conception of neo- and palaeo-cerebellum. *Schweiz. Arch. Neurol. Psychiatr*, 13:684–702.

The Olivopontocerebellar Atrophies, edited by R.C. Duvoisin and A. Plaitakis. Raven Press, New York © 1984.

The Neuropathology of Olivopontocerebellar Atrophy

Arnulf H. Koeppen and Kevin D. Barron

Neurology Service, Veterans Administration Medical Center, and Department of Neurology, Albany Medical College of Union University, Albany, New York 12208

HISTORY OF OLIVOPONTOCEREBELLAR ATROPHY

In 1891, under the title of "Contribution to the knowledge of the hereditary ataxias and cerebellar atrophy," Menzel (37) described the pathology of a hereditary case of olivopontocerebellar atrophy (OPCA). The term "atrophie olivo-ponto-cérébèlleuse," however, was first used in 1900 by Dejerine and Thomas (9) for a sporadic case with similar clinical and pathologic manifestations. In their extensive review of several forms of OPCA, Konigsmark and Weiner (33) cited articles by Pierret (42) and Royet and Collet (47) as possible earlier descriptions of OPCA; but a review of these papers raises doubt about the diagnosis because of atypical clinical and pathologic features and incomplete or inadequate examination of the pathologic specimens.

The mother, a brother, and two sisters of the patient in Menzel's report were ataxic. Also, one of the patient's seven children had been diagnosed as having hereditary ataxia. This child was only 8 years old when the patient of the report died. By current criteria, the mode of transmission was autosomal dominant, and the early affliction of a young child constituted anticipation. This phenomenon was observed in many large pedigrees published subsequently.

The examination of the brain of Menzel's patient showed gross atrophy of the pons and cerebellum. Microscopic examination revealed widespread loss of Purkinje cells, although tonsils, flocculus, and vermis were much less seriously affected. Surviving Purkinje cells and the molecular and granular layers appeared normal. The neuronal population of the dentate nuclei was unchanged, although the nerve cells appeared reduced in overall size. On Pal-Weigert myelin stains, the white matter of the cerebellar folia was greatly depleted, while fibers exiting from the hilum of the dentate nuclei were preserved. In the midbrain, the neurons of the substantia nigra were reduced in number. The basis pontis revealed sweeping loss of neurons. The transverse pontine fibers were greatly reduced, and the middle cerebellar peduncles were small. The normal myelin staining of the superior cerebellar peduncles stood out in stark contrast to the brachia pontis. In the medulla oblongata, the inferior olivary nuclei showed loss of neurons and olivocerebellar fibers. The periolivary fibers were similarly depleted. External arcuate, dorsal spinocerebellar, and myelinated fibers in the nuclei of Goll and Burdach were reduced. The inferior cerebellar peduncles were shrunken to about one-fourth their normal size. The spinal cord showed dorsal column degeneration and root fiber loss at all levels. There was also reduced staining of the dorsal spinocerebellar tracts and, to a smaller extent, of the pyramidal tracts. Anterior horn cells appeared smaller than normal and reduced in number. Menzel's description of Clarke's column is somewhat inconclusive. He described "fatty-pigmentary degeneration" but did not specifically state that these nerve cells were fewer than normal.

Dejerine and Thomas (9) gave clinical descriptions in two patients with progressive ataxia and autopsy findings in one. There was no family history, and the autopsied case was accepted by subsequent authors as a typical case of sporadic OPCA. Findings in the brain were similar to the observations in Menzel's specimen. They included gross atrophy of pons and cerebellum and, on microscopy, sweeping loss of Purkinje cells, near total loss of neurons in the basis pontis, with atrophy of the middle cerebellar peduncles, and neuronal depletion of the inferior olivary nuclei. The authors also specifically mentioned the disappearance of the arcuate nuclei of the medulla oblongata and the reduced size of the inferior cerebellar peduncles. As in Menzel's case, dentate nuclei and superior cerebellar peduncles were preserved. With the exception of some anomalous anterior horn gray matter at the fifth and sixth cervical level and an unexplained wedge-shaped defect of myelin staining in the cervical anterolateral white matter, the spinal cord was normal. Dejerine and Thomas (9) emphasized the integrity of Clarke's column in an apparent reference to spinal cord findings in Friedreich's ataxia.

These early publications have been followed by a steady stream of reports of similar cases. Almost all descriptions include autopsy data, because OPCA was principally an autopsy diagnosis before neuroradiologic methods permitted the detection of pontine and cerebellar atrophy during life. All major reviews of OPCA include pathologic descriptions (6,14–16,33). Subclassification of OPCA was attempted (33) but did not gain wide acceptance. Greenfield (22) devoted a chapter to OPCA in his monograph on spinocerebellar degenerations. In some reviews of hereditary forms of ataxia, OPCA was considered but not as a nosologic entity (49).

NEUROPATHOLOGIC FINDINGS IN THE UNDERSTANDING OF THE GENETICS OF OPCA

In his patient with clearly autosomal dominant OPCA, Menzel (37) found dorsal column degeneration, dorsal root fiber depletion, reduction in the number of anterior horn cells, degeneration of the dorsal spinocerebellar tracts and, to some extent, of the pyramidal tracts, and the more typical lesions in the inferior olivary nuclei, basis pontis, and cerebellum. In the sporadic case of OPCA reported by Dejerine and Thomas (9), the spinal cord was unaffected. Based on these early observations, Becker (5) suggested that involvement of the spinal cord was more common in hereditary OPCA than in the sporadic forms. The spectrum of lesions is so wide, however, that inspection of a microscopic slide of spinal cord alone cannot reliably distinguish between hereditary and sporadic cases (26). While the diagnosis of OPCA is principally based on neuropathologic features, a genetic diagnosis still depends on the collection of adequate data in a family study.

Prior to Marie's paper on "l'hérédo-ataxie cérébèlleuse" (36), all forms of hereditary ataxia were assigned to Friedreich's ataxia, which is a typical autosomal recessive disorder with juvenile onset and early progression to serious disability. Although Marie's "hérédo-ataxie cérébèlleuse" is now known to be a heterogenous group of disorders, his article led to the important separation of juvenile and adult onset cases. Among the latter, OPCA constitutes a large percentage. By definition, OPCA of the Menzel type is autosomal dominant. The true prevalence of hereditary OPCA among all cases of OPCA is not known, because sporadic cases are less likely to be reported than are cases of OPCA with definite family histories.

In his extensive reviews of OPCA types, Eadie (14–16) did not discuss the possibility that OPCA may be inherited via a recessive mode of transmission with the existence of asymptomatic carriers (heterozygotes) and an expected affection rate of 25%. Konigsmark and Weiner (33) accepted patients reported by Fickler (18) and Winkler (57) as belonging to the recessive variety of OPCA. In a recent review of 117 cases, Berciano (6) retained Fickler's patient among the recessive cases and added six additional cases from the literature (4,38,40,44,46,55). These six patients, drawn from a total of 54 hereditary cases, constitute a percentage of 11.1. Several cases were listed as indeterminate, including the one by Winkler (57), which had been accepted as an example of recessive transmission by Konigsmark and Weiner (33). Originals of the six cited papers (4,38,40,44,46,55), which suggested the existence of recessive transmission, were reexamined for this review.

In his *Études de Pathologie Nerveuse* in 1910, Raymond (44) devoted two chapters to hereditary ataxia, i.e., Friedreich's ataxia and "l'hérédo-ataxie cérébèlleuse." The patient identified as Mélie F. was described as a case of Friedrich's disease in the first chapter, but Berciano (6) erred in assigning her a diagnosis of OPCA. Mélie F. had a similarly affected sister. The parents were not obviously diseased, but the father died at the age of 41 years in a mental hospital while also suffering from complications of alcoholic neuropathy. The mother died from apoplexy at an unspecified menopausal age. Mélie F. showed first signs of ataxia at the age of 18 years and died at age 36 after recurrent attacks of cardiac arrhythmia and asystole. The description of the heart at autopsy is somewhat superficial but leaves no doubt about a nonatheromatous cardiomyopathy. Examination of the nervous system showed thinning of the spinal cord and an overall smallness of the brain. The peripheral nerves were also thin. On microscopic examination, the spinal cord revealed fiber loss in the dorsal and anterolateral funiculi, dorsal root atrophy, and neuronal loss in Clarke's column. The cerebellar cortex was reduced in overall thickness, and Purkinje cells were few in number. The dentate nuclei were normal, as were the superior cerebellar peduncles. In contrast, middle and inferior cerebellar peduncles were shrunken. The nuclei of the basis pontis were atrophic, but the neuronal population of the inferior olivary nuclei was not mentioned separately. The myelinated fibers of gracile and cuneate nuclei were grossly depleted, and "interolivary" fibers were reduced.

Although this case shared features of both Friedreich's ataxia and OPCA, Raymond (44) chose not to include it among the latter. Rather, he pointed out that involvement of the cerebellum may be substantial in otherwise typical Friedreich's ataxia. The juvenile onset, rapid progression, and cardiac disease also favor the diagnosis of Friedreich's disease. Although recessive inheritance was likely despite the early death of the father, the case has too many atypical clinical and pathologic features to warrant acceptance as an example of OPCA.

The two patients described by Fickler (18) were brother and sister. The brother suffered from epilepsy beginning at age 9 months. The seizure disorder became intractable after age 10 years, and he had daily convulsions after the age of 20 years. The pathologic description of the brain indicates that neuronal loss in the basis pontis and inferior olivary nuclei was minor, although transverse pontine and olivocerebellar fibers were depleted. Purkinje cell loss was quite variable; many were oriented in a bizarre fashion parallel to the cortical surface. What Fickler interpreted as possible Purkinje cell displacement into the granular layer probably were normal Golgi cells. The patient's sister was also ataxic but had suffered an unexplained right hemiplegia at age 8 months. There is sufficient doubt on clinical and pathologic grounds that these two patients were examples of recessive OPCA.

In Aring's case (4), the patient's mother had died during childbirth at an unknown age. The two affected siblings were brother and sister. The postmortem examination on the brother revealed OPCA, but also widespread cystic degeneration of the basal ganglia. There was no autopsy on the sister, who died from a similar illness. The study of this family is insufficient for inclusion among recessive OPCA.

Rosenhagen's patient 9 (46) had normal parents, but cousins were said to have a similar illness. The pathology of case 9 was earlier reported by Welte (56) (as case 4) and revealed so many atypical features that, in retrospect, the diagnosis of OPCA does not apply. The cerebellar cortex and basis pontis were not seriously affected. The main cerebellar lesion lay in the dentate nucleus, which showed neuronal loss and depletion of its efferent fibers. The diagnosis of a Friedreich variant was considered because of degeneration of dorsal and anterolateral columns, sweeping loss of nerve cells in Clarke's columns, and some loss of anterior horn cells. The overall lesion was similar to the dyssynergia cerebellaris myoclonica of Hunt (25). Hunt's two patients were brothers who had normal parents, so that recessive transmission may be accepted.

The siblings described by Titica and van Bogaert (55) had hereditary ballistic movements. Autopsy in the brother showed a near normal basis pontis and minor lesions of the inferior olivary nuclei and cerebellar cortex. In contrast, the dentate nuclei were severely affected. In addition, the brain showed neuronal loss in the substantia nigra, subthalamic nuclei, red nuclei, pallidum, and putamen. The authors did not intend to include this case as one showing OPCA and only discussed a possible relationship.

The patient described by Norman and Urich (40) had cerebellar hypoplasia with pontine and olivary changes. The only suggestion of heredity was a brother who had died at age 2½ years with mental retardation and microcephaly. In the case illustrated by Neumann and Cohn (38), the lesions were not those of OPCA. The neuronal population of the basis pontis, cerebellar cortex, and dentate nuclei was normal. Olivary neurons were reduced in number. Despite normal pontine neurons, the transverse fibers of the pons were pale on myelin stains and accompanied by gliosis. The patient also had lesions of the long tracts of the spinal cord and loss of anterior horn cells. The authors did not conclude that this case represented OPCA but a combined degeneration of spinocerebellar and olivopontocerebellar pathways.

Of all the cases discussed above, the patient of Neumann and Cohn (38) comes closest to a recessive form of OPCA. In the majority of patients reported under this designation, the evidence for this mode of transmission is insufficient. Most reported hereditary cases of OPCA are clearly autosomal dominant. It is possible that recessive cases of OPCA have been improperly classified as sporadic, because family histories frequently remain incomplete; at present, one can only speculate on this point.

GROSS NEUROPATHOLOGY OF OPCA

The gross appearance of the brain in fully developed OPCA is highly characteristic (Figs. 1 and 2). The cerebellum is small, and its hemispheres are far from the occipital poles (Fig. 1). Despite the reduction in volume, the surface may appear compact (Figs. 1 and 2), without expansion of the interfolial spaces. However, the cisterna magna and the ambient cistern are expanded due to shrinkage of the vermis and adjacent hemispheres. The size of the pons is greatly diminished (Figs. 1 and 2). The normal protuberance is lost, and the cerebral peduncles seem to connect directly with the medullary pyramids. Cranial nerves 3, 5, 6, 7, and 8 are especially prominent, because the basis pontis has receded. The basilar artery lies loose in a widened prepontine subarachnoid space. The surface of the remaining basis pontis frequently shows transverse folds as though corrugated, and it appears that the pulsations of the basilar artery have left a longitudinal groove. The middle cerebellar peduncles are shrunken (Fig. 2). The bulge of the inferior olivary nuclei is not generally reduced, but the medulla oblongata may appear smaller than normal.

Total brain weight may be normal but is commonly reduced. In the hereditary case illustrated in Fig. 4, the brain weight was only 900 g. Such massive reduction in weight cannot be explained by atrophy of brainstem and cerebellum alone. In the illustrated case, the size of the cerebrum was harmonically reduced, without gross lesions in a specific lobe. After removal of the cerebrum, the brainstem and attached cerebellum weigh much less than the approximate 10% of whole brain weight, or about 80 to 100 g in adults with OPCA.

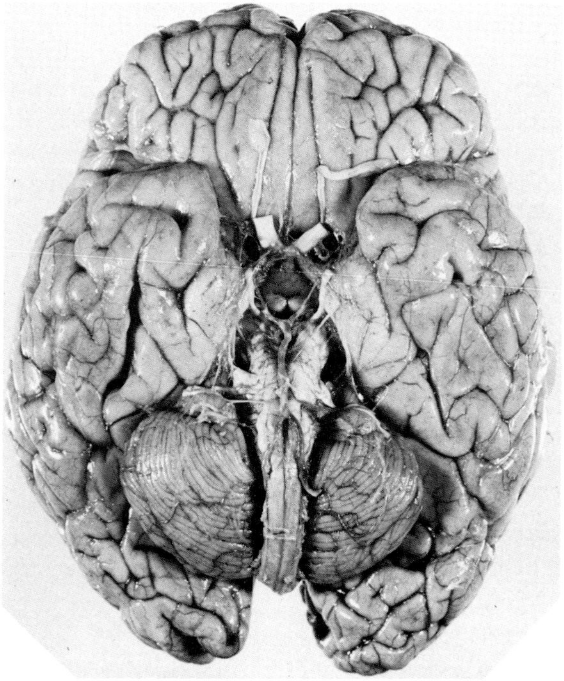

FIG. 1. Hereditary case of OPCA. Brainstem and cerebellum are greatly reduced in size. There is no recognizable bulge of the basis pontis, and the basilar artery lies in widened subarachnoid space. (From ref. 29.)

As a rule, the superior cerebellar peduncles are of normal size, and the dentate nuclei reveal no gross abnormalities. White matter atrophy in the cerebellar folia may be apparent to the naked eye. The midbrain frequently shows some pigment loss in the substantia nigra. Serial sections of the pons confirm the atrophy of the base and preservation of the tegmentum. In the medulla, the delicate meandering bands of the inferior olivary nuclei may be replaced by plumper structures.

The spinal cord is generally normal in size. Serial sections reveal gross lesions only in some of the advanced cases, in the atypical cases in which spinal lesions are especially severe, and those that represent transitional forms between Friedreich's ataxia and OPCA (44,46,56).

OPCA occurs in association with idiopathic orthostatic hypotension (45,50,51) and striatonigral degeneration (2,53). In some patients, idiopathic orthostatic hypotension, striatonigral degeneration, and OPCA may exist at the same time (39,51). The term multiple system atrophy (51) is appropriate for this condition. These unusual cases are not discussed further here, but useful reviews can be found in references 45 and 51.

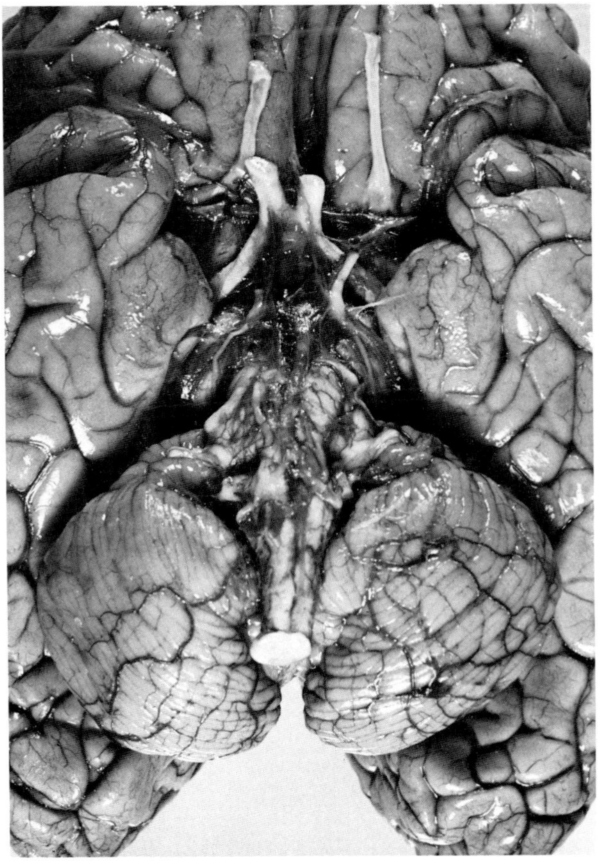

FIG. 2. Sporadic case of OPCA. In addition to atrophy of the cerebellum and pons, thinning of the middle cerebellar peduncles is apparent.

MICROSCOPIC NEUROPATHOLOGY OF OPCA

Cerebellum

The outstanding feature in the cerebellum is the loss of Purkinje cells; it may be so sweeping that none can be found. In other cases, Purkinje cell loss is less dramatic and not equal throughout the cerebellar cortex (Fig. 3a). Bergmann glia are commonly increased. Silver stains (Fig. 3b,c) show numerous empty baskets where Purkinje cells have disappeared (Fig. 3b), but in long-standing cases, baskets may also be absent. Expansions of Purkinje cell axons (torpedos) in the granular layer are also variable (Fig. 3c). The molecular layer is thinned, but the granular layer in many cases appears well preserved. Although Golgi cell counts have not been reported, these cells appear unaffected in OPCA. The white matter in the

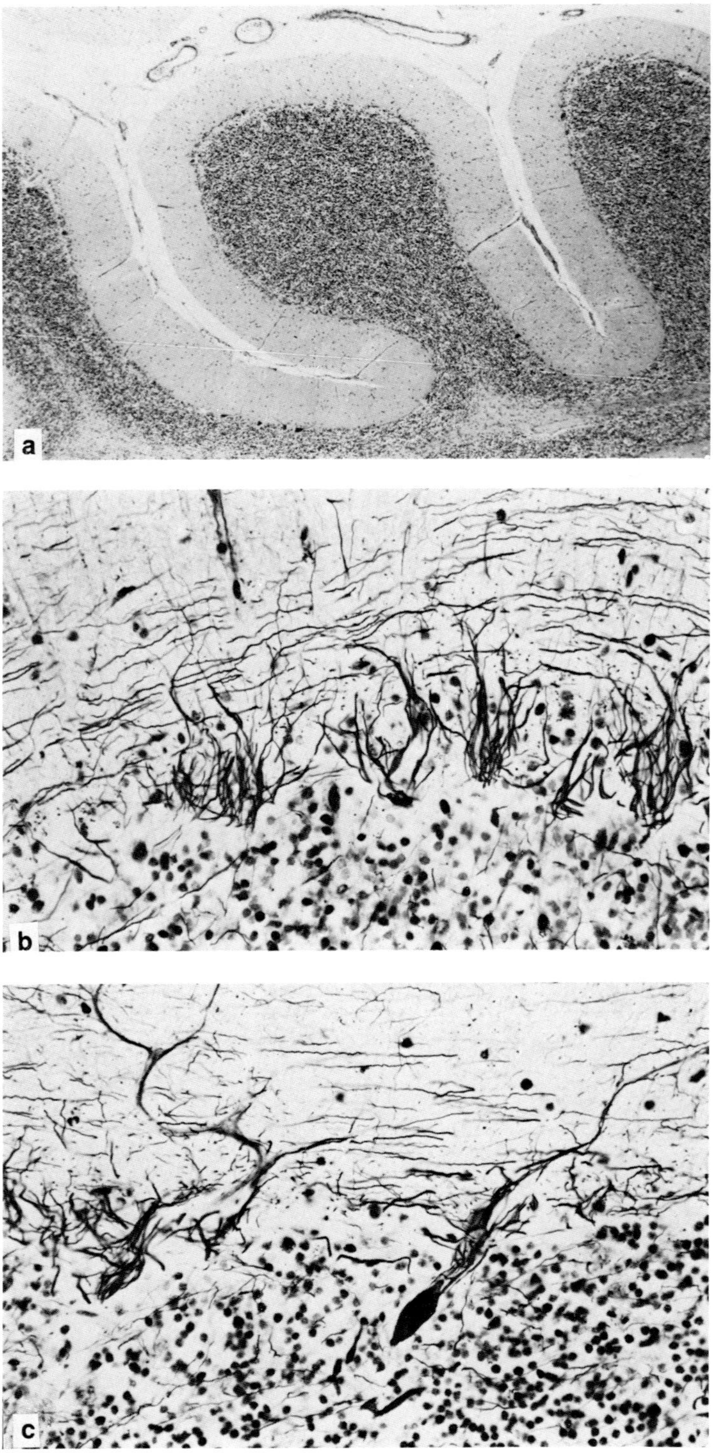
a
b
c

folia is distinctly depleted but better preserved around the dentate nuclei. Loss of myelin is matched by depletion of axons. Glial stains show a dense gliosis of fibrils, but astrocytic perikarya are not large. The dentate nuclei are generally well preserved, and their efferent fibers in the cerebellum, superior cerebellar peduncles, and midbrain stain normally.

Pons

The grossly visible loss of substance in the basis pontis is due to disappearance of pontine nuclei and transverse pontine fibers (Fig. 4). Myelinated fibers in the tegmentum and descending pontine fiber tracts are well preserved. Glial stains, such as the Holzer method, reveal small cell fibrous gliosis, which fills in some of the spaces left by the degenerating transverse fibers and shrunken neuronal groups.

Medulla Oblongata

Neuronal loss in the inferior olivary nuclei is variable and ranges from minor to complete (Fig. 5). Periolivary fibers and fibers of the amiculum are reduced. The remaining olivary nerve cells are smaller than normal when compared to control tissue. Axonal loss matches the fiber depletion shown by myelin stains (Fig. 5). The arcuate nuclei are commonly so atrophic that they can no longer be identified. Myelinated fibers terminating in the gracile and cuneate nuclei are degenerated, but the lesion depends on the severity of dorsal column degeneration in the spinal cord.

Spinal Cord

Changes in the spinal cord are variable. When present, degeneration of the dorsal columns is the most prominent finding (Fig. 6). The anterolateral funiculi show less serious fiber loss than the tracts of Goll and Burdach, but both dorsal spinocerebellar and lateral corticospinal tracts are affected. Neuronal loss in Clarke's column is suggested by some reports, but the depletion rarely reaches the degree seen in Friedreich's ataxia. Dorsal root fiber loss occurs occasionally but is generally mild, so that degeneration of the dorsal column should not be viewed as a mere result of radiculopathy. Anterior horn cells may be quite reduced in number, as in the cases with fasciculations described by Koeppen et al. (30) (family 1, Figs. 5 and 6 of ref. 30).

Degenerative changes of the cerebellum, pons, and medulla oblongata constitute the microscopic hallmark of OPCA. However, involvement of the central nervous system outside the three structures cited appears to be almost invariable (26).

FIG. 3. **a:** Thinning of molecular layer and loss of Purkinje cells. Cresyl Violet; original magnification, × 10. **b:** Cerebellar cortex. Numerous empty baskets are present in the Purkinje cell layer. Bodian; original magnification, × 100. **c:** Cerebellar cortex. Empty baskets, Purkinje cell dendrites, and an axonal torpedo (granular layer) are present. Bodian; original magnification, × 100.

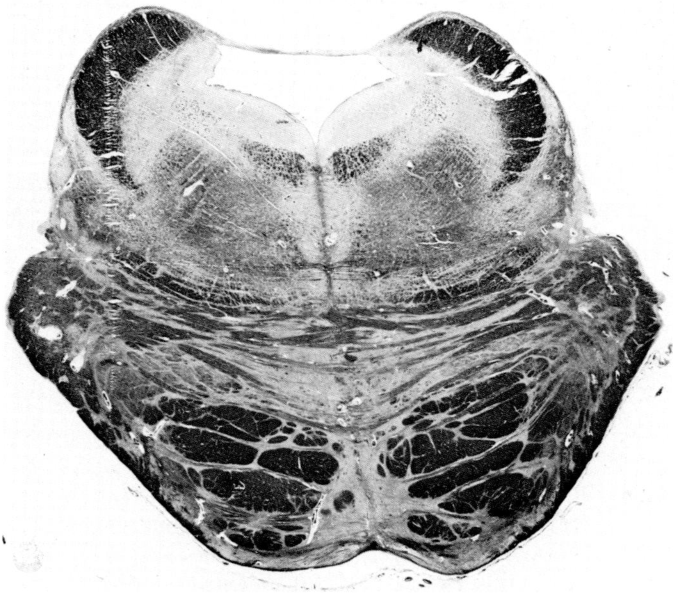

FIG. 4. Hereditary OPCA. The ventrodorsal diameter of the basis pontis is greatly reduced. Transverse pontine fibers stain poorly. Structures in the pontine tegmentum, notably the superior cerebellar peduncles, stain normally. Luxol Fast Blue-periodic acid Schiff stain; enlarged macrophoto. (From ref. 30.)

Jellinger and Tarnowska-Dziduszko (26) examined 20 cases of OPCA and listed affected nuclear groups and white matter. A partial list of such "associated lesions" is reproduced here, without implying frequency of involvement: (a) medulla oblongata: vestibular nuclei, dorsal motor nuclei of the vagus nerves, hypoglossal nuclei, neurons of the gracile and cuneate nuclei, pyramidal tracts; (b) pons and midbrain: oculomotor nuclei, red nuclei, substantia nigra, including pars reticularis, locus ceruleus, reticular formation; (c) diencephalon: thalamus, subthalamic nuclei, zona incerta; (d) cerebral hemispheres: subcortical white matter, cortex, caudate nuclei, putamen, globus pallidus.

Some patients with OPCA have disturbances of ocular motility, including frank ophthalmoplegia (for review, see ref. 33 and Chokroverty, *this volume*) and supranuclear ophthalmoplegia (29). The neuropathologic descriptions in the literature do not always specify how the corresponding nuclei of the nerves to the eye muscles are affected. The morphologic substrate for the supranuclear eye movement disturbance is not known but has been tentatively assigned to the paramedian reticular formation of the brainstem.

The retina was studied in several cases from hereditary OPCA (for reviews, see refs. 33 and 48), where pigmentary retinal degeneration was present. The lesion is thought to begin in the pigment epithelium and to involve the photoreceptor layers in consequence. Lesions in the choriocapillaris are probably also secondary.

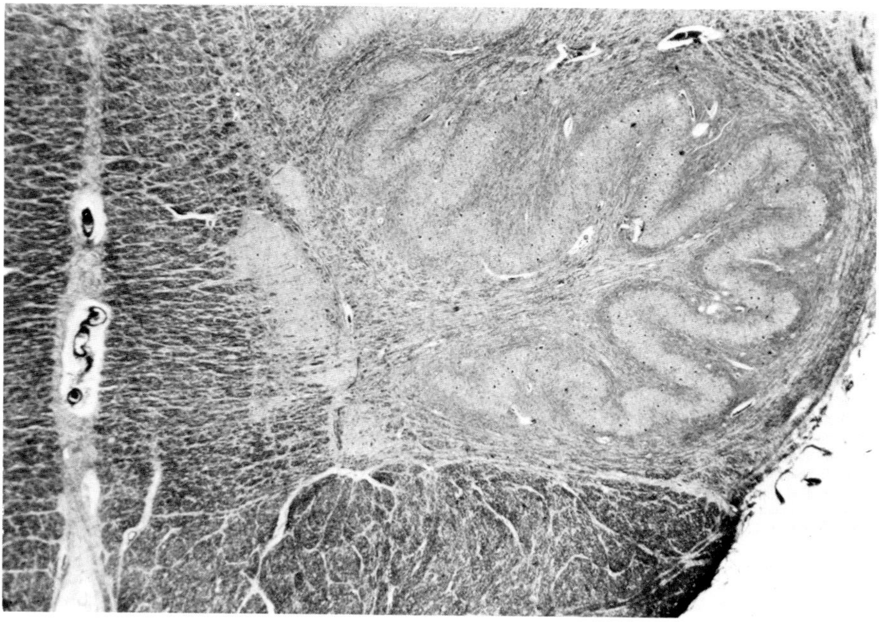

FIG. 5. Hereditary OPCA, same case as in Fig. 4. The chief inferior olivary nucleus and accessory olivary nuclei show neuronal loss and depletion of olivocerebellar and periolivary fibers. Luxol Fast Blue-periodic acid Schiff stain; original magnification, × 6.4. (From ref. 30.)

ENZYME HISTOCHEMISTRY OF OPCA

In 1981, a patient with autosomal dominant OPCA (patient VI, 7 of ref. 29) died from causes unrelated to his neurologic illness. Autopsy was performed 1 hr after death, and slices of cerebellum, pons, and medulla oblongata were processed for the histochemical demonstration of selected hydrolases. In Figs. 7–13, the activity of acetylcholinesterase and carboxylesterase (nonspecific esterase) is illustrated. For acetylcholinesterase, Gomori's modification (21) of the method of Koelle and Friedenwald (28) was used. Activity of nonspecific esterase was visualized by the technique of Lehrer and Ornstein (35). In the procedure for nonspecific esterase, ambenonium chloride and eserine sulfate were used as inhibitors of acetylcholinesterase.

Cerebellum

In the normal human cerebellum, the molecular layer shows intense diffuse reaction product for acetylcholinesterase (Fig. 7a). Neuronal cell bodies are not outlined. In the granular layer, the reaction is much less intense although still present, and the perikarya of some cells are stained. These cells have been tentatively identified as Golgi cells. Purkinje cells remain unstained. Dentate neurons and neuropil stain clearly (Fig. 7b). These observations are similar to earlier studies

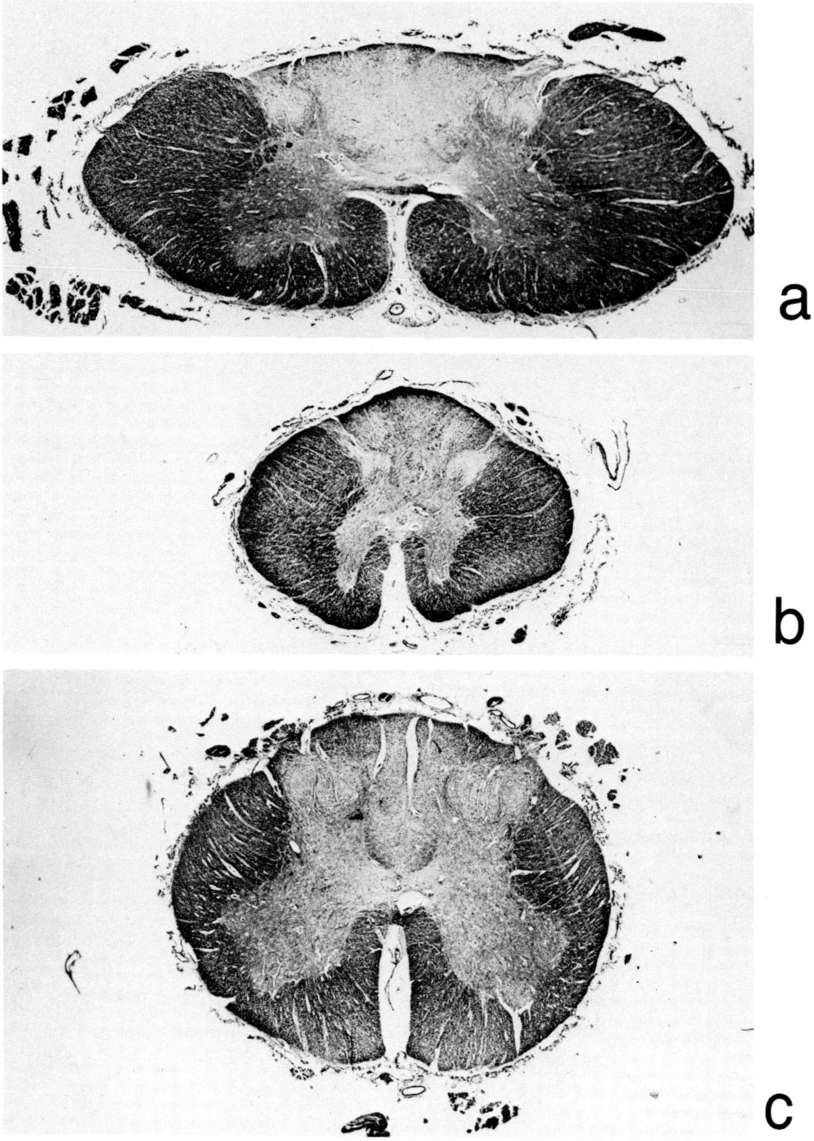

FIG. 6. Hereditary OPCA. Spinal cord sections at cervical, thoracic, and lumbosacral levels. The dorsal columns show depletion of myelinated fibers. Luxol Fast Blue-periodic acid Schiff stain; original magnification, × 4.

of acetylcholinesterase in human cerebellum (1,10,19). In the case of hereditary OPCA (Fig. 7c), there is near total loss of acetylcholinesterase activity in the cerebellar cortex, while dentate neurons have the expected density of reaction product. The almost total loss of acetylcholinesterase activity in the molecular layer is surprising, because typical cell stains do not suggest a similarly serious alteration. The findings point to a depletion of efferents to the molecular layer, more likely from the granule cells than from the climbing fibers of olivary origin.

Stains for nonspecific esterase also show a dramatic difference between OPCA and control cerebellum (Fig. 8). Purkinje cell perikarya and dendrites are well shown in the normal cerebellum by the Lehrer-Ornstein method. In OPCA, the technique reveals the loss of the Purkinje cell bodies and their dendrites (Fig. 8b) and a depletion of reactivity in the granular layer. Golgi cell reactivity appears preserved (Fig. 8b).

Pons

Both methods for acetylcholinesterase reveal a dramatic loss of reactivity in the basis pontis (Fig. 9). Neuronal groups with reaction product are greatly thinned in OPCA (Fig. 9b). Higher resolution shows the perikarya of some preserved neurons (Fig. 10b) but little reaction product in dendrites. The nerve cells are "rounded-off" rather than stellate, as in normal brain (Fig. 10a). Neuropilar reaction product is somewhat amorphous in OPCA (Fig. 10b), while dendritic shafts are outlined in controls (Fig. 10a). The stains for nonspecific esterases largely confirm neuronal loss and reduction of neuropilar reactivity (Figs. 11 and 12).

Medulla Oblongata

The inferior olivary nuclei in controls show dense acetylcholinesterase reaction product in neurons and neuropil and in a crisp outline of the capillary wall (Fig. 13a). In OPCA, the perikarya of the remaining olivary neurons (Fig. 13b,c) are smaller and do not stain well. Capillary staining is irregular but surprisingly dense if the relative lack of neuronal reaction product is considered. Acetylcholinesterase in capillary walls of the inferior olivary nuclei is thought to arise exclusively by neuronal "secretion" from olivary neurons (32). We suggest that acetylcholinesterase protein in the inferior olivary neurons of OPCA is not being retained adequately but instead is released into the interstitial space and capillary basement membranes, where it accumulates. Nonspecific esterase reactions of the inferior olivary nuclei confirm the neuronal loss.

The described enzyme-histochemical data supplement cell stains and highlight complex neuronal alterations, which await further studies, including Golgi impregnation and electron microscopy. Neuronal loss is shown quite readily by methods for acetylcholinesterase and nonspecific esterase. The remaining neurons are also abnormal, however, in that they appear rounded-off and devoid of dendritic processes. These static images suggest that dendritic loss precedes and accompanies disappearance of the neuronal cell body.

Recently, Purkinje cells in a case of hereditary OPCA were examined by a Golgi technique (20). The results confirmed vast dendritic alterations ranging from improper direction to frank loss. The remaining dendritic trunks showed sweeping loss of spiny branchlets, but spines and unusual knob-like protrusions occurred on primary dendrites and the nerve cell body. Purkinje cells were better preserved in parts of the vermis; but even here, the Golgi procedure revealed substantial loss of spiny branchlets.

ELECTRON MICROSCOPY OF OPCA

Biopsy (34,41) and autopsy (41) tissues from OPCA cerebellum have been examined with the electron microscope. Two patients in the report by Landis et al. (34) and one of three in the study by Petito et al. (41) were affected by hereditary OPCA and had cerebellar biopsies. In two additional patients (41), a family history was either not available, or the case was truly sporadic.

When the observations of these two groups of investigators are compared, it becomes apparent that at the ultrastructural as at the light microscopic level, involvement by OPCA is variable. Petito et al. (41) reported a marked reduction in cerebellar afferent fibers, including synaptic terminals of climbing fibers and mossy fibers. The synapses on stellate and basket cells also were greatly reduced. Synaptic connections between parallel fibers and Purkinje cells appeared normal, but glial processes lined much of the dendritic surface where other synapses would normally occur. Electron microscopy confirmed the paucity of Purkinje cells and their dendrites. Unusual cytoplasmic inclusions and vacuoles were present in Purkinje cell dendrites. In the granular layer, the lack of mossy fiber terminals was the most characteristic change. Some granule cells showed nonspecific cytoplasmic alterations. Although not specifically discussed, the only change in Golgi cells was an increase of lipofuscin.

In the two patients of the same family with OPCA reported by Landis et al. (34), degenerative changes in Purkinje cells were more prominent. Increased cytoplasmic and nucleoplasmic density was associated with many free ribosomes and the accumulation of peculiar lamellar bodies. Dendritic membranes of Purkinje cells revealed plaque-like thickenings and vesicular profiles nearby. Some axons in the molecular layer showed inclusions of tubular and membranous profiles and crystalloid structures. Some granule cells showed degenerative changes in their

FIG. 7. Enzyme histochemistry for acetylcholinesterase, cerebellum. Original magnification, × 4. **a:** Normal brain. The method produces dense diffuse reaction product in the molecular layer and less in granular layer and cerebellar white matter. **b:** Normal brain. Staining of neurons and neuropil in the normal dentate nucleus. **c:** Hereditary OPCA. Cerebellar cortex and dentate nucleus are present in the same section. There is essentially no reaction product in the cerebellar cortex or cerebellar white matter. The dentate nucleus stains normally.

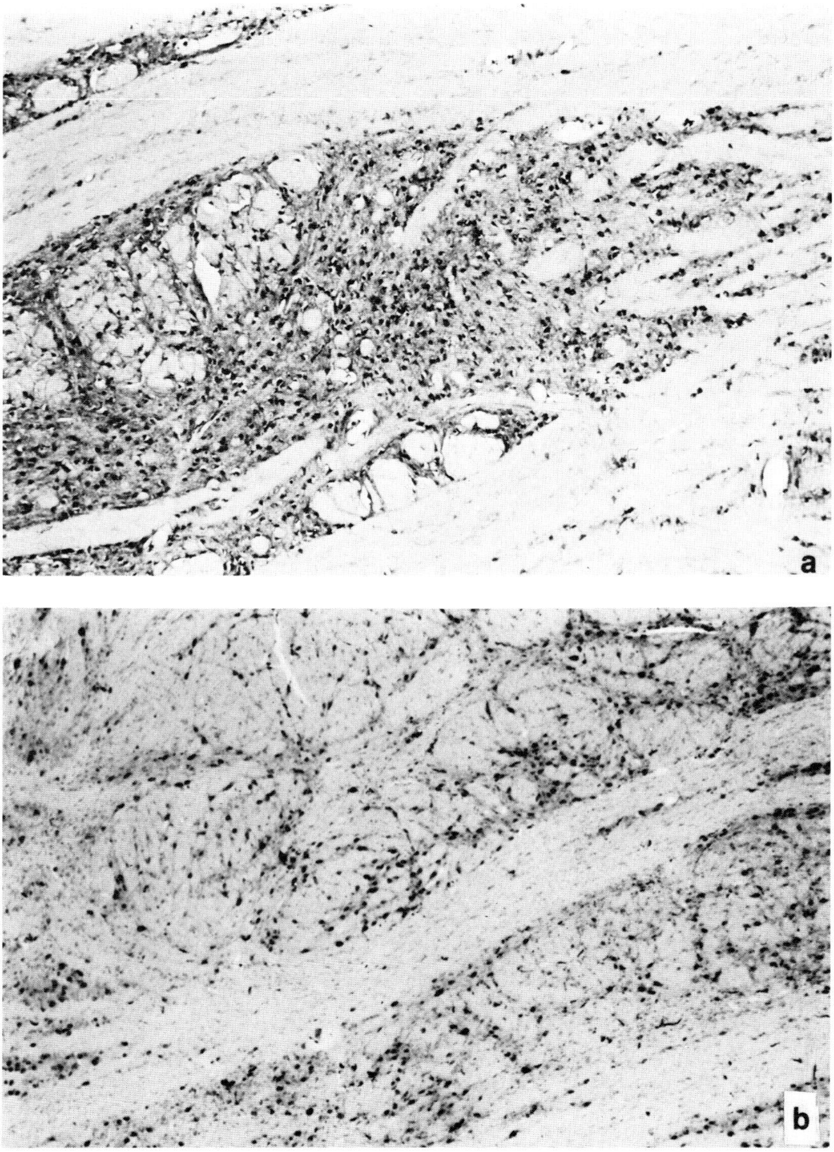

FIG. 11. Enzyme histochemistry for nonspecific esterase, basis pontis. Original magnification, × 10. **a:** Normal brain. Reaction product shows normal neuronal population and diffuse neuropilar activity. **b:** Hereditary OPCA. Nerve cells are greatly reduced in number, and neuropilar reaction product is sparse or absent. Compare perineuronal reaction product with staining intensity of surrounding white matter bundles.

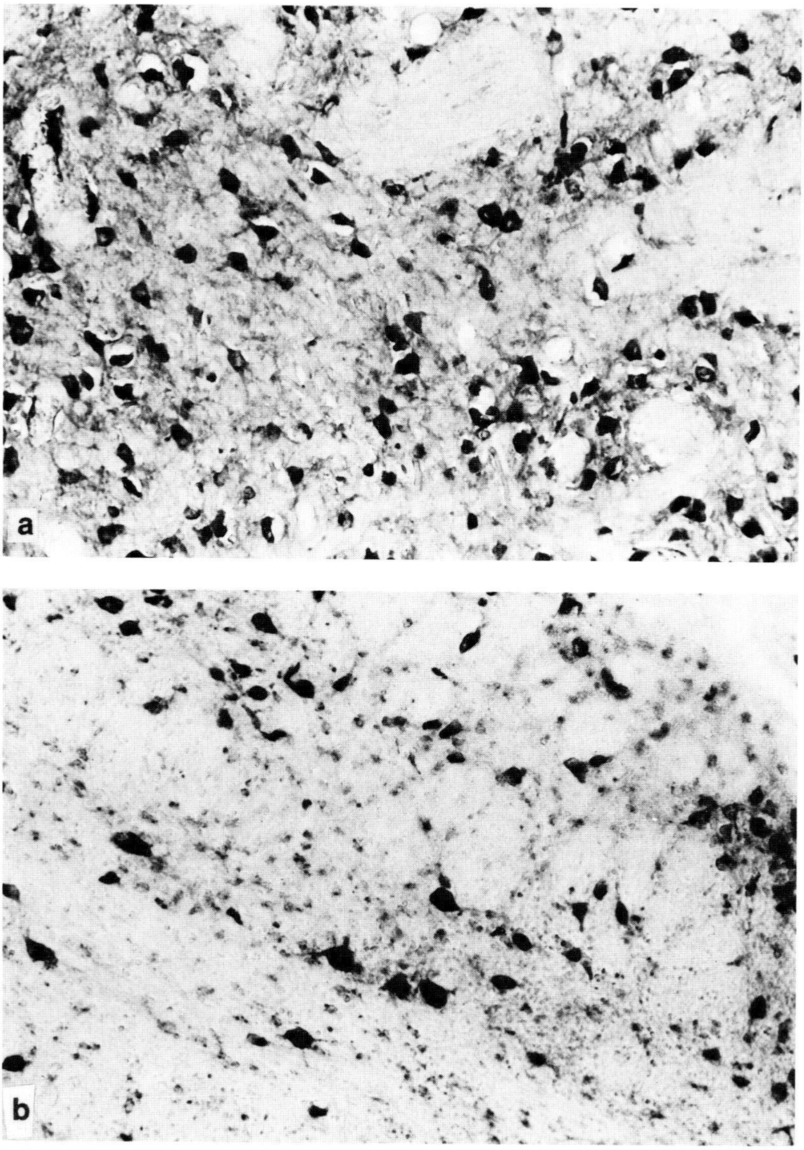

FIG. 12. Enzyme histochemistry for nonspecific esterase, basis pontis. Original magnification, ×40. **a:** Normal brain. Reaction product outlines cell bodies and delicate dendrites. Neuropilar reaction product can be recognized. **b:** Hereditary OPCA. Overall neuronal loss is apparent. In addition, dendrites are sparse and, when visualized, appear plump and stubby. Diffuse neuropilar reaction product is absent.

cytoplasm, but Golgi cells were not abnormal. Synaptic boutons were described as shrunken, and some axons were abnormally dense. The data did not allow the conclusion that afferent cerebellar connections were especially vulnerable in this form of familial OPCA, perhaps the only remarkable difference in the two reports. Retention of normal Golgi cells and hypertrophy of glial processes were present in all cases. None of the observations could be considered pathognomonic for OPCA. Many of the described membranous inclusions likely relate to artifact of fixation and autolytic change.

PATHOGENESIS OF OPCA

The pathogenesis of OPCA is not known. Canine hereditary ataxia (8,11) does not show OPCA but offers avenues for further study. In the autosomal recessive ataxia of Gordon setters reported by Cork et al. (8), the lesion was restricted to the cerebellar cortex. DeLahunta and Averill (11) described hereditary ataxia in Kerry Blue terriers. In early stages of the disease, only the cerebellar cortex was affected. Later, lesions occurred in the inferior olivary nuclei, substantia nigra, and caudate nuclei; the pons was spared.

Experimental lesions of the inferior olivary nuclei and some other brainstem nuclei can be produced by systemic administration of 3-acetylpyridine (for review, see ref. 12); however, this nicotinamide antagonist does not affect the basis pontis or cerebellar gray matter (13). The inferior olivary lesion is primary in contrast to OPCA, where it is thought to be due to the loss of Purkinje cells (see below).

Winkler (57) suggested that the involvement of pontine gray matter, inferior olivary nuclei, and arcuate nuclei, a constant feature of OPCA, related to the "cellbands of Essick." Essick (17) showed that the nuclei of the basis pontis arise by medial migration of neuroblasts from the lateral rhombic lip. Simultaneously, cells destined to become inferior olivary nuclei and arcuate nuclei migrate medially on a more ventral and superficial route. Winkler (57) implied that these three cell groups shared a "primary deficiency" that made them "less able to resist the struggle for life." His contemporaries accepted this concept of "abiotrophy," but it is rarely used today. According to Winkler's postulate, the loss of Purkinje cells is secondary, or transneuronal in more current terminology. Several observations make this mechanism unlikely. In parenchymatous cerebellar degeneration of sporadic or familial type (3,23,24,27,54), the inferior olivary nuclei are affected, while pontine nuclei are not. There is little question that the cortical cerebellar disease in these cases is primary. Holmes (24) and others thought that the olivary changes were secondary.

Koeppen et al. (31) reported a patient with sporadic cerebellar cortical degeneration in which the neurons of the dentate nuclei were also depleted. The anterior lamina of the inferior olivary nuclei showed neuronal loss, but the remaining nerve cells were enlarged, contained vacuoles, and gave rise to elaborate dendritic expansions (glomeruloid structures). The astrocytic response was of large cell type.

This process was identical to the olivary hypertrophy that follows lesions of the dentate nuclei or central tegmental tracts. The dorsal lamina and the accessory olivary nuclei also showed neuronal loss, but the surviving nerve cells were small. Gliosis consisted of proliferated small astrocytes. The authors interpreted the olivary hypertrophy as evidence of transneuronal degeneration (dentate lesion) and the changes in the dorsal lamina and accessory nuclei as retrograde atrophy (cerebellar cortical lesion). It was suggested that the dentate lesion preceded the cortical cerebellar disease, and that inferior olivary neurons responded to deafferentation first and to Purkinje cell death later. It should be recalled, however, that loss of Purkinje cells theoretically only removes the synaptic target of olivocerebellar fibers and does not interrupt their axons. The result is retrograde neuronal degeneration that differs by its slowness from a similar neuronal response to frank destructive lesions of the cerebellum.

The mixture of transneuronal and retrograde atrophy strongly suggests that the inferior olivary nuclei react to cerebellar lesions in a predictable manner. The lack of a similar response in pontine neurons in cases of parenchymatous cerebellar degeneration militates against the concept that olivary and pontine neurons share specific vulnerabilities. It is important to recall that the nuclei of the basis pontis project mostly to the granule cell layer and not directly to Purkinje cells. Synaptic terminals of the neurons in the basis pontis are removed by one or more interneuron from any changes that take place in Purkinje cells.

Pontine neurons may go on to atrophy without accompanying changes in cerebellar cortex or inferior olives, such as in spinopontine atrophy (7,43,52). The described cases with this condition share autosomal dominant transmission with familial OPCA, but their lesion centers on the basis pontis, the middle cerebellar peduncles, and the spinal cord. Cerebellar involvement is minor (43,52); when present, however, it is accompanied by proportional olivary degeneration. Pogacar et al. (43) actually suggested that spinopontine atrophy was a variant of OPCA. These cases further strengthen the idea that olivary changes are indeed secondary to the cortical cerebellar lesion that characterizes OPCA.

Histochemical visualization of acetylcholinesterase and nonspecific esterase (Figs. 7–13) shows a much more complex lesion than could be reconciled by a single common denominator. It is not apparent how the loss of reaction product for acetylcholinesterase in the neurons of the basis pontis and the pontine neuropil can give rise to depletion of enzyme activity in the molecular layer. While a primary cerebellar and pontine disease process is made likely by the cited observations, the individual steps toward the full picture of OPCA remain obscure.

FIG. 13. Enzyme histochemistry for acetylcholinesterase, inferior olivary nuclei. Original magnification, ×40. **a:** Normal brain. The reaction visualizes the nerve cell bodies and capillary walls. **b:** Hereditary OPCA. The dorsal lamina of the inferior olivary nucleus shows sparse and irregular reaction product in small surviving neurons. Irregular capillary wall staining is present. **c:** Hereditary OPCA. The ventral lamina of the inferior olivary nucleus shows reduction of nerve cell size and overall poor staining of the perikaryon. Capillary wall staining is irregular and appears excessively dense.

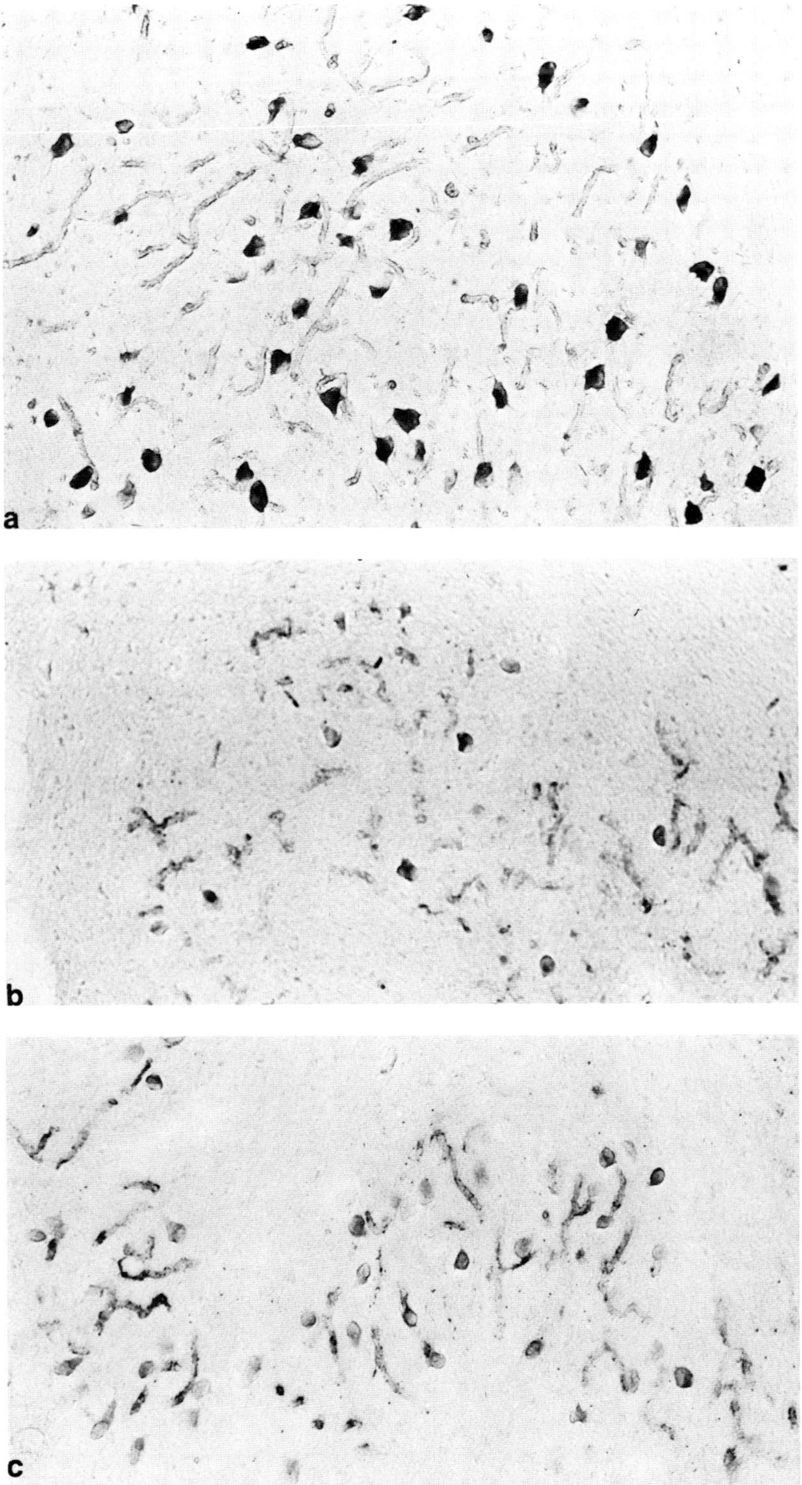
a
b
c

ACKNOWLEDGMENTS

This work was supported in part by the Veterans Administration, the National Ataxia Foundation, the Alexander von Humboldt Foundation, and the Robert W. Graves Fund of the Department of Neurology, Albany Medical College.

REFERENCES

1. Adams, C. W. M. *(editor)* (1965): Histochemistry of the cells in the nervous system. In: *Neurohistochemistry*, pp. 253–331. Elsevier, Amsterdam.
2. Adams, R., van Bogaert, L., and van der Eecken, H. (1961): Dégénérescences nigro-striées et cérébello-nigro-striées. *Psychiatr. Neurol. (Basel)*, 142:219–259.
3. Akelaitis, A. J. (1938): Hereditary form of primary parenchymatous atrophy of the cerebellar cortex associated with mental deterioration. *Am. J. Psychiatry*, 94:1115–1137.
4. Aring, C. D. (1940): Degeneration of the basal ganglia associated with olivo-ponto-cerebellar atrophy. *J. Nerv. Ment. Dis.*, 92:448–470.
5. Becker, P. E. *(editor)* (1966): Krankheiten mit hauptsächlicher Beteiligung des spino-zerebellaren Systems (Erbliche Ataxien). In: *Humangenetik. Ein kurzes Handbuch in fünf Banden, Vol. 5/1*, pp. 208–313. Thieme, Stuttgart.
6. Berciano, J. (1982): Olivopontocerebellar atrophy. *J. Neurol. Sci.*, 53:253–272.
7. Boller, F., and Segarra, J. M. (1969): Spino-pontine degeneration. *Eur. Neurol.*, 2:356–373.
8. Cork, L. C., Troncoso, J. C., and Price, D. L. (1981): Canine inherited ataxia. *Ann. Neurol.*, 9:492–499.
9. Dejerine, J., and Thomas, A. (1900): L'atrophie olivo-ponto-cérébèlleuse. *Nouv. Iconogr. Salpêt.*, 13:330–370.
10. DeGiacomo, P. (1962): Distribution of cholinesterase activity in the human central nervous system. In: *Proceedings of the Fourth International Congress of Neuropathology, Rome*, edited by H. Jacob, pp. 198–205. Thieme, Stuttgart.
11. DeLahunta, A., and Averill, D. R. (1976): Hereditary cerebellar cortical and extrapyramidal nuclear abiotrophy in Kerry Blue terriers. *J. Am. Vet. Med. Assoc.*, 168:1119–1124.
12. Desclin, J. C., and Escubi, J. (1974): Effects of 3-acetylpyridine on the central nervous system of the rat, as demonstrated by silver methods. *Brain Res.*, 77:349–364.
13. Desclin, J. C. (1974): Histological evidence supporting the inferior olive as the major source of cerebellar climbing fibers in the rat. *Brain Res.*, 77:365–384.
14. Eadie, M. J. (1975): Olivo-ponto-cerebellar atrophy (Dejerine-Thomas type). In: *Handbook of Clinical Neurology, Vol 21*, edited by P. M. Vinken and G. W. Bruyn, pp. 415–431. North Holland, Amsterdam.
15. Eadie, M. J. (1975): Olivo-ponto-cerebellar atrophy (Menzel type). In: *Handbook of Clinical Neurology, Vol. 21*, edited by P. J. Vinken and G. W. Bruyn, pp. 433–449. North Holland, Amsterdam.
16. Eadie, M. J. (1975): Olivo-ponto-cerebellar atrophy (variants). In: *Handbook of Clinical Neurology*, Vol. 21, edited by P. J. Vinken and G. W. Bruyn, pp. 451–457. North Holland, Amsterdam.
17. Essick, C. R. (1912): The development of the nuclei pontis and the nucleus arcuatus in man. *Am. J. Anat.*, 13:25–54.
18. Fickler, A. (1911): Klinische und pathologisch-anatomische Beiträge zu den Erkrankungen des Kleinhirns. *Dtsch. Z. Nervenheilk.*, 41:306–375.
19. Friede, R. L., and Fleming, L. M. (1964): A comparison of cholinesterase distribution in the cerebellum of several species. *J. Neurochem.*, 11:1–7.
20. Fujisawa, K., and Nakamura, A. (1982): The human Purkinje cell. A Golgi study in pathology. *Acta Neuropathol.*, 56:255–264.
21. Gomori, G. (1952): *Microscopic Histochemistry*. University of Chicago Press, Chicago.
22. Greenfield, J. G. (1954): *The Spinocerebellar Degenerations*. Blackwell, Oxford.
23. Hall, B., Noad, K. B., and Latham, O. (1941): Familial cortical cerebellar atrophy. *Brain*, 64:178–194.
24. Holmes, G. (1907): A form of familial degeneration of the cerebellum. *Brain*, 30:466–488.
25. Hunt, J. R. (1921): Dyssynergia cerebellaris myoclonica—primary atrophy of the dentate system: A contribution to the pathology and symptomatology of the cerebellum. *Brain*, 44:490–538.

26. Jellinger, K., and Tarnowska-Dziduszko, E. (1971): Die ZNS-Veränderungen bei den olivo-ponto-cerebellären Atrophien. *Z. Neurol.*, 199:192–214.
27. Jervis, G. A. (1950): Early familial cerebellar degeneration. *J. Nerv. Ment. Dis.*, 111:398–407.
28. Koelle, G. B., and Friedenwald, J. S. (1949): A histochemical method for localizing cholinesterase activity. *Proc. Soc. Exp. Biol. Med.*, 70:617–622.
29. Koeppen, A. H., and Hans, M. B. (1976): Supranuclear ophthalmoplegia in olivopontocerebellar degeneration. *Neurology*, 26:764–768.
30. Koeppen, A. H., Hans, M. B., Shepherd, D. I., and Best, P. V. (1977): Adult-onset hereditary ataxia in Scotland. *Arch. Neurol.*, 34:611–618.
31. Koeppen, A. H., Barron, K. D., and Cassidy, R. J. (1979): Transneuronal degeneration of the inferior olivary nuclei in system atrophy. *Acta Neuropathol.*, 47:155–158.
32. Koeppen, A. H., Barron, K. D., and Dentinger, M. P. (1980): Olivary hypertrophy: Histochemical demonstration of hydrolytic enzymes. *Neurology*, 30:471–480.
33. Konigsmark, B. W., and Weiner, L. P. (1970): The olivopontocerebellar atrophies: A review. *Medicine*, 49:227–241.
34. Landis, D. M. D., Rosenberg, R. N., Landis, S. C., Schut, L., and Nyhan, W. L. (1974): Olivopontocerebellar degeneration. Clinical and ultrastructural abnormalities. *Arch. Neurol.*, 31:295–307.
35. Lehrer, G. M., and Ornstein, L. (1959): A diazo coupling method for the electron microscopic localization of cholinesterase. *J. Biophys. Biochem. Cytol.*, 6:399–406.
36. Marie, P. (1893): Sur l'hérédo-ataxie cérébèlleuse. *Sem. Med.*, 13:444–447.
37. Menzel, P. (1891): Beitrag zur Kenntnis der hereditären Ataxien und Kleinhirnatrophie. *Arch. Psychiatr. Nervenkr.*, 22:160–190.
38. Neumann, M., and Cohn, R. (1955): Progressive familial ataxia. *J. Neuropathol. Exp. Neurol.*, 14:398–415.
39. Nick, J., Contamin, R., Escourolle, R., Guillard, A., and Marcantoni, J. P. (1967): Hypotension orthostatique idiopathique avec syndrome neurologique complexe a prédominance extrapyramidale. *Rev. Neurol.*, 116:213–227.
40. Norman, R. M., and Urich, H. (1958): Cerebellar hypoplasia associated with systemic degeneration in early life. *J. Neurol. Neurosurg. Psychiatry*, 21:159–166.
41. Petito, C. K., Hart, M. N., Porro, R. S., and Earle, K. M. (1973): Ultrastructural studies of olivopontocerebellar atrophy. *J. Neuropathol. Exp. Neurol.*, 32:503–522.
42. Pierret, M. (1871): Note sur cas d'atrophie périphérique du cervelet avec lésion concomitante des olives bulbaires. *Arch. Physiol. Norm. Pathol.*, 4:765–770.
43. Pogacar, S., Ambler, M., Conklin, W. J., and O'Neil, W. A. (1978): Dominant spinopontine atrophy. *Arch. Neurol.*, 35:156–162.
44. Raymond, F. (1910): *Études de Pathologie Nerveuse*. Delarue, Paris.
45. Roessmann, W. (1975): Primary orthostatic hypotension. In: *Handbook of Clinical Neurology, Vol. 22*, edited by P. J. Vinken and G. W. Bruyn, pp. 231–242. North Holland, Amsterdam.
46. Rosenhagen, H. (1943): Die primäre Atrophie des Brückenfusses und der unteren Oliven (dargestellt nach klinischen und anatomischen Beobachtungen). *Arch. Psychiatr. Nervenkr.*, 116:163–228.
47. Royet, H., and Collet, J. (1893): Sur une lésion systematisée du cervelet et de ses dépendences bulbo-protubérentielles. *Arch. Neurol. (Paris)*, 26:353–374.
48. Ryan, S. J., Knox, D. L., Green, W. R., and Konigsmark, B. W. (1975): Olivopontocerebellar degeneration. Clinicopathologic correlation of the associated retinopathy. *Arch. Ophthalmol.*, 93:169–172.
49. Schut, J. W. (1954): The hereditary ataxias. *Proc. Assoc. Res. Nerv. Ment. Dis.*, 33:293–324.
50. Schwarz, G. A. (1975): Dysautonomic syndromes in adults. In: *Handbook of Clinical Neurology, Vol. 22*, edited by P. J. Vinken and G. W. Bruyn, pp. 243–280. North Holland, Amsterdam.
51. Spokes, E. G. S., Bannister, R., and Oppenheimer, D. R. (1979): Multiple system atrophy with autonomic failure. *J. Neurol. Sci.*, 43:59–82.
52. Taniguchi, R., and Konigsmark, B. W. (1971): Dominant spinopontine atrophy. *Brain*, 94:349–358.
53. Takei, Y., and Mirra, S. S. (1973): Striatonigral degeneration: A form of multiple system atrophy with clinical parkinsonism. In: *Progress in Neuropathology, Vol. 2*, edited by H. M. Zimmerman, pp. 217–251. Grune & Stratton, New York.
54. Thorpe, F. T. (1935): Familial degeneration of the cerebellum in association with epilepsy. *Brain*, 58:97–114.

55. Titica, J., and van Bogaert, L. (1946): Heredodegenerative hemiballismus. *Brain*, 69:251–263.
56. Welte, E. (1939): Die Atrophie des Systems des Brückenfusses und der unteren Oliven. *Arch. Psychiatr. Nervenkr.*, 109:649–698.
57. Winkler, C. (1923): A case of olivo-pontine cerebellar atrophy and our conception of neo- and palaeo-cerebellum. *Schweiz. Arch. Neurol. Psychiatr.*, 13:684–702.

The Olivopontocerebellar Atrophies, edited by
R. C. Duvoisin and A. Plaitakis. Raven Press,
New York © 1984.

Morphological Changes of Olivopontocerebellar Atrophy in Computed Tomography and Comments on Its Pathogenesis

Yun Peng Huang and *Andreas Plaitakis

*Department of Radiology, Neuroradiology Section, and *Department of Neurology, Mount Sinai School of Medicine, City University of New York, New York, New York 10029*

DEFINITION

Although the term *olivopontocerebellar atrophy* (OPCA) was introduced in 1900 by Dejerine and André-Thomas (17) to describe 2 sporadic cases of the disease, Menzel in 1981 (35) was the first to report the pathological features of a similar disorder with autosomal dominant transmission. Currently included under OPCA are various types of closely related degenerative neurological disorders. These share certain common pathological features, such as atrophy of the inferior olives, cerebellar cortex, pontine nuclei, transverse pontine fibers, and the middle cerebellar peduncles. Other areas of the central nervous system (CNS), such as nuclei of the lower cranial nerves, the basal ganglia, and the spinal cord, may also be involved in some types of OPCA (12,22,25,27,55). The clinical picture may vary considerably; however, the majority of patients show a progressive cerebellar syndrome that is associated with other neurological features, such as corticospinal deficits, extrapyramidal signs (parkinsonism, dystonia, or chorea), oculomotor disturbances, bulbar dysfunction, spinal cord involvement, and/or peripheral neuropathy (19,46).

As a result of a special interest in spinocerebellar degeneration at our institution, we have had the opportunity to evaluate a large number of patients with various types of OPCA during the past few years. Most of these patients were examined neurologically. Some were members of well-known pedigrees in which OPCA had been documented by postmortem studies (6,55). As part of the evaluation of these patients, CT scan of the head was obtained routinely. The availability of such characteristic cases encouraged us to study clinico-pathologico-radiological (CT) correlations in OPCA. Demonstration by pneumoencephalography or by CT of the gross pathological features of OPCA, such as cerebellar and pontine atrophy, has been described by others (1–3,5,24,26,28,29,30,32,41,53,54). However, a systematic attempt to study radiologically in depth the various types of OPCA has not been made in the past. The CT characteristics of 5 distinct types of OPCA are reported in this chapter.

METHODS

Types of OPCA Studied

The nosology of OPCA remains confusing to this date. It is, however, clear that this entity represents a heterogeneous group of neurological disorders. Although many classifications of OPCA have been proposed, based on clinico-pathologic and genetic features, none of these is satisfactory. As suggested by Refsum and Skre (50), the final classification of various spinocerebellar degenerations should be based on the demonstration of gene-dependent, fundamental biochemical defects. Despite the recent progress in biochemistry of OPCA,[1] specific biochemical abnormalities have not been found in the majority of these afflictions.

Studying these disorders, one still has to use conventional criteria for classification in addition to the available biochemical markers. In the present study, we evaluated the following 5 different types of OPCA which were diagnosed and classified using biochemical and heredoclinical criteria:

1. Recessive OPCA associated with GDH deficiency
2. Sporadic OPCA associated with orthostatic hypotension
3. Dominant OPCA—"S" family (55)
4. Dominant OPCA—"W" family (spinopontine variety) (6,48)
5. Dominant OPCA associated with slow saccades

The first type includes 11 patients with *recessive OPCA associated with deficiency of glutamate dehydrogenase (GDH)* (42–47). These patients were affected by slowly progressive cerebellar and extrapyramidal syndromes of a late adult onset (5th–7th decades). Associated neurological manifestations were bulbar dysfunction, oculomotor disturbances (nystagmus, impaired pursuit or volitional saccades, etc.), corticospinal deficits, anterior horn cell signs, and/or peripheral neuropathy (see chapter by Plaitakis, *this volume*). The diagnosis was made by demonstrating reduced GDH activity in leukocytes isolated from peripheral blood of these patients.

Placed in the second type are 4 patients with *sporadic OPCA associated with orthostatic hypotension* (4,39,46). Similar to GDH-deficient cases, these patients showed progressive cerebellar and extrapyramidal syndromes of a late adult onset (5th–6th decades), associated with bulbar dysfunctions and corticospinal deficits. Characteristic clinical features of this entity, however, were symptoms and signs of progressive autonomic failure, such as orthostatic hypotension, sexual impotence, and incontinence, occurring early in the course of the illness (4,46). In constrast to the more indolent course experienced by the patients of the first type, these patients showed a quicker clinical deterioration, ending in incapacitation or death within 1 to 4 years. There was no associated GDH deficiency in this group.

The third type includes 5 members of a large family affected by *dominant OPCA*, known as the *"S" family* (55). They suffered from cerebellar syndrome of early adult onset (2nd–3rd decades), associated with mild corticospinal deficits, oculomotor disturbances (broken-up pursuit, ocular dysmetria), and peripheral neurop-

---

[1]See chapters by Perry, by Plaitakis, by Maruyama and Yamaguchi, and by Duvoisin and Chokvoverty, *this volume*.

athy. Bulbar symptoms, such as dysarthria, dysphagia, atrophy of the tongue, and facial weakness, as well as slowing of the saccadic eye movements and anterior horn cell signs, were usually seen in an advanced stage of the illness.

Included in the fourth type is a patient from another *dominant OPCA* family, known as the *"W" family* (6,48). This patient experienced diplopia at the age of 20 and, subsequently, progressive gait disturbances, spastic legs, and incoordination of hand movements. Positive neurological findings were marked gait and limb ataxia, severe leg spasticity with hyperreflexia and extensor plantar responses, bilateral facial weakness, oculomotor deficits, palatal myoclonus, and dysarthria. Because the pathology found in some of the deceased members of this family was more or less limited to the spinal cord and pons, this disorder was designated as spinopontine atrophy (6,59). However, more recent pathological studies in an additional member of the same family have shown that the cerebellum was also affected, suggesting that this disorder is an OPCA variant (48).

Finally, the fifth type consists of 4 patients with a form of *dominant OPCA* associated *with slow saccades* (47a). In these patients, there were characteristic slow, but full-ranged, volitional saccadic eye movements, as described in 1971 by Wadia and Swami (62) (see also chapter by Wadia, *this volume*). Other clinical features were cerebellar ataxia, corticospinal deficits, bilateral facial weakness (of a lower motor neuron type), and peripheral neuropathy.

These 5 types of OPCA were selected for this study because their diagnosis and classification could be made with reasonable certainty. Thus, the first type was associated with a specific biochemical defect and the second with the characteristic clinical features of autonomic failure. The remaining 3 were disorders with clear dominant transmission. Of the latter, the first 2 types were classified according to their family and are expected to be genetically (and therefore biochemically) homogeneous; whereas, the last type was separated on the basis of specific clinical manifestations.

Patients with suspected OPCA who could not be classified with certainty were excluded from this study. It should also be noted that our series does not cover the full spectrum of OPCA that may include rare types not available to us.

For the purpose of comparison, 2 patients with dominantly inherited cerebello-olivary atrophy (COA) were also studied; their findings are described here. Both were affected by an adult onset cerebellar ataxia not associated with any other neurological abnormalities (18).

Disease Stages

At present, no satisfactory staging system has been proposed for OPCA. Because the disorder has a variety of neurological manifestations which can occur in various combinations and severities, staging of the disease is expected to be far more difficult than that of other neurological disorders where only one neuronal system is predominantly involved (e.g., Parkinson's disease). Despite these considerations, the majority of OPCA patients are known to present with gait disturbances. Furthermore, deterioration in the patient's ability to walk correlates with the degree of disability. In view of this, the staging system used in this study was based on the degree of gait disturbances (Table 1).

TABLE 1. *Staging of OPCA based on ability to ambulate*

Stage	Degree of impairment	Characteristics
I	Slight	Detectable only on running, turning fast, hopping on one foot, or walking in tandem
II	Moderate	Gait clearly unsteady; able to ambulate independently without support
III	Marked	Able to ambulate only with support
IV	Severe	Wheelchair-bound or bedridden

Controls

The controls had no known degenerative neurological disorder. They were subjected to CT scanning because of various neurological symptoms and signs, such as possible transient ischemic attacks, seizure disorder, headache syndrome, impaired vision, decreased hearing, possible brain tumor, and trigeminal neuralgia. All CT scans showing a gross pathology, such as cerebral vascular accidents and brain tumors, were excluded. Also eliminated were patients with long-standing seizure disorders associated with cerebellar dysfunction secondary to phenytoin (Dilantin®) toxicity and with gait disturbances of unknown etiology. Controls were divided into 5 groups. Each group included 10 to 12 individuals of the same decade of life from approximately 30 to 80 years of age. The 30- to 39-year-old group was taken as baseline and compared with each group to evaluate the effect of aging on morphological changes of the brain.

Computerized Tomographic Investigations

The type of CT scanner utilized was the GE 8800, except in 5 cases in which an EMI 1010 was used. Of the latter, 3 cases had dominant OPCA (S family); the other 2 had sporadic OPCA with orthostatic hypotension and recessive OPCA with GDH deficiency, respectively. The majority of the CT images were obtained by sectioning parallel to a plane located between the orbitomeatal and inferior orbitomeatal planes. Small adjustments were made in measured values from CT images taken in the superior orbitomeatal plane. Five to ten percent was subtracted from the values in measuring the brainstem and the fourth ventricle in the anteroposterior direction. No adjustments were made in transverse measurements on CT images taken with different inclinations. All measurements were made directly from the films and converted to actual distances using the CT scan scale provided. In a few cases, these values were compared to the actual "distance-measurement" with a CT cursor. Measurements taken by each method were compatible. Figure 1 illustrates

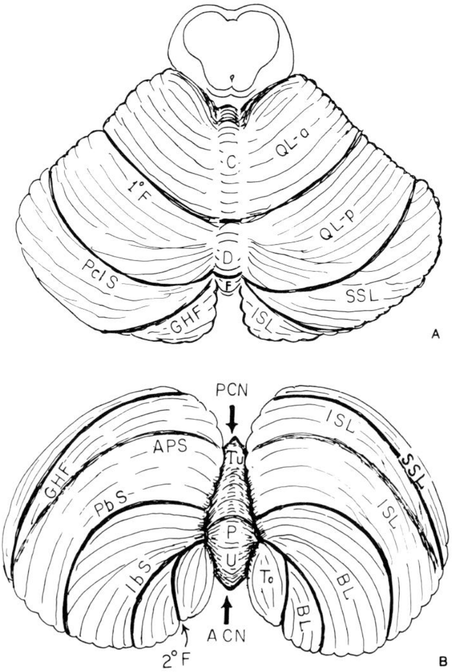

FIG. 1. Diagram of the cerebellum showing its major lobules and sulci. **A:** Superior surface. Labeled are culmen (C) and declive (D) of the vermis, folium (F), great horizontal fissure (GHF), inferior semilunar lobule (ISL), anterior (QL-a) and posterior parts (QL-p) of the quadrangular lobule, superior semilunar lobule (SSL), and primary fissure (1°F) of the cerebellum. The postclival sulcus (Pcl S), also called the posterior superior fissure, is also labeled. **B:** Inferior surface. The brainstem has been removed in order to show both the anterior (ACN) and posterior cerebellar notches (PCN). Labeled are ansoparomedian sulcus (APS), biventral lobule (BL), great horizontal fissure (GHF), intrabiventral sulcus (IbS), inferior semilunar lobule (ISL), pyramid (P), prebiventral sulcus (PbS), superior semilunar lobule (SSL), tonsil (To), tuber (Tu), uvula (U) and secondary fissure (2°F). The paravermian sulci on either side of the vermis are clearly shown.

normal surface anatomy of the cerebellum. Figures 2A to 2F show the modes of measurement of various parts of the brain: the ventricular cavities and the subarachnoid spaces, including the basal cisterns (in a 72-year-old control).

RESULTS

CT Changes with Aging in the Control Groups

With aging (in the controls) there was an increase in the size of the subarachnoid spaces, cisterns, and ventricles. As shown in Fig. 3, the greatest changes occurred in the size of the third ventricle, the sylvian fissures, and the intercaudate distance

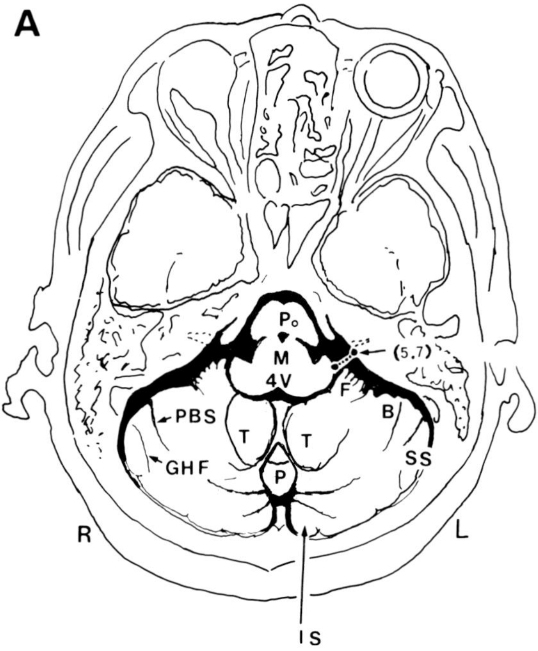
A
Po
M
4V
(5.7)
F
PBS
B
T
T
GHF
SS
P
R
L
IS

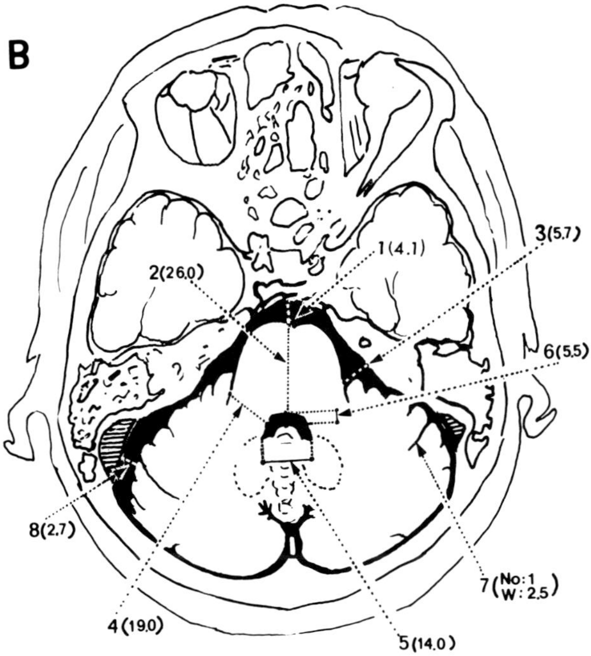
B
3(5.7)
1(4.1)
2(26.0)
6(5.5)
8(2.7)
7(No:1 W: 2.5)
4(19.0)
5(14.0)

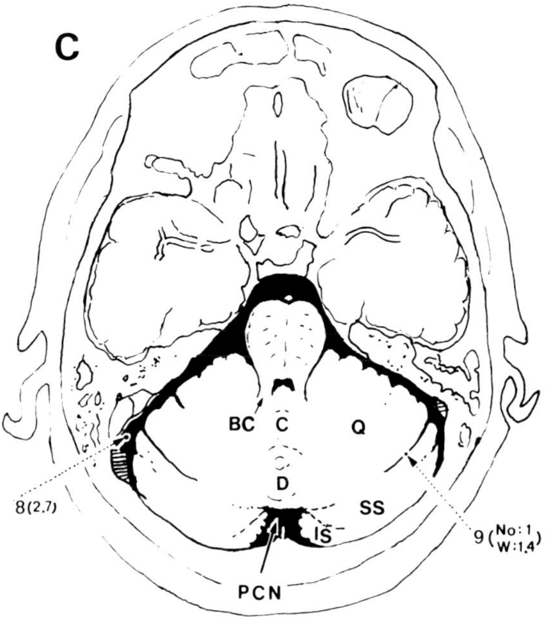

FIG. 2. A–F: Schematic drawings of CT sections with approximately 5° to 7° extension from the orbitomeatal plane, based on CT scans of a 72-year-old control (see Methods). A control of this age was selected for easy drawing because the cerebrospinal fluid spaces are more prominent in elderly individuals. Numbers in parentheses indicate the actual size (mean value expressed in millimeters) of anatomical structures, subarachnoid spaces, or ventricles found in the 70- to 79-year-old control group. **FIG. 2A.** Section through the internal auditory canals showing the cisterns of the cerebellopontine angle. Accurate measurement of various parts of the brainstem at the level of the pontomedullary junction is difficult because of poor delineation of the anatomical structures. This is due to artifacts derived from the petrous pyramids and the adjacent air cells. The averge depth of the cerebellopontine angle cistern *(dotted line)* was 5.7 mm in the control group (70- to 79-year-old control group). Labeled are biventral lobule (B), flocculus (F), great horizontal fissure (GHF), inferior semilunar lobule (IS), medulla oblongata (M), pons (Po), (preventral sulcus), (PBS), pyramid (P), superior semilunar lobule (SS), tonsil (T), and fourth ventricle (4V). Right (R) and left (L) are also indicated. **FIG. 2B.** Section through the mid-pons. Labeled are pontine cisterns *(1)*, anteroposterior diameter of the pons *(2)*, cisterns of the cerebellopontine angle *(3)*, brachium pontis *(4)*, transverse *(5)*, and anteroposterior *(6)*, diameters of the fourth ventricle, prebiventral sulcus *(7)*, and lateral angle cistern *(8)*. The average number (No) and width (W) are indicated in millimeters for the cerebellar hemispheric sulci *(7)*, measured at the level of the lateral angle cistern *(8)*, in the 70- to 79-year-old control group. **FIG. 2C.** Section through the upper pons. Labeled are lateral angle cistern *(8)*, postclival sulcus *(9)*, brachium conjuntivum (BC), culmen (C), declive (D), inferior semilunar lobule (IS), posterior cerebellar notch (PCN), quadrangular lobule (Q), and superior semilunar lobule (SS). The lateral angle cistern *(8)*, (adjacent to the lateral angle of the cerebellar hemisphere) is usually measured at or immediately below this level. The visualized cerebellar peduncle at this level is not the brachium pontis but the brachium conjuntivum (BC). At this level, the wall of the posterior cerebellar notch is formed laterally by the superior and inferior semilunar lobules and anteriorly by the declive, folium, and tuber.

D

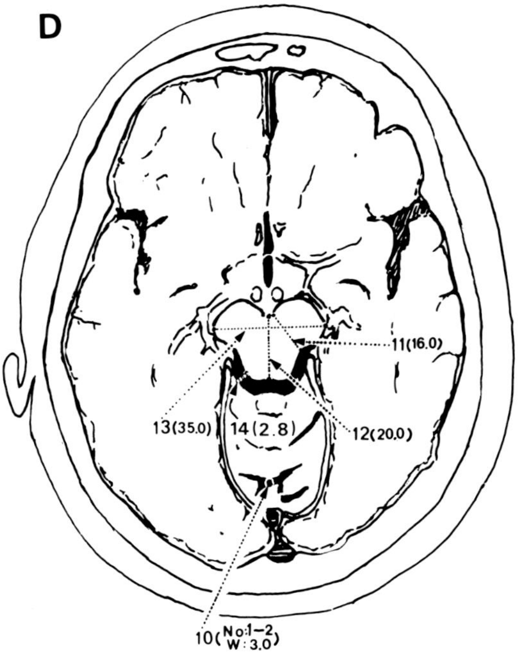

FIG. 2D. Section through the midbrain. Labeled are vermian sulci *(10)*, transverse diameter of the basis pendunculi *(11)*, and anteroposterior *(12)* and transverse diameters *(13)* of the mesencephalon. Because of the diverging bases of the cerebral peduncle, the transverse diameter *(13)* of the mesencephalon varies slightly depending on the level of section. The quadrigeminal cistern *(14)* was measured at the level of posterolateral portion of the mesencephalon.

E

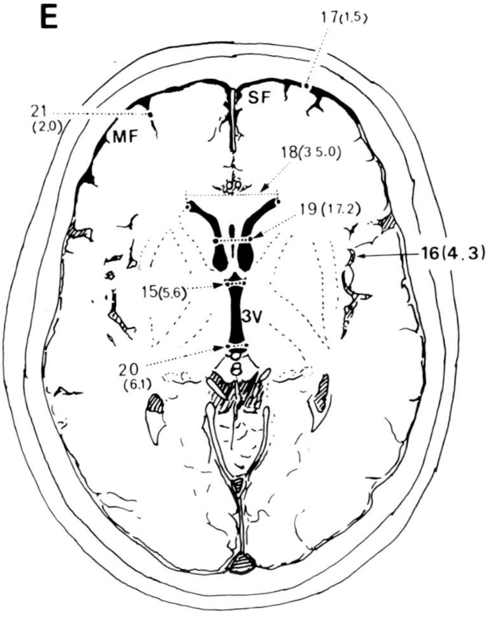

FIG. 2E. Section through the midlevel of the third ventricle and the pineal gland. Labeled are sylvian fissure *(16)*, subarachnoid space *(17)* of the frontal convexity, bifrontal cornuate distance *(18)* (measured between the widest portion of the two frontal horns), intercaudate distance *(19)*, transverse width of anterior *(15)*, posterior *(20)* parts of the third ventricle (3V), and anterior frontal sulci *(21)*. The superior frontal (SF) and the middle frontal gyri (MF) are also labeled.

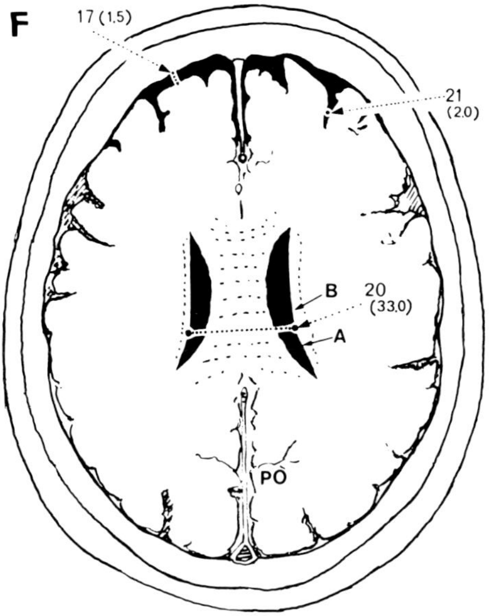

FIG. 2F. Section through the roof of the lateral ventricle. Labeled are subarachnoid space of the frontal convexity *(17)*, biparietal ventricular distance *(20)* at the junction of the body (B) and the atrium (A) of the lateral ventricle, and frontal sulci *(21)*. The parieto-occipital fissure (PO) is also indicated.

(between the medial aspects of the heads of the caudate nuclei). To a lesser degree the transverse widths of the lateral ventricles were also increased significantly at the level of the body (cella media) and at the anterolateral ends of the frontal horns (frontal bicornuate distance). The fourth ventricle, however, did not show a transverse widening until after 70 years of age.

With respect to the cerebellum, the visible sulci of the cerebellar hemispheres likewise increased in number, although little alteration was noted in their width with aging (Fig. 4A). The number and width of the vermian sulci, however, showed little change with aging. In addition, the size of the frontal sulci and the frontal subarachnoid space increased with aging in control groups (Fig. 4B).

CT Changes in Various Types of OPCA

Recessive OPCA Associated with Glutamate Dehydrogenase Deficiency

The most striking CT change was the dilatation of the anterior (233% of the control, $p < 0.0005$) and posterior (184% of the control, $p < 0.005$) third ventricle in transverse measurement (Fig. 4C; Table 2). Frequently, the enlarged third ventricle became oblong-shaped on transaxial section and ballooned on coronal section (Figs. 5–7). The enlargement appeared proportionally more pronounced

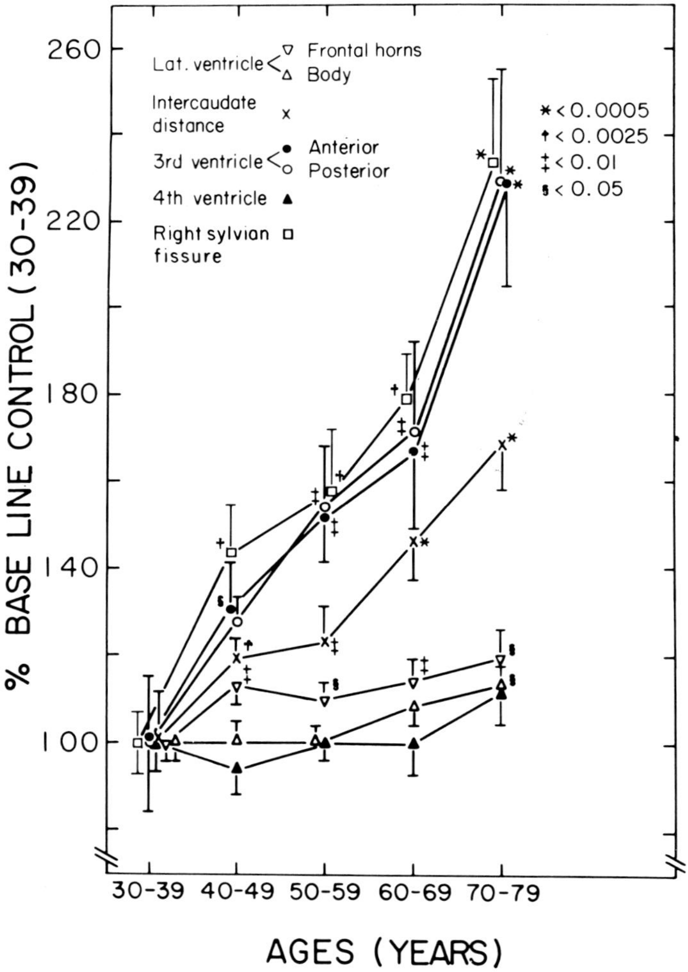

FIG. 3. Effect of aging on the sizes of the ventricles, the intercaudate distance, and the right sylvian fissure in nondegenerative controls. The frontal horns represent the frontal bicornuate distance (Fig. 2E). The body of the lateral ventricle was measured at the level of its roof (Fig. 2F), the intercaudate distance at its narrowest point (Fig. 2E), and the sylvian fissure at a level 5 mm below the section shown in Fig. 2E. The third and fourth ventricles (transverse diameter) were measured at their midlevels (Figs. 2B,2E). As shown here, the greatest changes were in the sizes of the sylvian fissure, the anterior and posterior third ventricle, and the intercaudate distance. A small, but significant, increase occurred in the size of the frontal horns in all age groups compared with baseline values (30- to 39-year-old age group). However, the size of the body of the lateral ventricle was increased significantly only in the 70- to 79-year-old age group. Symbols represent mean values for each age group. The values of the 30- to 39-year-old age group were used as a baseline. Each age group consists of 10 to 12 controls.

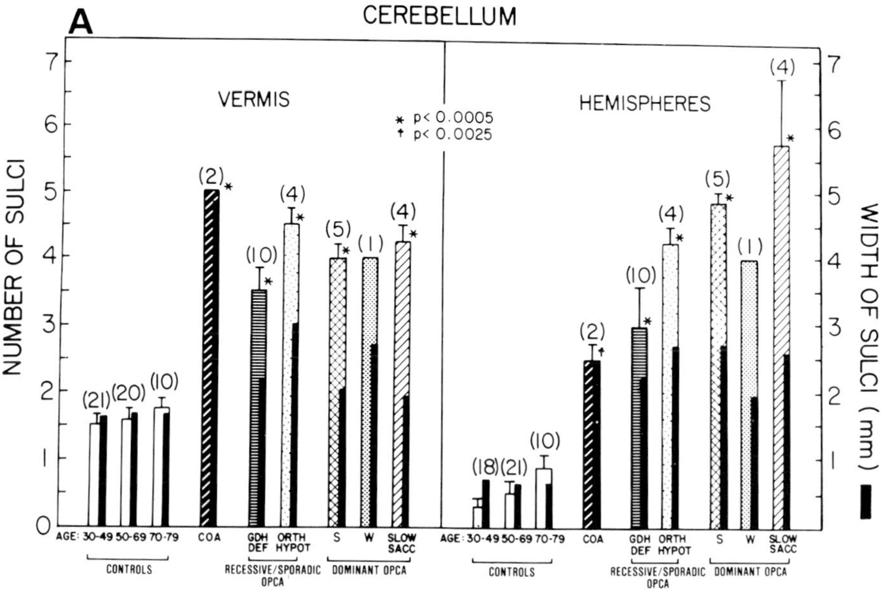

FIG. 4. A–G: Size of selected anatomical structures, ventricles, and subarachnoid spaces: COA, cerebello-olivary atrophy; GDH DEF, recessive OPCA associated with GDH deficiency; ORTH HYPOT, sporadic OPCA associated with orthostatic hypotension. S, dominant OPCA—"S" family (all 5 patients were members of the family described by Schut and Haymaker, ref. 55); W, another form of dominant OPCA—"W" family: a member of W family described as a spino-pontine variant (6,48); SLOW SACC, another form of dominantly inherited OPCA associated with slow saccadic eye movements. Number of individuals studied, given in parentheses. Full size columns indicate the mean number of sulci; brackets, standard errors. The solid black columns indicate the width (in millimeters) of the measured sulci.

Each category of patients was compared to the matching control age group. Thus, the 2 patients with cerebelloolivary atrophy (COA) (ages 59–67) were compared to 20 patients of 50 to 69 years of age. The 11 patients with GDH-deficient OPCA (GDH DEF) (ages 62–78) were compared to 20 controls of 60 to 79 years of age. The 4 patients with sporadic OPCA associated with orthostatic hypotension (ORTH HYPOT) (ages 54–72) were compared to 20 controls of 50 to 69 years of age. The 5 patients with dominant OPCA of the Schut and Haymaker type (S) (ages 30–42) were compared to 20 controls of 30 to 49 years of age. The patient from the "W" family (W) (age 31) as well as the 4 OPCA patients with slow saccades (SLOW SACC) (ages 30–38) were compared to 10 controls whose age ranged from 30–39. Occasionally, in cases of artifacts, measurements of certain anatomical structures were omitted. For details about measurements, see Methods (Figs. 2A–F). **A** *(above)*: Degree of cerebellar atrophy quantified by the number and width of the cerebellar sulci in patients with various types of OPCA. The number and width of the cerebellar sulci shown here and the width of the frontal sulci (see Fig. 4G) of three control groups are also included for comparison. **B:** Degree of frontal atrophy graded by the width of the frontal sulci and the frontal subarachnoid space in patients with various types of OPCA and nondegenerative controls. **C:** Size of the anterior and posterior third ventricle in patients with various subtypes of OPCA. **D:** Size of the fourth ventricle in patients with various types of OPCA. **E:** The size of the pons (anteroposterior diameter) and brachium pontis (width) in patients with various types of OPCA. **F:** Size of the mesencephalon in patients with various types of OPCA. **G:** Intercaudate distance and the size of the right sylvian fissure in patients with various types of OPCA.

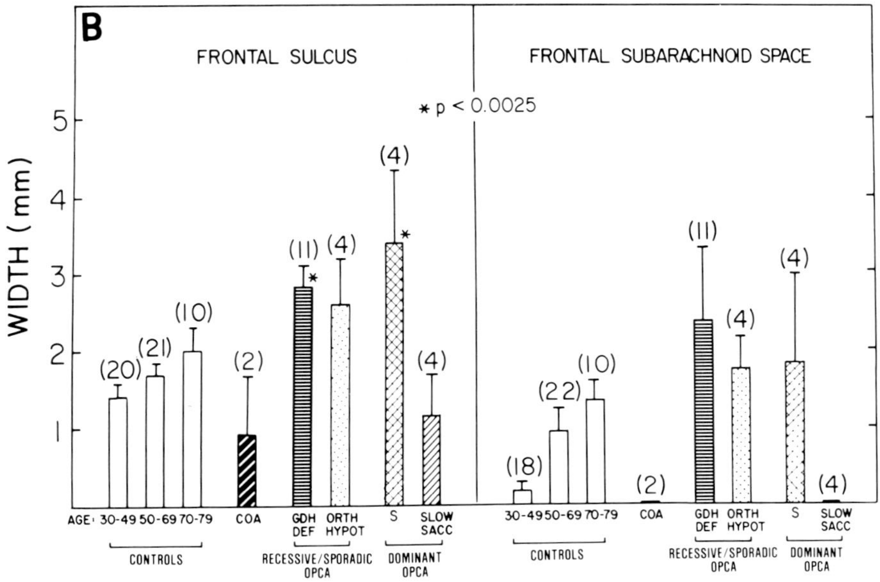

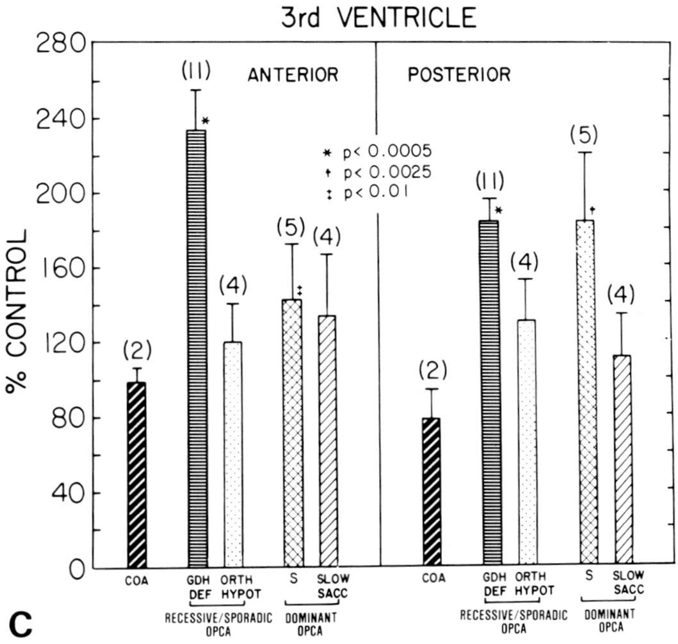

FIG. 4. *(Continued). (See legend on p. 49.)*

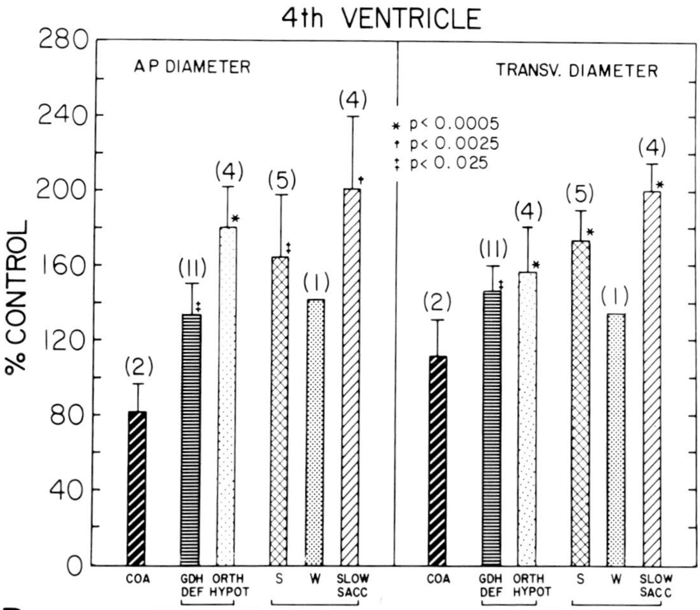

D

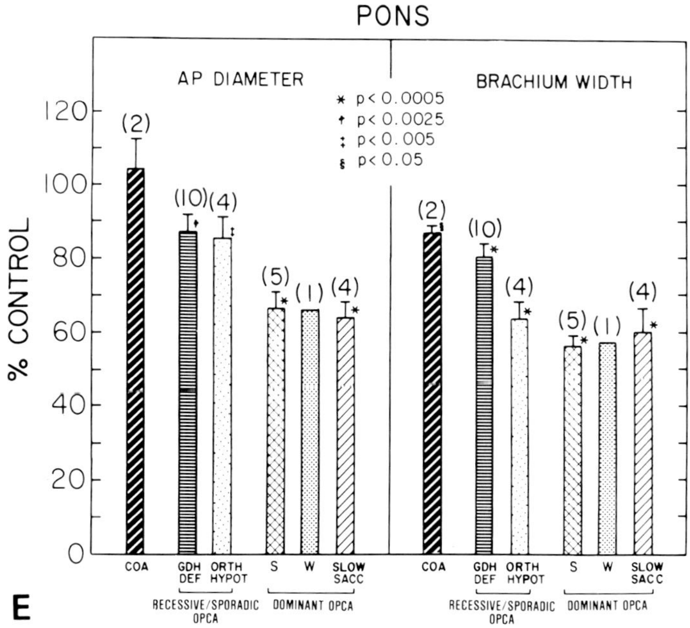

E

FIG. 4. *(Continued). (See legend on p. 49.)*

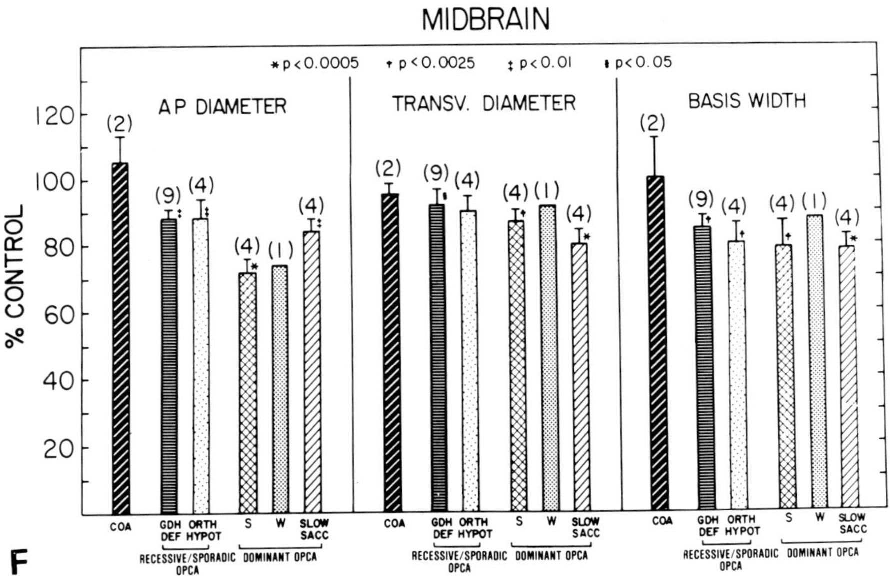

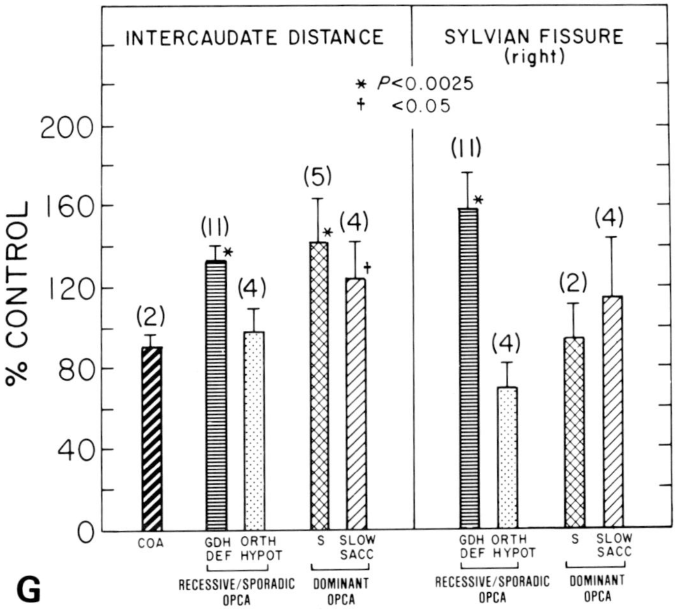

FIG. 4. *(Continued). (See legend on p. 49.)*

anteriorly, reflecting atrophy of the hypothalamus and thalamus (Fig. 7E). The fourth ventricle was slightly enlarged transversely (148%, $p<0.025$) and anteroposteriorly (135%, $p<0.025$) (Figs. 4D, 5A, 7E). The brainstem showed atrophy. Thus, the anteroposterior diameter of the pons decreased to 87% of the control ($p<0.0025$), the width of the brachium pontis to 80% ($p<0.005$) (Fig. 4E). The anteroposterior diameter of the midbrain also decreased to 88% of the control ($p<0.01$) (Fig. 4F). A variable degree of cerebellar cortical atrophy was noted, particularly in the semilunar lobules and, to a lesser extent, in the vermis (Figs. 4A, 5). Some degree of frontal cortical atrophy is evidenced by the increased width of the frontal sulci and subarachnoid spaces (Figs. 4B, 6A, 6C). The sylvian fissures were dilated (Figs. 4G, 5C, 6A, 7D, 7E), and the intercaudate distance (Figs. 4G, 6A, 7D) increased reflecting atrophy of the putamen (and perhaps the temporal lobe) and the caudate nucleus (4). The degree of atrophy of the cerebellum, brainstem, and supratentorial structures varied considerably among these patients. Thus, some patients showed a predominant cerebellar and brainstem atrophy with less pronounced changes in the supratentorial structures.

In one case (Fig. 7), there was marked atrophy of the brainstem and cerebellum, with morphological features reminiscent of those found in patients with dominant OPCA with slow saccades (see below). The differences between this case and cases of dominant OPCA with slow saccades were the presence of the enlarged third ventricle and the widened sylvian fissures. An additional distinction between these two categories of OPCA was the pattern of cerebellar atrophy. Thus, as described below, patients with slow saccades showed a severe degree of pancerebellar wasting, particularly in the anterior lobe, whereas patients with GDH deficiency showed atrophic changes most pronounced in the semilunar lobules (Figs. 5A, 5D).

TABLE 2. *CT features of various types of OPCA and of COA*

Disorder	CT findings
OPCA	
GDH deficient	Enlarged third ventricle (anterior > posterior); cerebellar atrophy (vermis + hemispheres), frontal atrophy, enlarged fourth ventricle, pontine and mesencephalic atrophy
OPCA with orthostatic hypotension	Cerebellar atrophy (vermis + hemispheres), frontal atrophy, enlarged fourth ventricle, pontine atrophy (brachium pontis > pons) and mesencephalic atrophy
Dominant OPCA (S Family)	Cerebellar atrophy, pontine atrophy (brachium pontis >pons), enlarged fourth ventricle, enlarged third ventricles, midbrain atrophy, frontal atrophy
Dominant OPCA (W Family)	Pontine atrophy (brachium > pons), cerebellar atrophy, midbrain atrophy, parietal atrophy
Dominant with slow saccades	Pancerebellar atrophy (especially anterior lobe) enlarged fourth ventricle, pontine atrophy (tegmentum), midbrain atrophy. Frontoparietal and or parieto-occipital convolutional atrophy
Cerebello-olivary atrophy (COA)	Cerebellar atrophy (vermis > hemispheres); brachium pontis atrophy

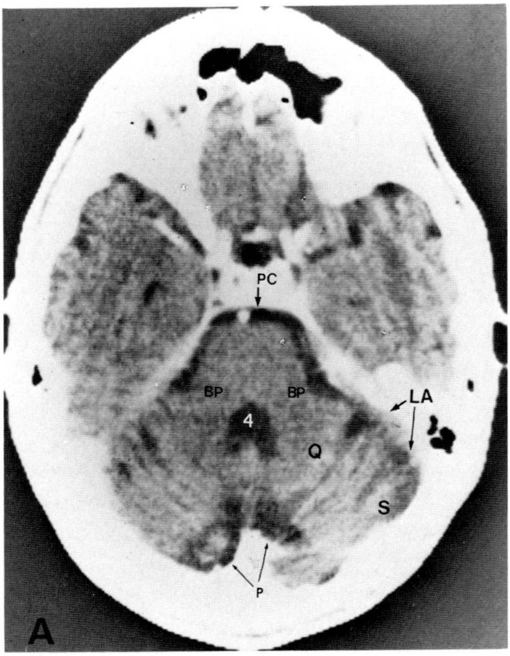

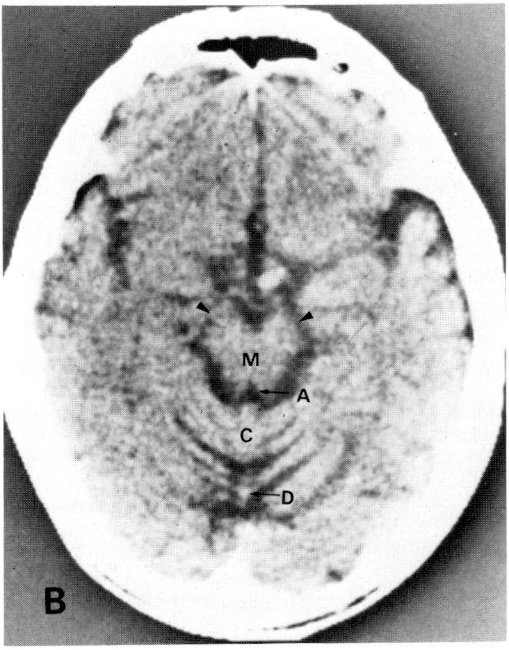

FIG. 5. A–D. *(Legend on p. 56.)*

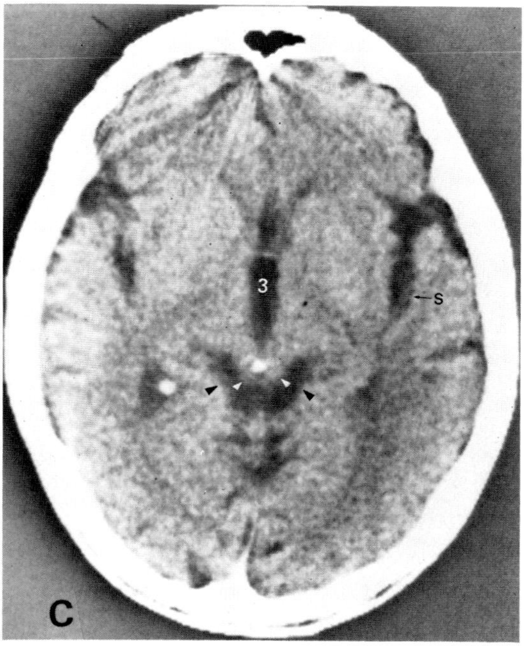
3
S
C

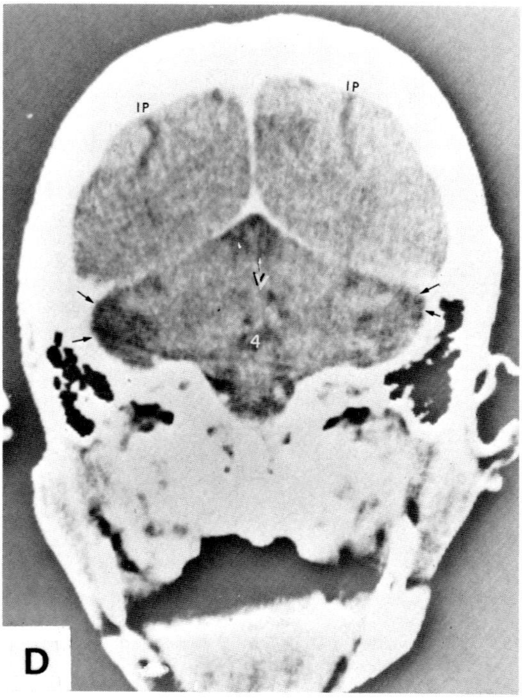
IP
IP
V
4
D

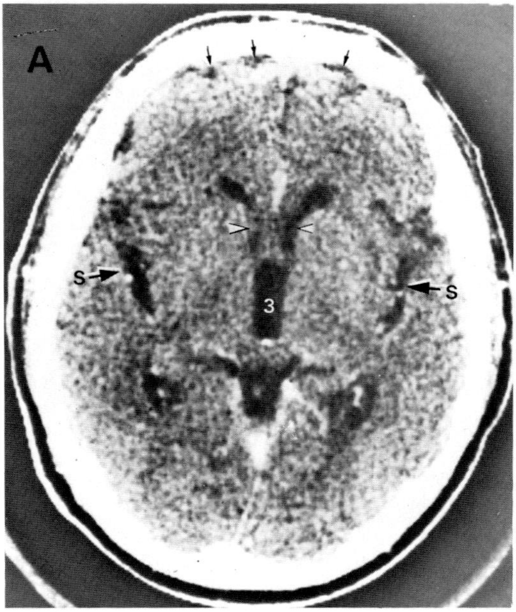

FIG. 6. **A–C:** Recessive OPCA associated with GDH deficiency (case 2). The patient is a 71-year-old man with a progressive neurological disorder characterized by cerebellar, extrapyramidal (parkinsonism), bulbar, and corticospinal deficits of 4 to 5 years duration (stage III). One of his brothers, age 70, has been similarly affected (CT scan not shown) (see Fig. 5, family C, chapter by Plaitakis, *this volume*). **A:** Section through the midlevel of the third ventricle (case 2). Note the marked rectangular enlargement of the third ventricle *(3)*. There is widening of the intercaudate distance *(white arrowheads)*, the sylvian fissures (S), and to a lesser extent the frontal sulci *(arrows)*. **B:** A modified coronal section through the anterior third ventricle. Note the enlarged diamond-shaped third ventricle *(3)*. The presumed locations of the hypothalamic sulci *(arrowheads)* are indicated. The sylvian fissures (S) are slightly prominent. The intraparietal sulci (IP) and lateral ventricles (LV) are labeled. **C:** Another modified coronal section through the anterior part of the frontal horns (case 2). The greatly widened superior *(1)*, middle *(2)*, and inferior *(3)* frontal sulci can be seen. The interhemispheric fissure *(arrow)* is also widened.

FIG. 5. **A–D** *(see pp. 54–55):* Recessive OPCA associated with GDH deficiency (case 1). The patient is a 65-year-old man with a progressive cerebellar disorder associated with extrapyramidal features, occulomotor disturbances, corticospinal deficits, dysarthria, anterior horn cell signs, and peripheral neuropathy of 16 years duration (stage III). One of his brothers, age 70, has been similarly affected since age 50 (CT scan not shown) (cases 2 and 3 in ref. 42). **A:** Section through the midpons (case 1). There is a moderate to extreme widening of the cerebellar sulci in the region of the semilunar (S) and the adjacent quadrangular lobules (Q). This results in widening of the lateral angle cistern (LA) and posterior cerebellar notch (P). Also note the slight atrophy of the brachia pontis (BP). The pontine cistern (PC) and the fourth ventricle *(4)* are labeled. **B:** Section through the mesencephalon (case 1). There is atrophy of the superior vermis, with the declive (D) being more affected than the culmen (C). Note the flattening of the anterolateral portion of the basis peduncli *(arrowheads)*, most likely reflecting atrophy of the underlying fiber tracts (corticospinal fibers, corticopontine fibers, etc.). The aqueduct (A) of the mesencephalon (M) is dilated. **C:** Section through the anteroinferior portion of the third ventricle (case 1). Note the enlargement of the anterior third ventricle *(3)* and the widening of the sylvian fissure (S). A slight shrinkage of the superior part of the tectum *(white arrowheads)* and enlargement of the quadrigeminal cistern *(black arrowheads)* are also visible. The left sylvian fissure (S) is prominent. **D:** Coronal section of the cerebellum through the posterior part of the fourth ventricle *(4)* (case 1). The superior vermis (V) exhibits moderate shrinkage, and the lateral parts of the cerebellar hemispheres show severe atrophic changes which extend deeply. This wasting is in the region of the superior and inferior semilunar lobules *(arrows)*. The intraparietal sulci (IP) are prominent.

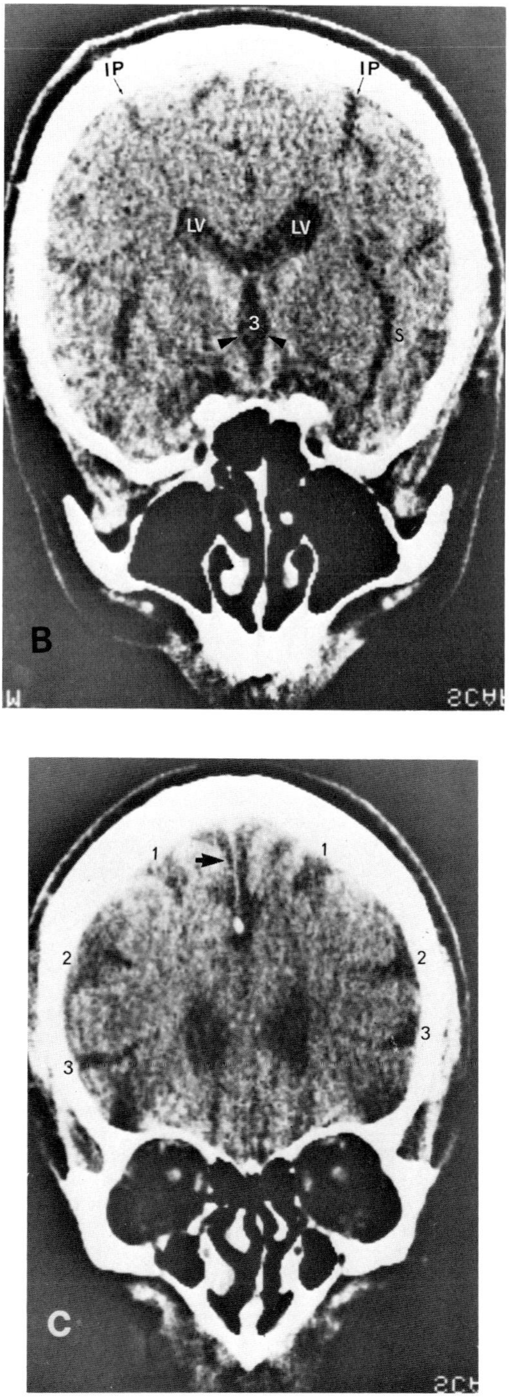

FIG. 6. (*Continued*). (*See legend on p. 56.*)

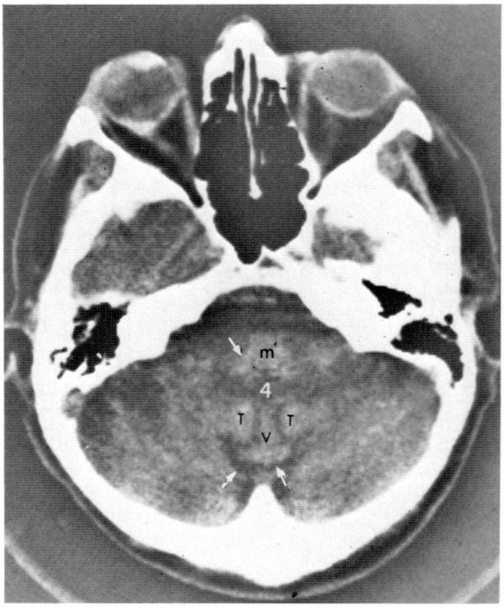

FIG. 7. A–F: OPCA associated with GDH deficiency (case 3). This 67-year-old woman has progressive gait ataxia, incoordination of hand movements, oculomotor disturbances, impaired smooth pursuit and saccadic eye movements, dysarthria, and parkinsonism of 12 years' duration (stage IV). (See chapter by Plaitakis, Fig. 2, *this volume*;) (case 1 of ref. 47.) **FIG. 7A:** Section through the pontomedullary junction. The atrophic restiform bodies *(black arrow)*, the small upper part of the medulla oblongata (m), the shrunken cerebellar tonsils (T), and the diminutive inferior vermis (V)—all surrounded by large subarachnoid spaces—are clearly seen. Widened cerebellar sulci anterolaterally and inferiorly are also clearly seen. The lower part of the fourth ventricle *(4)* and the suprapyramidal sulcus *(white arrows)* are labeled.

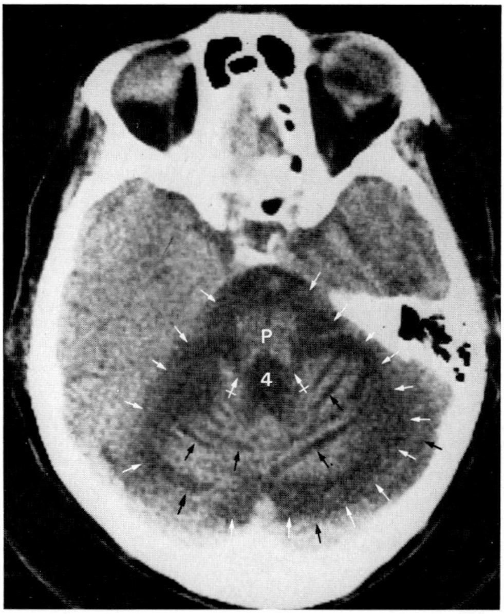

FIG. 7B. Section through the upper part of the midpons in the orbitomeatal plane (case 3). Marked atrophy of the brainstem and cerebellar folia is well demonstrated. The pons (P) and the brachia conjunctiva *(crossed white arrows)* show marked shrinkage and the floor of the fourth ventricle *(4)* has a concave appearance. The enormously enlarged subarachnoid space anterior to the pons, and around and above the superior aspects of the cerebellum is evidenced by the wide zone of decreased attenuation *(white arrows)* surrounding the cut surface of the cerebellum and the brainstem. The widened cerebellar sulci *(black arrows)* and small brachia conjunctiva are well demonstrated in this case. The brachia pontis in a lower cut are also markedly atrophic (not shown).

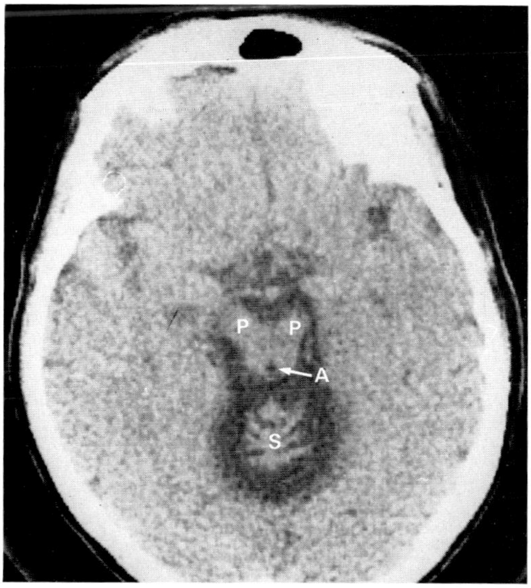

FIG. 7C. Section through the mesencephalon. The mesencephalon, particularly the bases peduncli (P) are atrophic on both sides. The interpeduncular fossa is therefore widened. The aqueduct (A) is large. The cut surface of the upper cerebellum near the apex or summit (S) shows atrophic folia and a widened subarachnoid space (zone of decreased attenuation) surrounding the shrunken cerebellum.

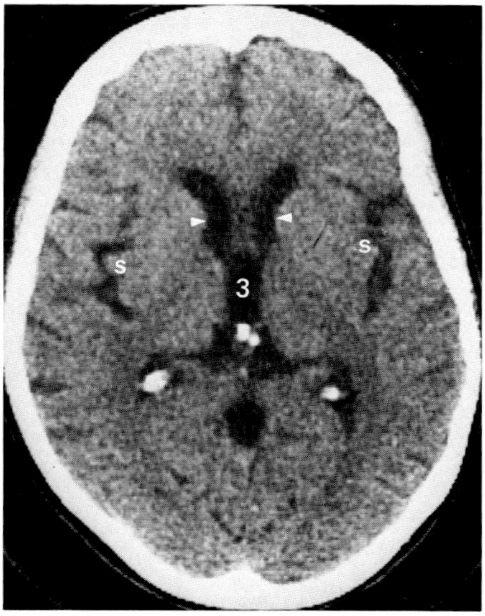

FIG. 7D. Section through the midlevel of the third ventricle. The third ventricle *(3)*, is enlarged and oblong-shaped. The intercaudate distance *(arrowheads)* is widened. The sylvian fissure (S) is enlarged on the left (the level of measurement of the sylvian fissures is usually 5 mm below this section; that of the frontal sulci is in general at 5 mm above this level). The frontal sulci are slightly widened at higher level (not shown).

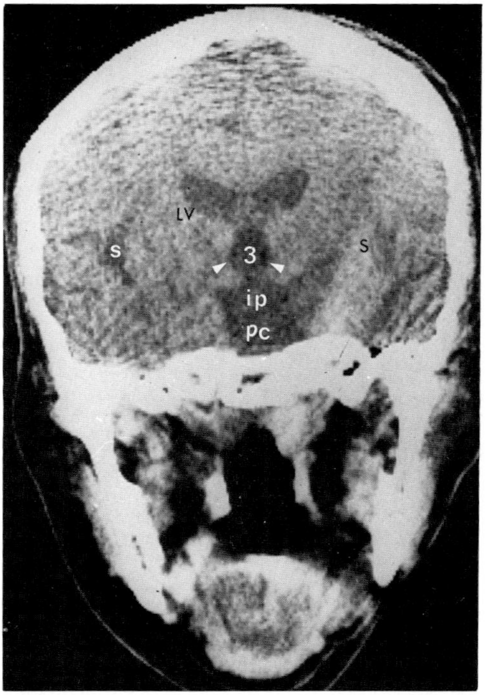

FIG. 7E. Modified coronal section through the third ventricle (case 3). Note the globular third ventricle *(3)* of the *ex vacuo* type in this section; the lower portion shows proportionally a greater involvement than the upper part. This appears to reflect the atrophy of the thalamus and hypothalamus. *Opposing arrowheads* correspond to the hypothalamic sulci. The dilated sylvian fissures (S) (partially obscured by an artifact) seem to echo involvement of the putamen and adjacent temporal lobe. The lateral ventricle (LV) and the interpeduncular (ip) and pontine cistern (pc) are labeled.

Sporadic OPCA with Orthostatic Hypotension

This type of OPCA has CT features clearly different from the GDH-deficient type. In all 4 patients studied, the size of the third ventricle and the intercaudate distances were normal (Figs. 4C, 4G, 8C). The sylvian fissures were also not enlarged (Figs. 4G, 8C). The abnormal findings were atrophy of the cerebellar hemispheres, vermis, and brainstem (particularly the pons and the brachia pontis) (Figs. 4, 8B, 8C). The fourth ventricle widened both anteroposteriorly (180% of the control, $p < 0.005$) and transversely (156% of the control, $p < 0.005$). Compared with the GDH-deficient cases, the degree of atrophy of the brainstem (particularly of the brachium pontis) was greater in this group (Fig. 4E). In 2 cases in which serial CT scans were obtained, rapidly advancing cerebellar atrophy was noted (CT scan not shown). This correlated well with the rapid downhill clinical course reported in these patients (46). Some less pronounced frontal cortical

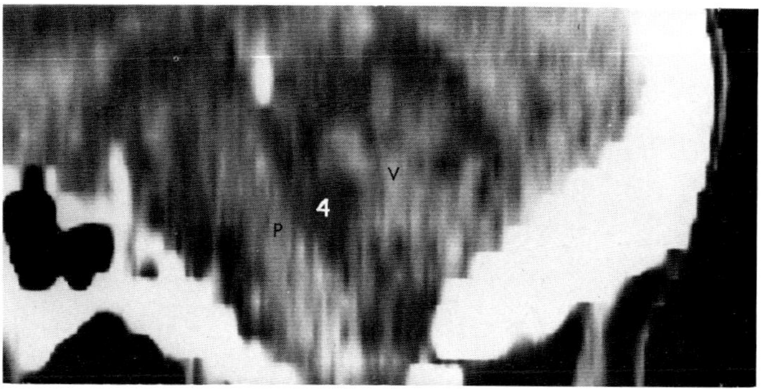

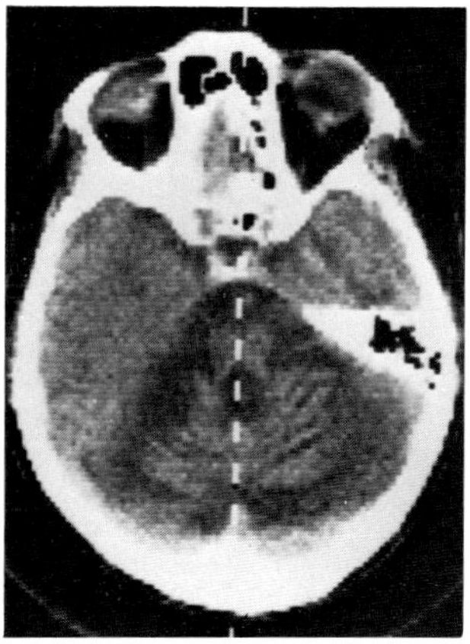

FIG. 7F. *(Above)* Midsagittal CT reconstruction showing the atrophic vermis (V), dilated fourth ventricle *(4)* markedly atrophic brainstem, particularly the pons (P). *(Left)* The *dotted line* shows the plane of CT section.

atrophy (Fig. 4B) was also noted in these cases similar to GDH-deficient OPCA cases.

Dominant OPCA

Both dominant and nondominant OPCAs have cerebellar and brainstem atrophy; however the dominant OPCA showed more severe brainstem atrophy (Figs. 4E, 4F) and more widespread cerebral, particularly parietal, convolutional atrophy.

"S" Family

The characteristic CT features in this type of OPCA were a severe atrophy of the brachium pontis (Fig. 4E) and, in contrast to nondominant types of OPCA, the cerebellar cortical atrophy was most pronounced in the anterior lobe and the superior part of the middle lobe of the cerebellum (Figs. 9, 10). Although atrophy appeared to begin in the brachia pontis and cerebellum in patients at an early stage (Fig. 9), the brainstem including the tegmentum showed severe atrophy in a late

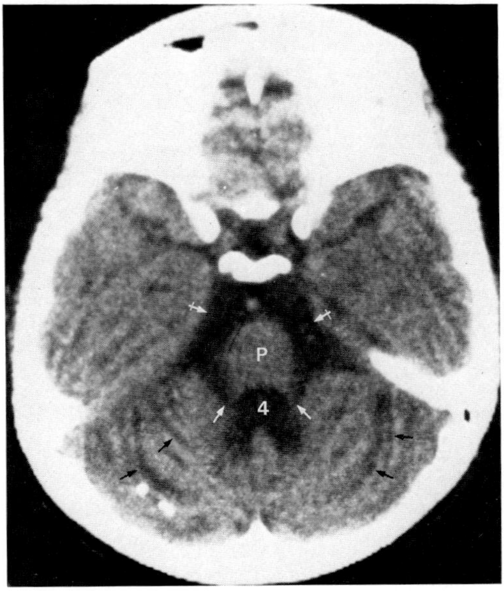

FIG. 8. A–D: Sporadic OPCA associated with orthostatic hypotension (case 4). There is no GDH deficiency. The patient is a 53-year-old Korean woman with a 4-year history of progressive cerebellar syndrome, associated with bulbar and corticospinal deficits, sphincter involvement, and orthostatic hypotension (over a 40 mm Hg fall in blood pressure from supine to erect position) (stage II). **FIG. 8A** *(above)*. Section through the center of the fourth ventricle (case 4). Note the markedly enlarged fourth ventricle *(4)*, atrophy of the pons (P), brachia pontis *(white arrows)*, and cerebellar hemispheres *(black arrows)*. The pontine cistern *(crossed white arrows)* is widened.

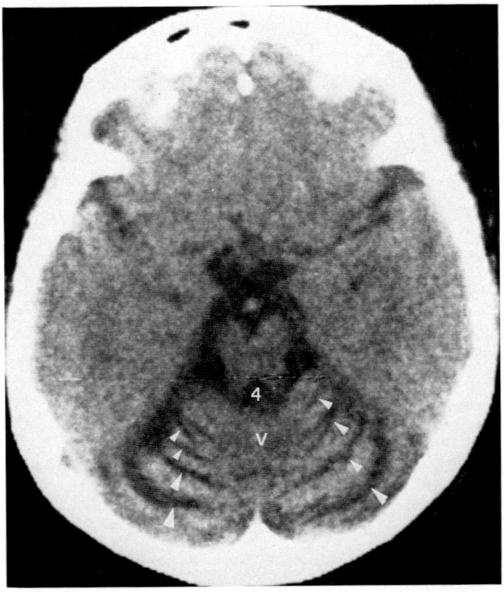

FIG. 8B. Section through the ponto-mesencephalic junction (case 4). Note the marked widened cerebellar sulci *(arrowheads)* due to atrophic cerebellar hemispheres. The vermis (V) is less affected. The subarachnoid space around the brainstem and cerebellum is notably increased. Note the superior extension of the enlarged fourth ventricle *(4)*. The brainstem is atrophic.

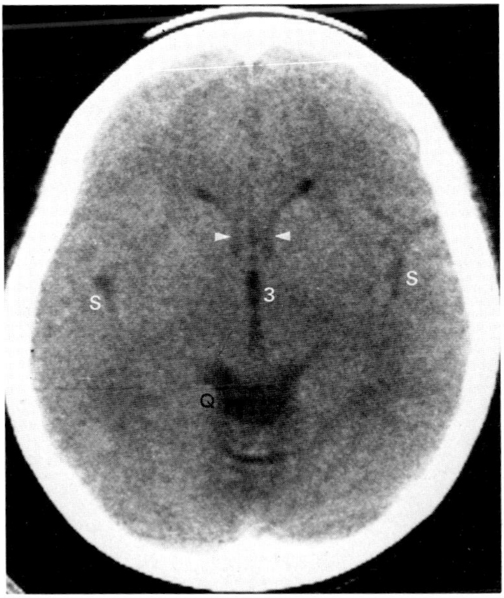

FIG. 8C. Section through the lower third ventricle (case 4). Note the normal intercaudate distance *(opposing arrowheads)*, third ventricle *(3)* and sylvian fissures (S). The quadrigeminal cistern (Q) is wide.

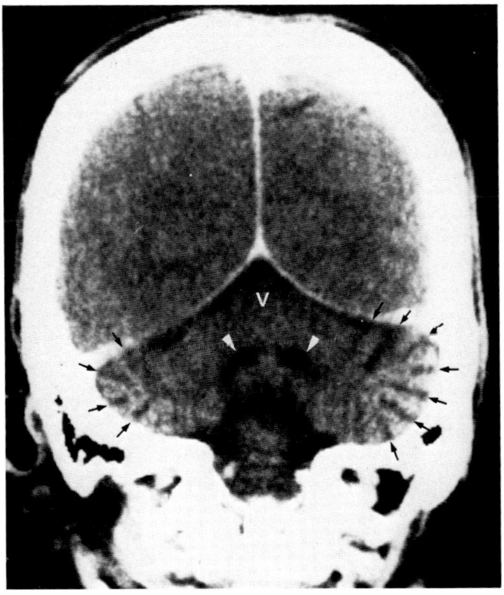

FIG. 8D. Coronal section through the fourth ventricle (case 4). Note atrophy of the cerebellar hemispheres *(black arrows)*. The enlargement of the fourth ventricle is evidenced by its dilated posterior superior recesses *(white arrowheads)*. The vermis (V) is relatively spared.

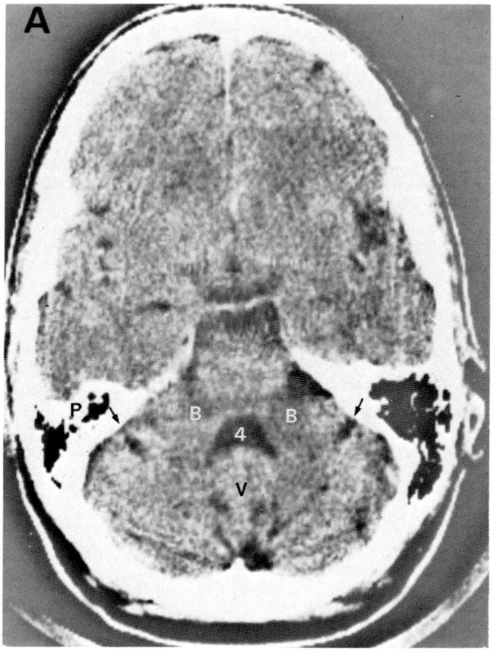

FIG. 9. A–B: Dominant OPCA—"S" family (case 5). This 30-year-old man has been affected since age 24 (stage II). (No detailed history available.)

FIG. 9A. Dominant OPCA—"S" family (case 5). This 30-year-old man has been affected since age 24 (stage II). (No detailed history available. Section through the midportion of the fourth ventricle (case 5). The fourth ventricle *(4)* is moderately enlarged. There is moderate to marked atrophy of the brachia pontis (B). The cerebellar sulci *(arrows)* are widened. The inferior vermis (V) shows slight degree of atrophy, particularly posteriorly. The anterior part of the primary fissure (P) is also labeled.

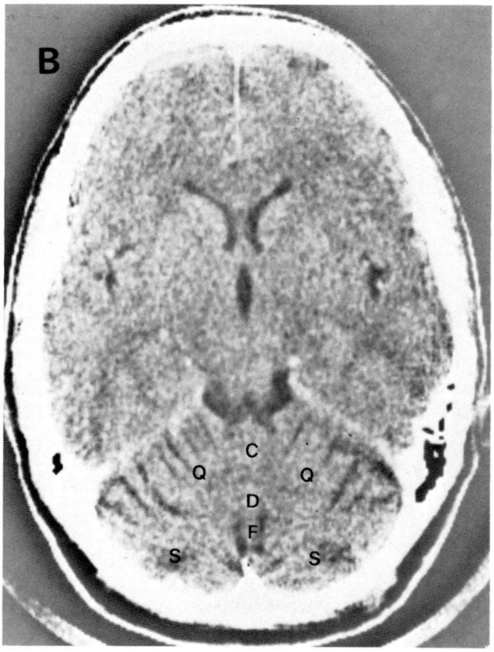

FIG. 9B. Section through the superior vermis, the superior colliculi, and the frontal horn (case 5). There is diffuse atrophy of the cerebellar cortex which is characteristically more prominent in the anterior lobe and in the upper part of the middle lobe. The atrophic cerebellar folia and the subjacent white matter create a coarse-comb appearance. The quadrangular lobule (Q) and declive (D) are markedly involved in the atrophic processes, whereas the semilunar lobules (S) and culmen (C) are relatively spared in the early stages. The folium (F) is labeled.

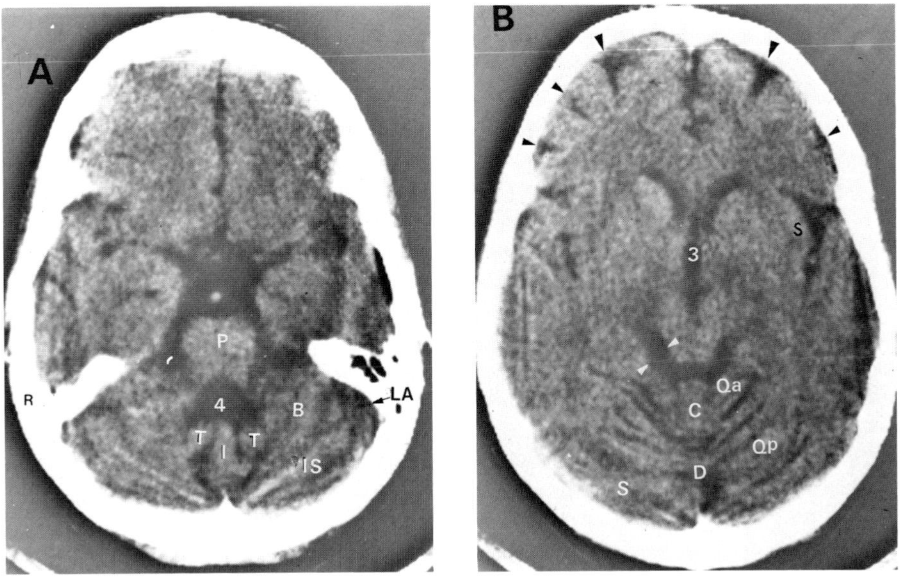

FIG. 10. Dominant OPCA—"S" family (case 6). This 42-year-old woman has been afflicted since age 29 (stage III). (No detailed history available.) **A:** Section through the fourth ventricle and midpons in the superior orbitomeatal plane (case 6). The brachia pontis and the brachia conjunctiva are severely atrophic. The inferior part (I) of the vermis and the cerebellar hemispheres, including the tonsils (T) and the biventral lobules (B), show wasting. The floor of the fourth ventricle *(4)* is concave. The inferior semilunar lobules (IS), lateral angle cistern (LA), and the right side (R) are labeled. **B:** Section through the superior colliculi (case 6). There is marked atrophy of culmen (C), declive (D) and anterior (Qa) and posterior (Qp) parts of the quadrangular lobules. The quadrigeminal cistern *(opposing arrowheads)* is widened. Note atrophy of the frontal lobes *(black arrowheads)*. The superior semilunar lobule (S) and third ventricle (3) are labeled.

stage (Fig. 10A). The anteroposterior diameter of the pons was reduced to 66% of the control ($p<0.0005$), the width of the brachium pontis to 58% ($p<0.0005$) (Fig. 4E). The fourth ventricle became enlarged; the transverse diameter increased to 176% of the control ($p<0.005$) and the anteroposterior diameter to 164% ($p<0.025$) (Fig. 4D). The floor of the fourth ventricle became concave, especially in advanced cases (Fig. 10A). Enlargement of the anterior (142% of the control, $p<0.01$) and the posterior third ventricle (184% of the control, $p<0.01$) was noted (Fig. 9B) but to a lesser degree than in GDH-deficient OPCA. The intercaudate distance was also significantly increased (Fig. 4G). Similar to tegmental involvement, atrophic changes of the supratentorial structures, including convolutional (frontal > parietal) atrophy (Figs. 4B, 10B), were seen only in advanced stages of the illness (Figs. 4B, 10B).

"W" Family

Although the study of this family was limited to one case, the CT features observed were rather striking: pontine atrophy with flattening of the anterior and

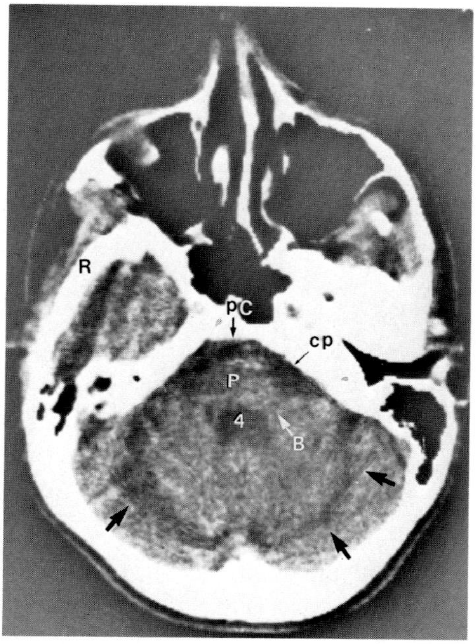

FIGS. 11. A–C: Dominant OPCA—"W" family (spinopontine variety) (case 7). This 31-year-old female has been affected since age 18 (stage III). Neurological findings included dysarthria, slight bilateral ptosis, nystagmus, facial weakness of lower motor neuron type, palatal myoclonus, gait and limb ataxia, and severe spasticity involving her legs. (Also reported by Pogacar, ref. 48, case 2). **FIG. 11A** *(above).* CT section through the mid to lower pons in the inferior orbitomeatal plane (case 7). There is severe wasting of the pons (P) and the brachia pontis (B), and widening of the pontine (PC) and the cerebellopontine angle (cp) cisterns. Note the moderately enlarged fourth ventricle (4) and the widened cerebellar sulci *(large black arrows)*, particularly in and adjacent to the postclival sulci. R, right side.

posterolateral aspects (Fig. 11A, 11B). The anteroposterior diameter of the pons was reduced to 64% of the controls and the width of the brachium pontis to 58%. There was also a marked atrophy of the vermis and, to a lesser extent, of the cerebellar hemispheres. Cerebral atrophy was noticeable in the parietal region (Fig. 11C).

OPCA with Slow Saccades

The pathology here appeared to begin in the tegmentum of the pons and anterior lobe of the cerebellum (Fig. 13). The most striking findings were (a) ballooning of the fourth ventricle of the *ex vacuo* type (enlarged to 200% of the control, $p < 0.025$ both anteroposteriorly and transversely) (Figs. 4D, 12A–C); (b) severe atrophy of the entire pons (the anteroposterior diameter of the pons decreased to

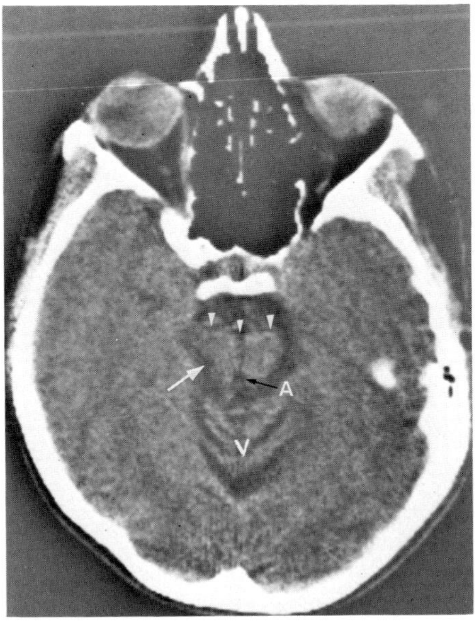

FIG. 11B. Section through the upper pons and superior vermis (case 7). The brainstem is atrophic and flat-pear–shaped. There is flattening *(triple arrowheads)* of the anterior aspect of the pons *(basis pontis)* and concavity of the posterolateral part of the tegmentum *(white arrow)*. The latter may result from atrophy of the brachia conjuctiva and pontis and the adjacent structures. The aqueduct (A) is dilated and the vermis (V) and cerebellar hemispheres are atrophic with dilated sulci.

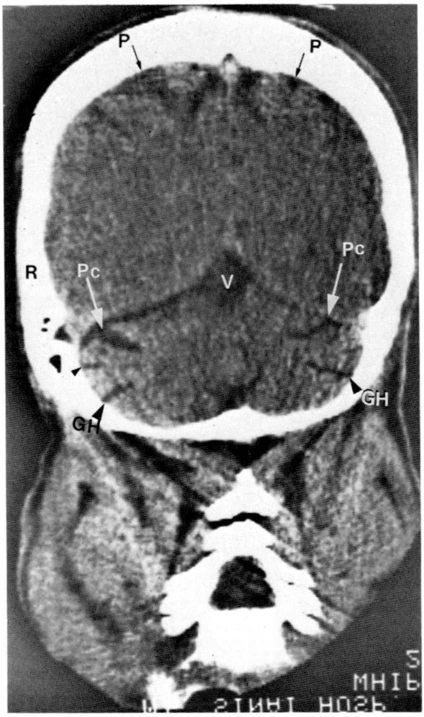

FIG. 11C. Coronal section through the vermis (case 7). Extreme widening of the postclival (Pc) and great horizontal (GH) fissures is noted. The superior vermis (V) and the parietal lobe are also atrophic. The intraparietal fissure (P) and right side (R) are labeled.

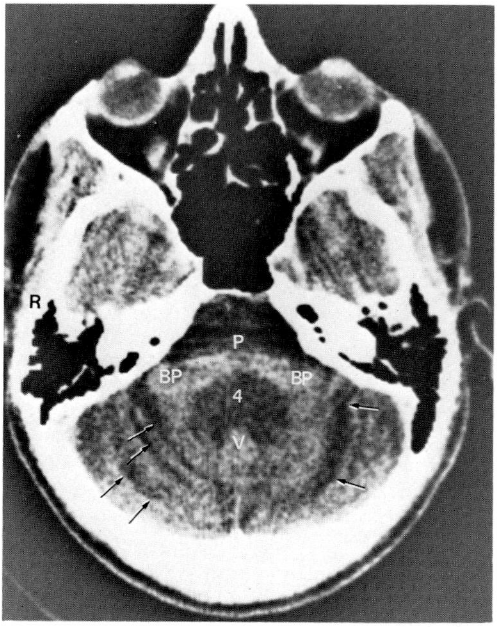

FIG. 12. A–E: Dominant OPCA with slow saccades (case 8). This 36-year-old man has been affected since age 26 (stage III). On neurological examination, the patient was found to have slow volitional saccadic eye movements (vertical > horizontal) with normal smooth pursuit, slight dysarthria, bilateral facial weakness of the lower motor neuron type, gait and limb ataxia, corticospinal deficit, and vibratory sensory loss of the lower extremities. Several family members, including his mother and a 31-year-old brother, have been similarly affected (47a).

FIG. 12A. Section through the midportion of the lower pons (case 8). The fourth ventricle *(4)* shows ballooning, owing to marked atrophy of the tegmentum of the pons (P), brachia pontis (BP), vermis (V), and the adjacent cerebellar hemisphere. The cerebellar sulci *(arrows)* (particularly the prebiventral and ansoparamedian sulci) are extremely widened and extend deeply into the juxtaventricular area, indicating both cortical and subcortical cerebellar atrophy (pancerebellar). R, right side.

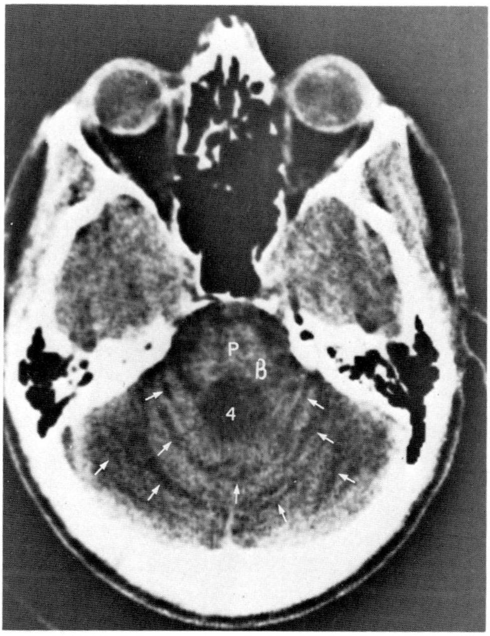

FIG. 12B. Section through the ballooned upper fourth ventricle of the *ex vacuo* type (case 8). Extreme widening of the cerebellar sulci *(arrowheads)* is obvious. The pons (P) shows marked, diffuse atrophy. The typical concave appearance of the floor of the fourth ventricle *(4)* is likely the result of marked atrophy of the pontine tegmentum, the middle cerebellar peduncles, and other neighboring structures. Note the extension of tissue wasting deep into the paraventricular area and severe atrophy of the anterior lobe—characteristic findings in this type of OPCA.

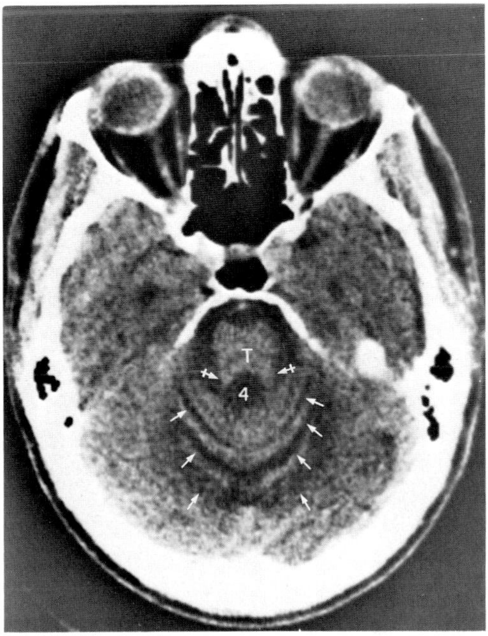

FIG. 12C. Section through the upper pons (case 8). Ballooning of the fourth ventricle *(4)* is also seen at this level. The brachia conjunctiva *(arrows)* and the tegmentum (T) show diminution in size particularly posteriorly. The lateral aspects of the pons are flattened. The atrophic brainstem therefore creates a "molar tooth" appearance with its atrophic roots projecting posteriorly. The cut surface of the cerebellum is severely atrophic *(crossed arrows)*.

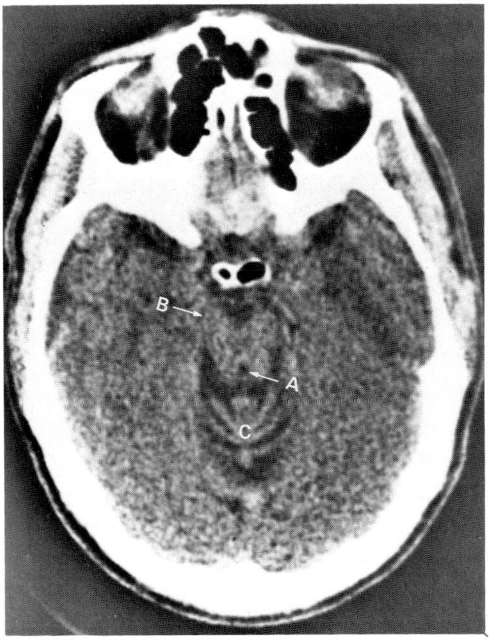

FIG. 12D. Section through the mesencephalon (case 8). Severe dilatation of the aqueduct (A) is likely the result of atrophy of the mesencephalon, especially in the periaqueductal area. This also appears to be an extension of the ballooned fourth ventricle. The bases (B) of the cerebral peduncles appear less affected. The atrophic cerebellar apex (C), indicating marked involvement of the anterior lobe, is labeled.

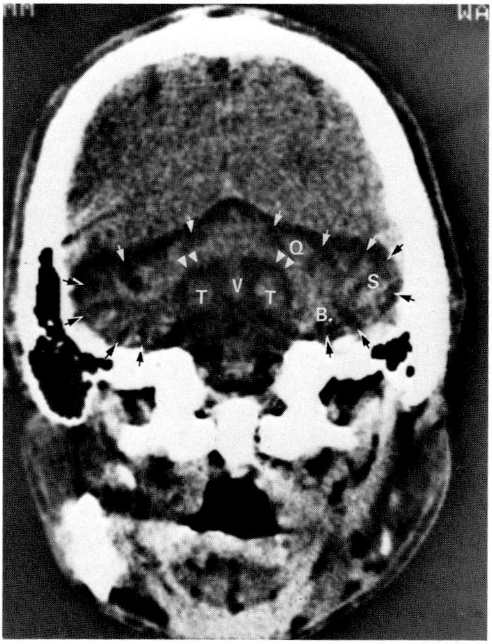

FIG. 12E. Modified coronal section through the vermis and the tonsils (case 8). There is severe atrophy of the entire cerebellum, including the inferior vermis (V), and the quadrangular (Q), semilunar (S), and biventral (B) lobules. The cerebellar tonsils (T) are small. Note the large subarachnoid spaces over the cerebellar surface and within the sulci *(single black and white arrows)*. The posterior superior recesses of the fourth ventricle are large *(double white arrowheads)*.

64% of the control, $p<0.0005$; the transverse width of the brachium pontis down to 58%, $p<0.0005$) (Figs. 4E, 12A–C, 13); and (c) shrinkage of the cerebellum (Figs. 4A, 12, 13). Characteristically atrophic changes of the pons were more prominent in the posterior and lateral aspects. Owing to excavation of the floor of the fourth ventricle and the diminished size of the brachia conjunctiva, the brainstem had the appearance of a "molar tooth" with its "roots" projecting posteriorly (Figs. 12C, 13). The cerebellar sulci were widened, most likely reflecting atrophy of the folia and the medullary body. The atrophy was most pronounced in the anterior lobe (Figs. 12, 13). Unlike other types of OPCA, the atrophic processes in this group extended into the inferior part of the cerebellar hemispheres, affecting the cerebellar tonsils and the adjacent biventral lobules (in addition to the semilunar and quadrangular lobules). These changes along with atrophy of the inferior vermis created a widening of the peritonsillar and paravermian subarachnoid spaces in CT scans (Fig. 12E). Often periventricular atrophy extends upward to involve the periaqueductal area, even to the rostral end (Fig. 12D).

Cerebello-olivary Atrophy

The most striking feature was marked atrophy of the vermis, with few gross anatomical changes in the cerebellar hemispheres (Figs. 4A, 14). A moderate degree of atrophy was, however, observed in coronal sections, involving the lateral parts

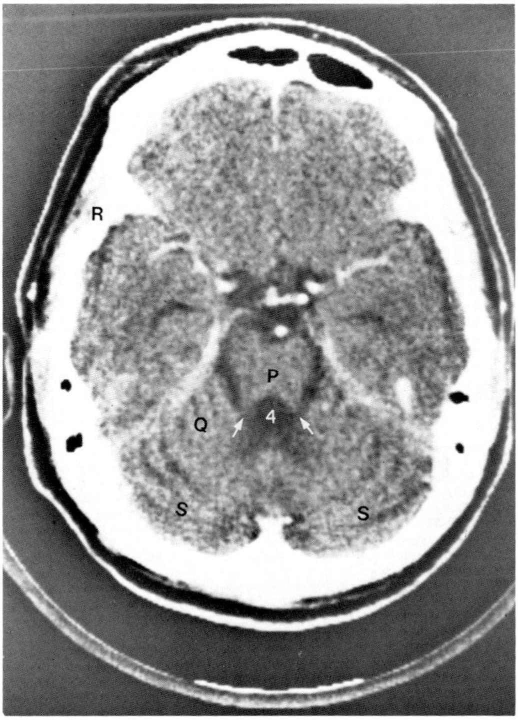

FIG. 13. Another case of dominant OPCA with slow saccades in the early stage of the disease (case 9). Section through upper pons. This 30-year-old man was seen because of gait disturbances commencing at the age of 18. Abnormal neurological findings included slow saccadic eye movements, normal smooth pursuit, slight gait ataxia, and bilateral facial weakness (stage I). The fourth ventricle *(4)* is enlarged and its floor is convex anteriorly. The brachia conjunctiva *(arrows)* are reduced in size. There is moderate to severe atrophy with widened sulci in the region of the quadrangular (Q) and semilunar (S) lobules. The pons (P) is labeled. It should be noted that in OPCA associated with slow saccades, early CT changes are atrophy of the cerebellum and pontine tegmentum and enlargement of the fourth ventricle with the anteriorly convex floor. R, right side.

of the semilunar lobules on both sides, maximally near the lateral angles of the cerebellum (Fig. 14C). The brachia pontis were slightly atrophic (Fig. 14A). The brainstem and the ventricular system, including the fourth ventricle, failed to show any appreciable abnormalities.

DISCUSSION

Evaluation of morphological changes of the brain with CT offers an advantage over an examination of the brain at autopsy. CT scanning allows the study of the

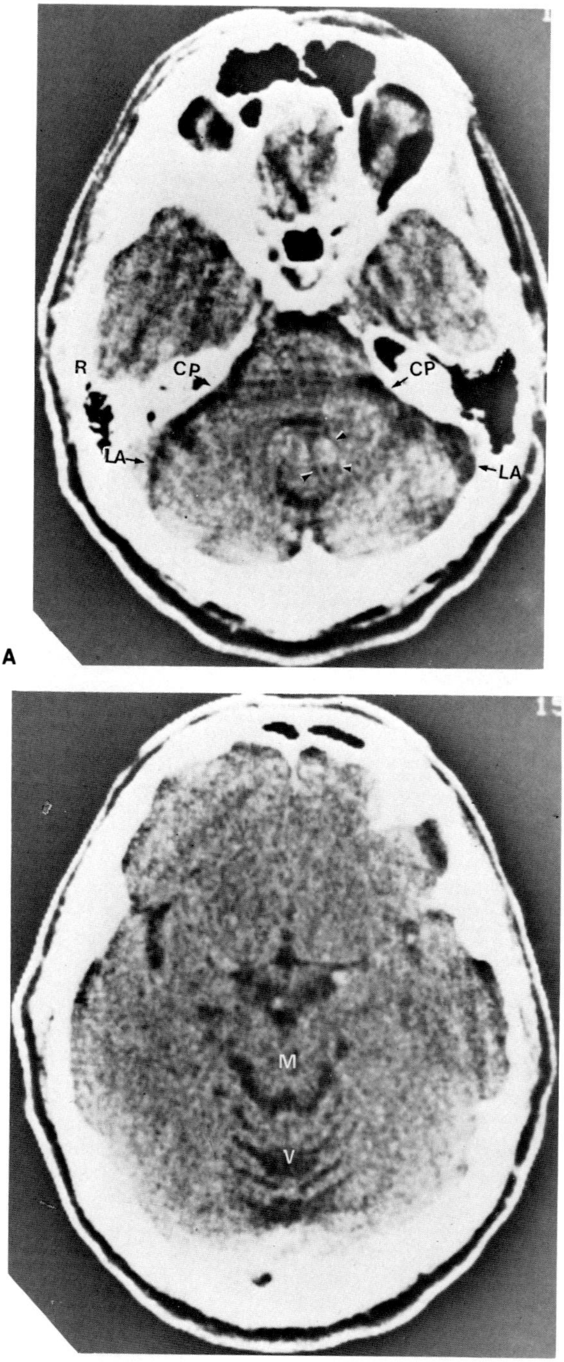

FIG. 14. (*Legend on p. 73.*)

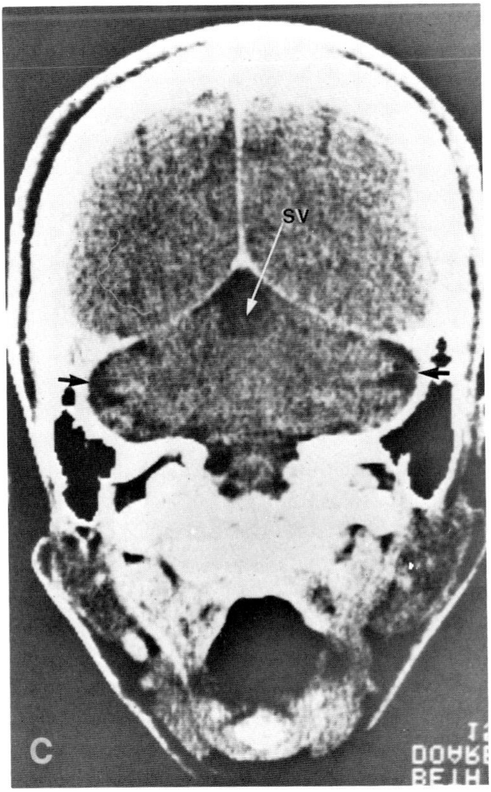

FIG. 14. A–C: Cerebello-olivary atrophy (case 10). This 59-year-old man has been afflicted by dominantly inherited progressive cerebellar ataxia since age 42 (stage II). Besides a slight degree of dysarthria, no other associated neurological manifestation was found (pure cerebellar syndrome clinically). **A:** CT section through the midpons in the orbitomeatal plane (case 10). The lateral angle cistern (LA) and, to a lesser extent, the cerebellopontine angle cistern (CP) show widening. The peritonsiller space *(arrowheads*—only labeled on the left) is also slightly widened. The pons appear to be of normal size and shape. **B:** CT section through the mesencephalon (case 10). A marked widening of the sulci of the superior vermis (V) is clearly seen. The mesencephalon (M) is normal. **C:** Coronal section of the cerebellum behind the fourth ventricle (case 10). Note the severe atrophy of the superior vermis (SV). The cerebellar hemisphere are less affected except for the lateral parts of the semilunar lobules *(arrows)*. The lateral angle cisterns are therefore widened.

brain *in vivo* and at different stages of illness. Pathology usually investigates the end stage of diseases, particularly in neurodegenerative disorders.

In this study, the CT characteristics of 5 different types of OPCA were analyzed in detail. Results showed that all forms share common CT features, such as varying degrees of cerebellar and brainstem atrophy and enlargement of the fourth ventricle. These were frequently correlated with the stage of the disease. However, the patterns of these atrophic changes appeared distinctive enough to be of value in the diagnosis and classification of these disorders.

CT features in *OPCA with GDH deficiency*, other than the atrophy of the posterior fossa structures, were enlargement of the third ventricle, increased intercaudate distance, and widening of the sylvian fissure and frontal sulci. This appeared to reflect atrophy of the hypothalamus–thalamus, caudate nucleus, putamen, and frontal lobe, respectively. Since no pathological studies have been obtained in any of the GDH-deficient cases at our institution, future pathological examinations are required to confirm the gross morphological changes demonstrated by CT. Also pathological examination would define the precise histological changes that occur in this disorder.

In *OPCA with orthostatic hypotension*, rapidly advancing cerebellar and brainstem atrophy was found usually in association with normal supratentorial structures in contrast to the GDH-deficient cases. Indeed, the third ventricle, the intercaudate distance, and the sylvian fissures were normal in these patients. Further comparison between these two entities showed that atrophy of the cerebellum, brachium pontis, and enlargement of the fourth ventricle were more marked in patients with orthostatic hypotension than with GDH deficiency.

Oppenheimer (39) reviewed 15 autopsied cases of multiple system atrophy (MSA) with progressive autonomic failure (PAF) from the literature and his own series. Histological features included a loss of the preganglionic cells in the intermediolateral column of the spinal cord (85% of the cases), substantia nigra (75%), striatum (56%), nuclei pontis (53%), inferior olive (53%), locus ceruleus (40%), cerebellar cortex (40%), dorsal vagal nuclei (26%), pyramidal tract (26%), anterior horn cells (13%), and sympathetic ganglia (6%). The hypothalamus has always been found to be normal in this disorder (39). These histologic findings somewhat agree with the CT demonstration of the cerebellar and brainstem atrophy and the normal-sized third ventricle found in our patients. However, the reported atrophy of the striatum (39) did not appear to be present in the CT scans of our series, possibly because the cases collected by Oppenheimer included 2 forms of MSA—the nigrostriatal degeneration (expected to show an involvement of the striatum) and OPCA—in contrast to our cases which included only clinically diagnosed OPCA associated PAF.

Therefore, this type of OPCA should be suspected when one encounters a progressive cerebellar and extrapyramidal syndrome of late adult onset, associated with orthostatic hypotension, with atrophy of the cerebellum and brainstem, and with a normal-sized third ventricle and sylvian fissures.

In the *dominant OPCA—"S" family*, the pathological changes described by Schut and Haymaker (55) include severe atrophy of the cerebellum and the 3 pairs of its peduncles, the inferior olives, the pons, the lower cranial nerve nuclei, the basal ganglia, the substantia nigra, the posterior columns, and the anterior horn cells of the spinal cord. In some cases there was convolutional atrophy of the frontal, frontoparietal, and temporal lobes. Most of these pathological changes were reflected in the CT scans evaluated in this study. Our CT studies further indicate that the brachia pontis and anterior lobe of the cerebellum were involved early in the course of the illness. In the advanced cases, one found severe atrophy of the pons (including its tegmentum), enlargement of the posterior third ventricle, increased intercaudate distance, and cerebral convolutional atrophy.

The above CT data are of particular interest since slow saccadic eye movements (which likely result from involvement of the pontine tegmentum—see below) were observed in the late stages of the illness.

In the *dominant OPCA—"W" family*, the pathological findings originally described in 1969 by Boller and Segarra (6) were neuronal degeneration of the basal ganglia (worst in the globus pallidus), cellular rarefaction of the nuclei, and demyelination of all 3 (particularly the middle) pairs of the cerebellar peduncles. Cerebellar involvement was relatively mild though microscopically the changes were definitely present. The lateral and anterior columns of the spinal cord were pale. The thoracic nucleus (Clarke's column) showed demyelination, whereas the cerebral cortex was reported to be well preserved.

As already described, Pogacar et al. (48) have recently shown that atrophy of the cerebellum and inferior olives was present in another member of this family at postmortum. Involvement of the cerebellum seen in CT scan in our patient favors the classification of this disorder as a form of OPCA, as suggested by Pogacar et al. The flattened bell-shaped upper pons seen in CT scan appeared to be the result of atrophy of the basis pontis and brachia conjunctiva. Atrophy of the pyramidal tracts may also contribute to the anterior flattening of the pons. It is of particular interest that this patient exhibited clinically severe spasticity which may correspond to the involvement of corticospinal tract as suggested by CT.

Since only one case was available for study in this group, it cannot be unequivocally concluded that these findings were specific to this disorder. Additional family members must be studied to determine if these CT features are consistent.

In *OPCA with slow saccadic eye movements* there was a greatly ballooned fourth ventricle of the *ex vacuo* type. Owing to excavation of the floor of the fourth ventricle, together with atrophy of the brachia pontis and conjunctiva, the brainstem showed, in CT scan, a "molar tooth" appearance with its "roots" projecting posteriorly. The ballooning of the fourth ventricle extended upward to cause an enlarged aqueduct. In the cerebellum, the severe wasting involved the entire cerebellum, particularly the anterior lobe. The atrophy also extended deeply to reach the paraventricular area (pancerebellar atrophy). This resulted in an enlargement of the subarachnoid spaces surrounding and extending deep into the cerebellum. Unlike other types of dominant OPCA, prominent cerebral convolutional atrophy with widened sulci and gaping sylvian fissures were usually not observed, at least in the early stage.

The pathological changes reported by Koeppen and Hans (25) (case 3 in their series) in this type of OPCA include marked atrophy of the pons and cerebellum, a degenerated Purkinje cells replaced by abundant Bergmann glia, an atrophic granular layer, demyelinated cerebellar white matter, and patchy neuronal loss of the dentate nucleus with involvement of its efferent fibers. There was a marked neuronal loss of the basis pontis, demyelination of the transverse pontine fibers, and atrophy of the inferior olivary nuclei. The parietal and occipital lobes showed atrophy of the subcortical white matter. The dorsal columns of the spinal cord were said to show moderate demyelination. The tegmentum of the pons, the central tegmental tract, and the medial longitudinal fasciculus were said to be normal.

The severe degree of cerebellar atrophy (including the white matter of the cerebellum) observed pathologically matches CT findings of our study. However, the marked atrophic changes involving the tegmentum of the pons (present even at the early stages of the illness) and shown by CT have not been previously described in pathological studies. This characteristic CT feature is of particular importance in understanding some of the neurological manifestations found in this disorder.

As described by Cohen et al. (11) and others (56), the paramedian zone of the pontine reticular formation (medial portion of the nucleus reticularis magnocellularis between the trochlear and abducens nuclei) (8) is the area where the fast phases of horizontal nystagmus or horizontal saccadic eye movements are generated. Neurons in this region of the reticular formation activate the motoneurons of eye muscles to produce quick saccadic eye movements during both volitional refixation and the fast saccadic components of caloric and optokinetic nystagmus. The rostral mesencephalic reticular formation (particularly the rostral interstitial nucleus of the median longitudinal fasciculus) appears to play a similar role in the generation of the vertical saccades (10). The smooth pursuit system appears to bypass these areas.

Since the patients showed defective volitional saccadic eye movements and absence of quick phases of the optokinetic and oculovestibular nystagmus (in the presence of intact pursuit eye movements), then the dysfunction in these patients must arise from the paramedian reticular formation of the brainstem (68). In view of these considerations, the CT evidence presented here, which indeed shows a wasting in this area of the brainstem, strongly supports the above hypothesis (Fig. 15). The likelihood of degeneration of interneurons of the reticular formation of these areas should therefore be investigated histologically, including careful counting of the cell population.

→

FIG. 15. A–B: Diagram of transaxial section of the midpons showing the paramedial zone of the pontine reticular formation and lateral reticular nuclei of the pons. **A:** Transaxial section of the midpons in a normal individual. Labeled are ansoparamedian sulci (APS), biventral lobule (BL), brachium pontis (BP), dentate nucleus (DN), great horizontal fissures (GHF), inferior paravermian sulcus (IPS), inferior semilunar lobules (ISL), inferior vermis (IV), lateral angle (LA) of the cerebellum, lateral leminiscus (LL), lateral reticular nuclei (LRN), medullary body (MB), medial leminiscus (ML), posterior angle (PA) of the cerebellum, post clival sulci (PclS), posterior cerebellar notch (PCN), paramedian zone of reticular formation (PMZRF), nuclei pontins (PN), the posterior part of the quadrangular lobule (QL-p), superior semilunar lobules (SSL) and cerebellar tonsils (T). The fourth ventricle (*4*V), the fifth (*5*N), sixth *(6)*, seventh (*7*N), and eighth (*8*N) cranial nerve nuclei are also labeled. **B:** Transaxial section of the midpons in a case of dominantly inherited OPCA associated with slow or defective saccadic eye movements and normal pursuit (case 8). Note the severe pancerebellar atrophy (extending deeply into the paraventricular area), the ballooned fourth ventricle with its concave floor, and the severe involvement of the tegmentum of the pons, as seen in Fig. 12B (case 8). The presumptive histological changes of the tegmentum have been based on the clinical evidence of involvement of the paramedian pontine reticular formation and the VII cranial nerves, with sparing of the vestibular nuclei and the VI cranial nerve. (See text discussion on OPCA associated with slow saccades). See Fig. 15A for abbreviations. The medial longitudinal fasciculus (MLF) is also indicated.

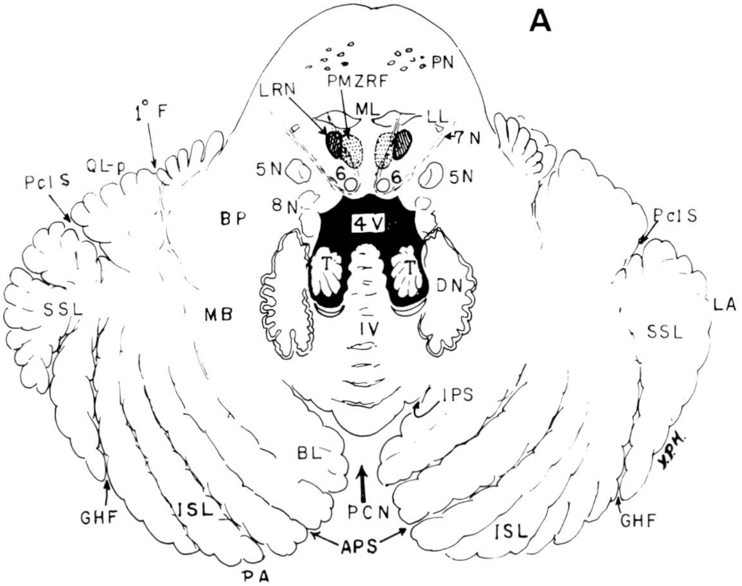

In summarizing the CT findings of the dominant types of OPCA, it should be noted that all 3 subtypes in their advanced stages showed a similar pattern of atrophy (cerebellum, brainstem, and cerebral convolutions). It is, therefore, not surprising to find that there were no remarkable pathological differences among subtypes of dominant OPCA at autopsy (see chapter by Koeppen and Barron, this volume). However, CT scans provided the opportunity to evaluate morphological changes of the brain at early stages of this illness, which were distinctly different

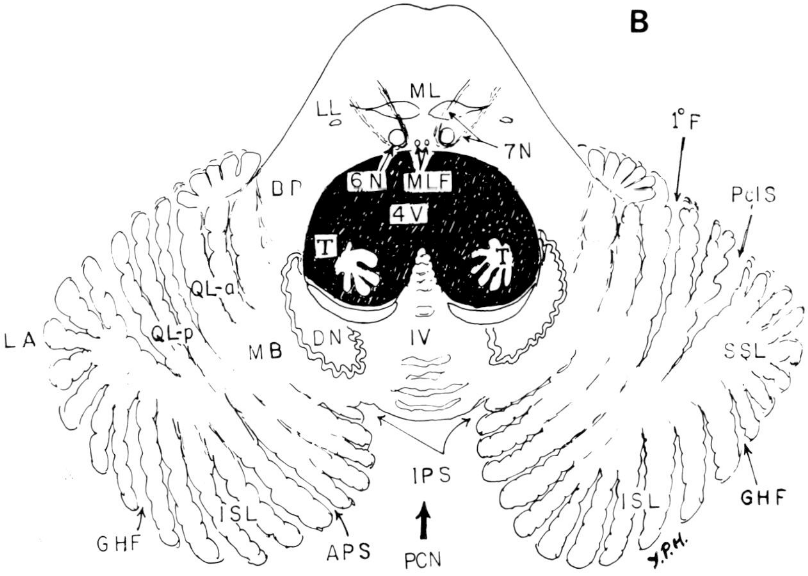

among these disorders. Therefore, CT scans appear to be of particular value in the diagnosis, classification, and understanding of the living pathology of OPCA.

Comment on the Pathogenesis of OPCA

Currently, the pathogenesis of the topographic abnormalities of the brain remains unknown in most cases of OPCA. This is primarily because these disorders have not been understood at the molecular level. On the other hand, CT findings in patients with GDH deficiency appear to suggest that the pattern of neuronal degeneration in these patients may be directly or indirectly related to the underlying biochemical abnormality as described below.

A number of investigations have demonstrated that certain acidic neurotransmitter amino acids, such as glutamate and aspartate (16,51), are potentially neurotoxic and can cause neuronal degeneration when present in excessive amounts in the nervous tissue (13,14,36–38). Experimentally, an intravenous or a subcutaneous injection of monosodium glutamate (MSG) produced retinal degeneration in rodents (31) and atrophic lesions in the hypothalamus of premature monkeys and rodents (36–38). In the latter case, this is particularly true in and adjacent to the arcuate nuclei where the blood-brain barrier is poorly developed, allowing a crossover of the glutamate into the nervous tissue. In addition, when these animals with neonatal MSG toxicity were allowed to reach their maturity, the third ventricle was found to be enlarged (7). The neurotoxicity of these substances may be related to their ability to cause hyperexcitation of the postsynaptic neurons (excitotoxic theory) (13,14,36–38). Since GDH may play an important role in glutamate oxidation, a genetic deficiency of this enzyme may cause an excessive accumulation of this amino acid transmitter in the brain of affected patients (45). Furthermore, since the enzyme may be involved in the glutamatergic transmission mechanisms, excessive accumulation of glutamate may occur at the synaptic cleft during neurotransmission (Fig. 16) with resultant degeneration of the postsynaptic neurons (45).

According to this excitotoxic theory, there should be degeneration of those structures that are innervated by glutamatergic fibers (14). For this reason, we have surveyed the literature concerning the areas of the brain that have been shown to receive putative glutamatergic innervation. The fibers that are thought to use glutamate as their excitatory transmitter are (a) the parallel fibers of granule cells of the cerebellum synapsing with the distal dendrites of the Purkinje cells (61,63,65), (b) the corticopontine fibers with the nuclei pontis (58,60,66); (c) the corticostriate fibers with putamen or with the caudate nuclei (15,33), (d) the corticothalamic fibers with the ventrolateral nucleus of the thalamus (9,20), (e) corticorubral fibers with the red nucleus (9,64), (f) the corticonigral fibers with the substantia nigra, and (g) the corticospinal fibers (66) ending in the fourth and seventh interneuron laminae of the spinal cord. In addition, the cortical pyramidal interneurons which make synapses with the Betz cells are said to be glutamatergic (58). Based on these considerations, we propose that most of the histologic changes found in OPCA, in particular the morphological changes of the brain reflected in CT in patients with GDH deficiency, may be explained by degeneration of the structures

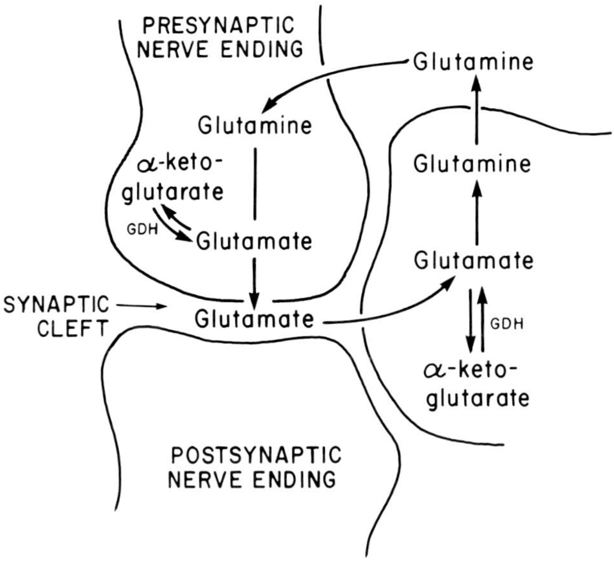

FIG. 16. Hypothetical glutamatergic synaptic junction based on the concept by McGeer and McGeer (34a). Glutamate is thought to be released into synaptic cleft during neurotransmission and to activate the postsynaptic nerve endings. This amino acid may be largely eliminated from the synaptic cleft by uptake into the neighboring glial cells. In these cells glutamate may be oxidized to α-ketoglutamate (via GDH) (67) or aminated to form glutamine (via glutamine synthetase). Glutamine in turn, is taken up by the presynaptic nerve terminals and is converted to glutamate (via glutaminase). Though the enzyme has been shown to be associated with nerve terminals, its exact role in this location has been poorly understood. Decreased glutamate oxidation expected to occur in GDH deficiency could lead to an excessive accumulation of the amino acid at the synaptic cleft with resultant degeneration of the postsynaptic neurons (45).

that receive direct glutamatergic innervation. Indeed, atrophy and eventual loss of postsynaptic cells, at the junctions between the parallel fibers of the granule cells and the distal dendrites of the Purkinje cells of the cerebellum, have been well established in OPCA (Fig. 17). Abnormal accumulation of the glutamate released by the terminals of the corticopontine fibers at the basis pontis could lead to degeneration of the postsynaptic nuclei pontis, the transverse pontine fibers, and therefore the middle cerebellar peduncles (Fig. 18). Similar considerations may also apply to the involvement of the caudate nucleus and putamen, and other structures known to receive most of the glutamatergic corticostriatal fibers (Fig. 18).

As already described, selective destruction of hypothalamic neurons with enlargement of the third ventricle has been produced experimentally by systemic administration of MSG to premature animals. In view of these data, the CT findings of this study, which show a marked enlargement of the anterior third ventricle in patients with GDH-deficient OPCA, are of particular interest. They reveal that anatomical correlates of glutamate toxicity may also exist in humans in a disease process associated with abnormal glutamate metabolism (see chapter by Plaitakis, *this volume*). Atrophy of the thalamus can be attributed to its glutamatergic inner-

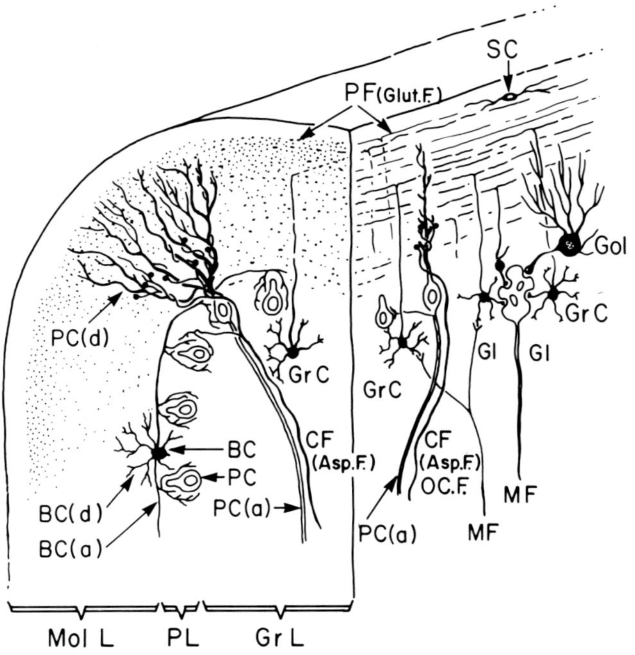

FIG. 17. Diagram of the cerebellar folium showing cytoarchitectures and their relationship to putative glutamatergic and aspartergic afferent fibers. The cerebellopetal fibers are the climbing fibers originating from the inferior olive and the mossy fibers which include all other incoming fibers. The latter, climbing fibers, synapse with the granule cells which in turn send the parallel fibers to the upper molecular layer of the cerebellar cortex. The parallel fibers conversely make synaptic contacts with the distal dendritic branches of the Purkinje cells. These granule cells and their parallel fibers are thought to use glutamate as their neurotransmitter. The climbing fibers, probably originating at the inferior olives, run through the restiform body of the opposite side to reach the cerebellar cortex where they form synapses with the proximal dendritic trees of the Purkinje cells.

vation by the corticothalamic tract. Whether involvement of the hypothalamus is related to a selective sensitivity to glutamate toxicity or to not-yet-discovered glutamatergic inputs to this area is not known at present. Based on the experimental evidence described above, it seems unlikely that the high levels of circulating glutamate in this disorder (45) could cause selective damage to the hypothalamic area in an adult individual unless this can occur after a chronic exposure of many years' duration.

The substantia nigra, red nucleus, and spinal cord, all thought to receive innervation by glutamatergic fibers, could not be identified by CT and therefore could not be studied. However, such clinical evidence as the frequently encountered signs of parkinsonism and spinal cord dysfunction suggests that the CNS regions in these patients with GDH deficiency are often affected. Similarly, involvement of the anterior horn cells, which may receive innervation by glutamatergic interneurons (66), could be manifested clinically as an atypical motor neuron disease (47).

With regard to the frontal convolutional atrophy observed in CT scans of patients with GDH deficiency, no apparent explanation is available. Whether this could

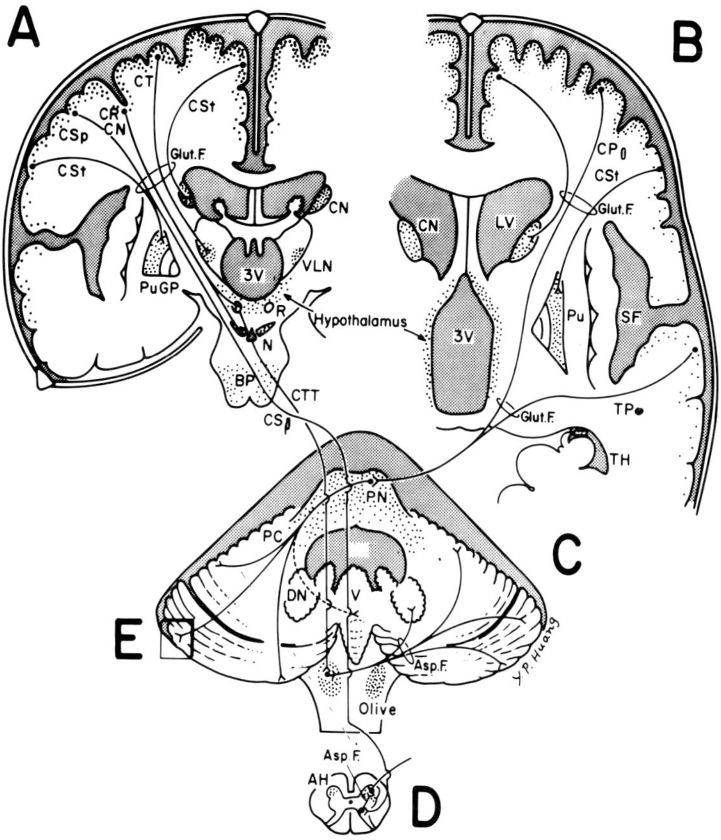

FIG. 18. Diagram showing putative glutamatergic corticofugal fibers and areas of morphological changes of the brain occurring in the GDH-deficient OPCA in the supra- *(A,B)* and infratentorial regions *(C)*, and in the spinal cord *(D)*. The boxed area *(E)* is shown in Fig. 17. The fiber systems thought to utilize glutamate as their excitatory transmitter (Glut. F) include the corticopontine tract (CPo), including frontopontine fibers and temporopontine fibers (TP_o); corticorubral fibers (CR); corticospinal tract (CSp); corticostriate fibers (CSt); and corticothalamic fibers (CT). Labeled also are anterior horn cells (AH), putative aspartergic climbing fibers (Asp. F), basis pontis (BP), caudate nucleus (CN), the central tegmental tract (CTT), the dentate nucleus (DN), the globus pallidus (GP), the lateral ventricle (LV), pontocerebellar fibers (PC), nuclei pontis (PN), putamen (Pu), substantia nigra (N), the red nucleus (R), the sylvian fissure (SF), the temporal horn (TH), the vermis (V), the ventrolateral nucleus of the thalamus (VLN) and the third (3V) and fourth ventricles. The coarsely dotted areas indicate brain regions which are directly innervated by the above glutamatergic fibers and which showed atrophic changes in CT. The neurotransmitter of the central tegmental tract (CTT) is not known at present. The spinal pyramidal tract interneurons are said to be either glutamatergic (66) or aspartergic (21).

result from retrograde transneuronal degeneration (14) or from an altered glutamatergic mechanism of cortical pyramidal interneurons (58) is not clear at present.

Finally, one must consider the involvement of the inferior olivary nuclei and their climbing fibers, a consistent finding in OPCA. Again, whether this is related to a transneuronal transynaptic degeneration (due to loss of the target Purkinje cells) or to an altered glutamatergic input in the medulla oblongata is not known at present.

Though additional studies are needed to test this hypothesis, these considerations may provide a logical explanation for the pathogenesis of CNS lesions occurring in GDH-deficient OPCA. Since other forms of OPCA have shown similar but distinctly different morphological features in CT, it is possible that they may be related to similar but alternate pathogenetic mechanisms (see chapter by Plaitakis, *this volume*).

Relationship to the Aging Process

With the aging process, there may be a slowly advancing widening of the sulci and diminution of the gyri, particularly in the frontal lobe and in the region of the sylvian fissures. In some cases, frank frontal atrophy may appear early (between 50 and 70 years of age), whereas in others cerebral atrophy does not occur until late in life (over 70 years). This study showed that a widening of the sylvian fissures occurred with aging. Cerebellar atrophy, on the other hand, was found to be less pronounced, frequently beginning after 60 to 80 years and becoming prominent after 80 years.

Figure 3 shows that the greatest changes occurring in nondegenerative controls with aging were widening of both the third ventricle and the sylvian fissure, an increase in the intercaudate distance, and frontal atrophy. Since these changes were somewhat similar to those found in GDH-deficient OPCA, it is possible that the disorder is a premature physiological senescence, as suggested by Raymond in 1908 (49).

Recent studies that show a decline in number of the Purkinje cells with aging appear to support this conjecture (D. V. Jeste, *personal communication*). Senescent cytoarchitectural degeneration of the Purkinje cells does not appear to be limited to the distal dendritic defoliation (the site of the synaptic contact between the parallel fiber and the Purkinje cell) for it is also seen in the more proximal part of the dendritic tree (the sites of the synapses between the climbing fibers and the Purkinje cells) (52). Elderly individuals may be more susceptible to glutamate toxicity because the K^+-evoked release of this amino acid has been found to increase linearly with age (57). Also, GDH activity has been shown to decline in the brains of aged animals (23). Neuroexcitotoxic amino acids may therefore be involved in the mechanism of physiological senescence in the human brain. Naturally, those with a genetic deficiency of GDH may be particularly predisposed to develop an accelerated neuronal degeneration of greater severity and earlier onset.

ACKNOWLEDGMENTS

This research was supported in part by NIH Grant NS-16861, and RR-71, NIH Division of Research Resources, General Clinical Center Branch. The authors are indebted to Dr. L. J. Schut for providing Figures 9 and 10 and some clinical information on the "S" family and to Dr. W. Yang for some of the CT scans included in this study. We are grateful to Dr. B. Cohen for his invaluable advice; to Mrs. Gwen Hanley, Mrs. Louisa Haigler, Mr. J. Huang, and Miss C. Huang for their help in preparing this manuscript.

REFERENCES

1. Abe, S., Miyasaka, K., Tashiro, K., Takei, H., Isu, T., and Tsuru, M. (1983): Evaluation of the brain stem with high resolution CT in cerebellar atrophic processes. *Am. J. Neuroradiol.*, 4:446–449.
2. Aita, J. F. (1978): Cranial computerized tomography and Marie's ataxia. *Arch. Neurol.*, 35:55–56.
3. Allen, J. H., Martin, J. T., and McLain, L. W. (1979): Computed tomography in cerebellar atrophic processes. *Radiology*, 130:379–382.
4. Bannister, R., and Oppenheimer, D. R. (1972): Degenerative diseases of the nervous system associated with autonomic failure. *Brain*, 95:457–474.
5. Bentson, J. R., and Keesey, J. C. (1974): Pneumoencephalography of progressive supranuclear palsy. *Radiology*, 18:77–79.
6. Boller, F., and Segarra, J. M. (1969): Spinopontine degeneration. *Europ. Neur.*, 2:356–373.
7. Bodnar, R. J. Abrams, G. M., Zimmerman, E. A., Krieger, D. T., Nicholson, G., and Kizer, J. S. (1980): Neonatal monosodium glutamate. *Neuroendocrinology*, 30:280–284.
8. Brodal, A. (1981): *Neurological Anatomy in Relation to Clinical Medicine*, 3rd Ed. Oxford University Press, Oxford.
9. Bromberg, M. B., Penney, J. B., Jr., Stephenson, B. S., and Young, A. B. (1981): Evidence of glutamate as the neurotransmitter of cortico-thalamic and cortico-rubral pathways. *Brain Res.*, 215:369–373.
10. Buttner-Ennever, J. A., Buttner, U., Cohen, B., and Baumgartner, G. (1982): Vertical gaze paralysis and the rostral interstitial nucleus of the medical longitudinal fasciculus. *Brain*, 105:125–149.
11. Cohen, B., Komatsuzaki, A., and Bender, M. B. (1968): Electro-oculographic syndrome in monkeys after pontine reticular formation lesion. *Arch. Neurol.*, 18:78–92.
12. Colon, R. V., Snead, O. C., and Cabollos, R. (1981): Olivopontocerebellar atrophy in children—A report of 7 cases in two families. *Ann. Neurol.*, 10:355–363.
13. Coyle, J. T., London, E. D., Biziere, K., and Zaczek, R. (1979): Kainic and neurotoxicity: Insights into the pathophysiology of Huntington's disease. In: *Advances in Neurology, Vol. 23: Huntington's Chorea*, edited by T. N. Chase et al., pp. 593–608, Raven Press, New York.
14. Coyle, J. T. (1982): Neurotoxic amino acids in Human degenerative disorders. *Trends Neurosci.*, 5:287–288.
15. Cowan, W. M., and Powell, T. P. S. (1966): Strio-Pallidal projection in the Monkeys. *J. Neurol. Neurosurg. Psychiatry*, 29:426–439.
16. Curtis, D. R., and Watkins, J. C. (1963): Acidic amino acids with strong excitatory actions on mammalian neurones. *J. Physiol.*, 166:1–14.
17. Dejerine, J., and André-Thomas, A. (1900): L'atrophie oliovoponto-cérébelleuse. *Nouv. Iconogr. Salpet.*, 13:330–370.
18. Eadie, M. J. (1975): Cerebello-olivary Atropy (Holmes type). In: *Handbook of Clinical Neurology*, Vol. 21, edited by P. J. Visken and G. W. Bruyn, pp. 403–414, North-Holland, Amsterdam.
19. Eadie, M. J. (1975): Olivo-ponto-cerebellar Atrophy. In: *Handbook of Clinical Neurology*, Vol. 21, edited by P. J. Visken and G. W. Bruyn, pp. 415–431, North Holland, Amsterdam.
20. Fonnum, F., Storm-Mathison, J., and Divac, I. (1981): Biochemical evidence for glutamate as neurotransmitter in cortico-striatal and corticothalamic fibers in rat brain. *Neuroscience*, 6:863–873.
21. Graham, L. T., Shank, R. P., Werman, R., and Aprison, M. H. (1972): Distribution of some synaptic transmitter suspects in cat spinal cord: Glutamic acid and γ-aminobutyric acid, glycine and glutamate. *J. Neurochem.*, 14:465–472.
22. Greenfield, J. G. (1954): *The Spino-cerebellar Degenerations*. Blackwell Scientific Publications, Oxford.
23. Kaur, G., and Kanungo, M. S. (1970): Alterations in glutamate dehydrogenese in the brain of rats of various ages. *Can. J. Biochem.*, 48:203–206.
24. Kennedy, P., Swash, M., and Wylie, I. G. (1978): The clinical significance of pneumographic cerebellar atrophy. *Neuroradiology*, 16:116–119.
25. Koeppen, A. H., and Hans, M. B. (1976): Supranuclear ophthalmoplegia in olivoponto-cerebellar degenerations. *Neurology*, 26:764–768.
26. Koller, W. C., Glatt, S. L., Perlik, S., Huckman, M. S., and Fox, J. H. (1981): Cerebellar atrophy demonstrated by computed tomography. *Neurology (NY)*, 31:405–412.
27. Konigsmark, B. W., and Weiner, L. P. (1970): The olivo-ponto-cerebellar atrophies: A review. *Medicine (Baltimore)*, 49:227–241.

28. Kuru, Y., Sumie, H., Kondo, T., and Kurokawa, S. (1978): Basiparallel cut by pneumoencephalography and cerebellar atrophy. *Neuroradiology*, 16:116–119.
29. Lee, S. H., and Toglia, J. U. (1978): Cerebellar atrophy: Pneumoencephalography and computerized tomography correlation. *Neurology*, 16:179–180.
30. LeMay, M., and Abramowicz, A. (1965): The pneumoencephalographic findings in various forms of cerebellar degenerations. *Radiology*, 85:284–290.
31. Lucas, D. R., and Newhouse, T. P. (1957): *AMA Arch. Ophthalmol.*, 58:193.
32. Maruyama, S., et al. (1976): Investigation of spinocerebellar degeneration patients with computerized tomography. Research committee on spinocerebellar degeneration in (Japanese), Report No. 1, pp. 119–129.
33. McGeer, P. L., McGeer, E. G., Scherer, U., and Singh, K. (1977): A glutamatergic corticostriatal path? *Brain Res.*, 128:369–373.
34. McGeer, E. G., McGeer, P. L., and Singh, K. (1978): Kainate-induced degeneration of neostriatal neurons: Dependency upon corticostriatal tract. *Brain Res.*, 139:38–383.
34a. McGeer, P. L., and McGeer, E. G. (1981): Amino acid neurotransmitters. In *Bone Neurochemistry*, edited by G. L. Siegel, R. W. Albers, B. W. Agranoff, and R. Katzman, pp. 233–268. Little Brown and Co., Boston.
35. Menzel, P. (1981): Beitrag zur Kenntnis der hereditaren ataxie und kleinhirnatrophie. *Arch. Psychiatr. Nervenkr.*, 22:160–190.
36. Olney, J. W., and Sharpe, L. G. (1969): Brain lesions in an infant rhesus monkey treated with monosodium glutamate. *Science*, 166:386–388.
37. Olney, J. W., Ho, O. L., and Rhee, V. (1971): Cytotoxic effects of acidic and sulfur containing amino acids of the infant mouse central nervous systems. *Exp. Brain Res.*, 14:61–76.
38. Olney, J. N. (1978): Neurotoxicity of excitatory amino acids. In: *Kainic Acid as a Tool in Neurobiology*, edited by E. M. McGeer, J. N. Olney, and P. L. McGeer, pp. 95–121. Raven Press, New York.
39. Oppenheimer, D. (1983): Neuropathology of progressive autonomic failure. In: *Autonomic Failure*, edited by R. Bannister, pp. 267–283. Blackwell, Oxford.
40. Parnavelas, J. G., and McDonald, J. K. (1983): The cerebral cortex. In: *Chemical Neuroanatomy*, edited by P. Emson, pp. 509–549. Raven Press, New York.
41. Pedersen, L., and Glydensted, C. (1978): Computerized tomography in hereditary ataxies. *Acta Neurol. Scand.*, 58:81–88.
42. Plaitakis, A., Nicklas, W. J., and Desnick, R. J. (1980): Glutamate dehydrogenase deficiency in three patients with spinocerebellar syndrome. *Ann. Neurol.*, 7:297–303.
43. Plaitakis, A., Berl, S., Nicklas, W. J., and Yahr, M. D. (1980): Glutamate dehydrogenase deficiency in spinocerebellar degenerations: Correlation with adult-onset recessive ataxia. *Tran. Am. Neurol. Assoc.*, 105:476.
44. Plaitakis, A., Berl, S., and Yahr, M. D. (1981): Amino acids as putative transmitters: The role of aspartate and glutamate in nervous system dysfunction and degeneration. In: *Neurology. Int. Congr. Ser 568*, pp. 259–273.
45. Plaitakis, A., Berl, S., and Yahr, M. D. (1982): Abnormal glutamate metabolism in adult-onset degenerative neurological disorders. *Science*, 216:193–196.
46. Plaitakis, A. (1982): The olivo-ponto-cerebellar atrophies. *Semin. Neurol.*, 2:334–342.
47. Plaitakis, A., Berl, S., and Yahr, M. D. (1984): Neurological disorders associated with deficiency of glutamate dehydrogenase. *Ann. Neurol. (in press).*
47a. Plaitakis, A., Huang, Y. P., and Rudolf, S. (1983): Clinical electrophysiological and CT findings in dominant olivo-ponto-cerebellar atrophy with slow saccades. *Neurology*, 33(Suppl 2):218.
48. Pogacar, S., Ambler, M., Conklin, W. J., O'Neil, W. A., and Yong Lee, H. (1978): Dominant spinopontine atrophy. Report of two additional members of family W. *Arch. Neurol.*, 35:156–162.
49. Raymond, F. (1908): The relationship of the so-called family disease to a premature physiological senescence localized to certain organic systems and considered with special reference to the nervous system. *Lancet*, 1:1859–1862.
50. Refsum, S., and Skre, H. (1978): Neurological approaches to the inherited ataxia. *Adv. Neurol.*, 21:1–13.
51. Roberts, P. J., Storm-Mathisen, J., and Johnston, G. A. R. (1981): Glutamate: Transmitter in the central nervous system. John Wiley, New York.

52. Rogers, J., Zornetzer, S. F., and Bloom, F. E. (1981): Senescent pathology of cerebellum Purkinje neuron and their parallel fiber afferents. *Neurobiol. Aging*, 2:15–25.
53. Rothman, S. L. G., and Glanz, S. (1978): Cerebellar atrophy: The differential diagnosis by computerized tomography. *Neuroradiology*, 16:123–126.
54. Savoiardo, M., Bracchi, M., Passerini, A., Visciani, A., DiDonato, S., and Cocchini, F. (1983): Computed tomography of olivopontocerebellar degeneration. *Am. J. Neuroradiol*, 4:509–512.
55. Schut, J. W., and Haymaker, W. (1951): Hereditary ataxia: Pathological study of 5 cases of common ancestry. *J. Neuropathol. Clin. Neurol.*, 1:183–213.
56. Spector, R. H., and Troost, B. T. (1981): The ocular motor system. *Ann. Neurol.*, 9:517–524.
57. Smith, C. C. T., Bower, D. M., and Davison, A. N. (1983): The evoked release of endogenous amino acids from tissue prisons of human neocortex. *Brain Res.*, 269:103–109.
58. Stone, T. S. (1973): Cortical pyramidal tract interneuromas and their sensitivity to L-glutamic acid. *J. Physiol.*, 233:211–225.
59. Taniguchi, R., and Konigsmark, B. W. (1971): Dominant spino-pontine atrophy. Report of a family through three generations. *Brain*, 94:349–350.
60. Thangnipon, W., and Storm-Mathisen, J. (1981): K^+-evoked Ca^{2+}-dependent release of D-[^{3}H]-aspartate from terminals of cortico-pontine pathway. *Neurosci. Lett.*, 23:181–186.
61. Truex, R. C., and Carpenter, M. B. (1973): *Human Neuroanatomy.* Waverly Press, Baltimore.
62. Wadia, N. H., and Swami, R. K. (1971): A new form of heredofamilial spinocerebellar degeneration with slow eye movements (nine families). *Brain*, 94:359–374.
63. Williams, P., and Warwick, R. (1975): *Functional Neuroanatomy of Man.* W. B. Saunders, Philadelphia.
64. Young, A. B., Bromberg, M. B., and Penney, J. B., Jr. (1981): Decreased glutamate uptake in subcortical areas differentiated by sensorimotor cortical ablation in the cat. *J. Neurosci.*, 1:241–249.
65. Young, A. B., Oster-Granite, M. L., Herndon, R. M., and Snyder, S. H. (1974): Glutamic acid: Selective depletion in hamster cerebellum. *Brain Res.*, 73:1–13.
66. Young, A. B., Penney, J. B., Dauth, G. W., Bromberg, M. B., and Gilman, S. (1983): Glutamate or aspartate as a possible neurotransmitter of the cerebral cortico-fugal fibers in the monkey. *Neurology (Cleveland)*, 33:1513–1516.
67. Yu, A. C., Schousboe, A., and Hertz, L. (1982): Metabolic fate of ^{14}C-labeled glutamate in astrocytes. *J. Neurochem.*, 39:954–960.
68. Zee, D. S., Optican, L. M., and Cook, J. D. (1976): Slow saccades in spinal cerebellar degeneration. *Arch. Neurol.*, 33:243–251.

The Olivopontocerebellar Atrophies, edited by
R. C. Duvoisin and A. Plaitakis. Raven Press,
New York © 1984.

Cerebellodiencephalic Interactions in Olivopontocerebellar Atrophy

Hirotaro Narabayashi

Department of Neurology, Juntendo University School of Medicine, Hongo, Bunkyo-ku, Tokyo 113, Japan

Olivopontocerebellar atrophy (OPCA) is a well-known chronic, progressive condition presenting cerebellar symptoms in the early stages of the disease, which are later followed and overlapped by a parkinsonian syndrome. For this reason, it has been classified under the term of multiple system degeneration (or atrophy). It is possible to see a stage of relatively pure cerebellar symptomatology and then a stage of mixed cerebellar and extrapyramidal manifestations. Hirayama et al. (4,5) analyzed the chronologic course of clinical symptomatology in terms of the appearance of cerebellar and extrapyramidal signs, by comparing OPCA with strionigral degeneration, dentatorubropallido-Luysian atrophy (DRPLA) and the Shy-Drager syndrome. The authors observed that in OPCA, the parkinsonian symptoms usually appeared 2 to 5 years after the onset of cerebellar signs, although the severity of the extrapyramidal signs was variable from case to case. In the later stages, with severe parkinsonian symptoms, the previously dominant cerebellar signs tended to disappear or to be replaced by the former; it was often difficult to identify signs of the original OPCA. These observations offer a means to understand the interrelationship between cerebellar and extrapyramidal signs.

Narabayashi (10) attempted a clinical analysis of the interrelationship between the cerebellar and extrapyramidal symptoms as a working hypothesis. The analysis started from the observation that extrapyramidal signs are present in any posture or movement when the patient is awake, even in a state of complete rest of the muscles and of no psychologic tension. This is commonly seen in chorea, hemiballism, dystonia, and parkinsonian tremor. Parkinsonian tremor is considered a diencephalic extrapyramidal symptom, since the tremor-generating mechanism is found in the ventral intermediate nucleus (VIM) of the thalamus, as previously described, although the site of the morphologic lesion is in the midbrain (9). On the other hand, cerebellar dysfunction is not characterized by any specific signs observable at rest, except some slight postural changes, such as a slight external rotation of the thigh when the patient is lying at rest. The muscular hypotonia of cerebellar disease is detectable only on passive manipulation. Most of the known cerebellar signs are evident only when the muscles are in action, i.e., in posture or movement.

According to this analysis, the coexistence of cerebellar and extrapyramidal signs tends to make the latter less apparent in the resting state. Examples are the intention or postural tremor of cerebellar disease, as in the DRPLA. In cases with intention or postural tremor, pathology is found or suspected in the cerebellum or in its projection to the cerebrum, but the neurophysiologic mechanism generating these tremors is presumed to be in the VIM of the thalamus (13). In this specific subnucleus, a group of neurons discharging synchronously with the peripheral tremulous movement of a certain part of the contralateral extremities is almost always detectable, as in the parkinsonian tremor through a thin microelectrode inserted during the course of stereotaxic surgery (13,14). Electrical stimulation of VIM through the same electrode immediately inhibits or modifies the corresponding tremor, and a small electrocoagulation of these neurons almost always abolishes the tremor dramatically (9,12). The neuronal mechanism generating these tremors within the thalamus reflects pathology in the cerebellothalamic projection (8). Thus the intention or postural tremor of cerebellar disease is understandable as a combination of diencephalic neuronal activities and a loss of cerebellar influence. In neurophysiology, the cerebellothalamic projection has been considered facilitatory in nature (2). A similar situation is proposed for DRPLA, in which the site of pathology is in both extrapyramidal and cerebellar structures. In this condition, the abnormal movement, mostly mild athetosis, is not clearly observable at rest but begins to appear when the muscles are activated in a voluntary effort to make a movement or maintain a certain posture.

To pursue these considerations, Narabayashi et al. (11) compared the effects of psychologic loading by using mental calculation and motor loading with minimal muscle contraction, such as flexing the elbow, which seems to require almost no psychologic effort. These two loading tests were done in the supine position in patients with abnormal movement. Two examples are shown in Fig. 1. In Fig. 1A, the choreic movements are increased under psychologic loading but not with motor loading. On the other hand, intention tremor in Fig. 1B is enhanced by the latter but not the former.

In summary, extrapyramidal abnormal movements due to diencephalic pathology are present at rest and are increased and enhanced by psychologic loading but not by motor loading. When cerebellar pathology is present, abnormal movements tend not to be observable in muscles at complete rest. They start to appear and become observable with motor loading but not with psychologic loading alone. When once present with motor loading, however, they can be enhanced by the addition of psychologic loading. This simple analysis suggests a facilitatory role of the cerebellothalamic projection on motor phenomena occurring at the diencephalic level.

AN ILLUSTRATIVE CASE OF OPCA

Figure 2 depicts the clinical course in a patient with typical OPCA who was observed for about 3 years before he died. The total course, which extended over 7 years, is divided into three stages: the first stage with cerebellar symptoms, the

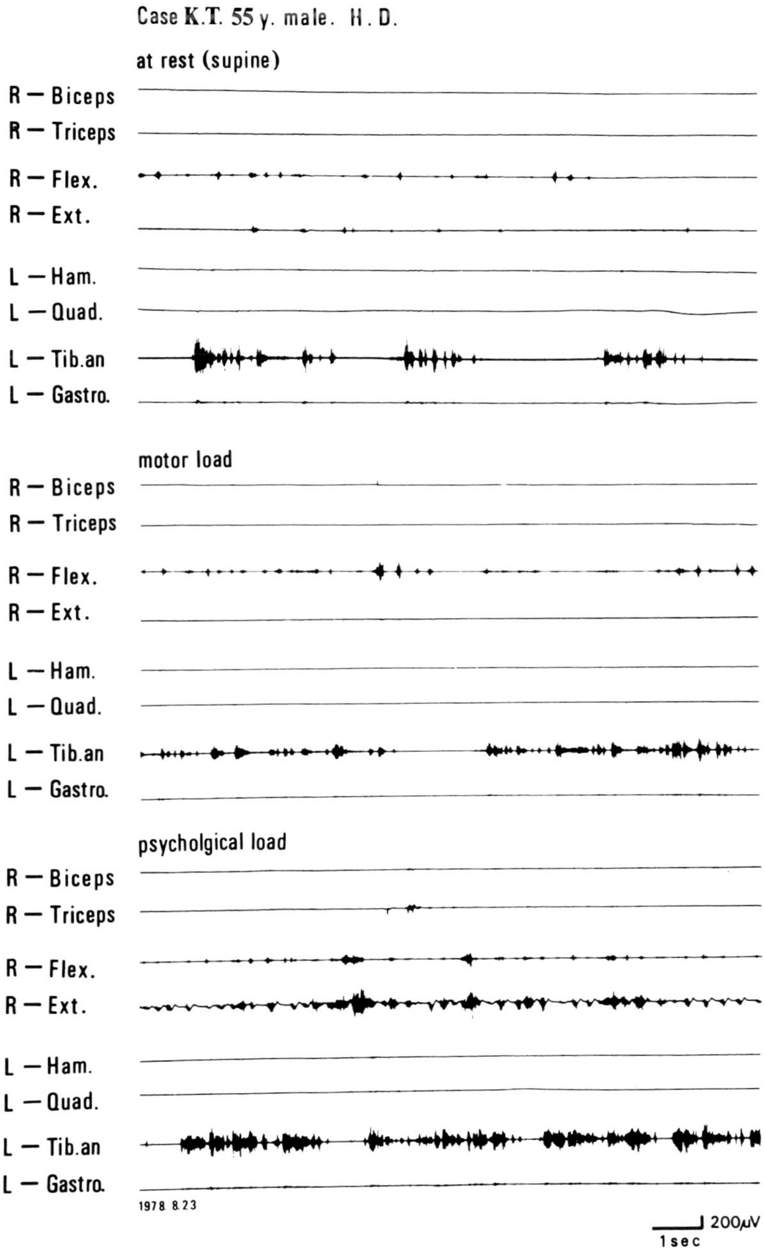

FIG. 1A. Effects of two loading tests on chorea in Huntington's disease by surface electromyography (see text).

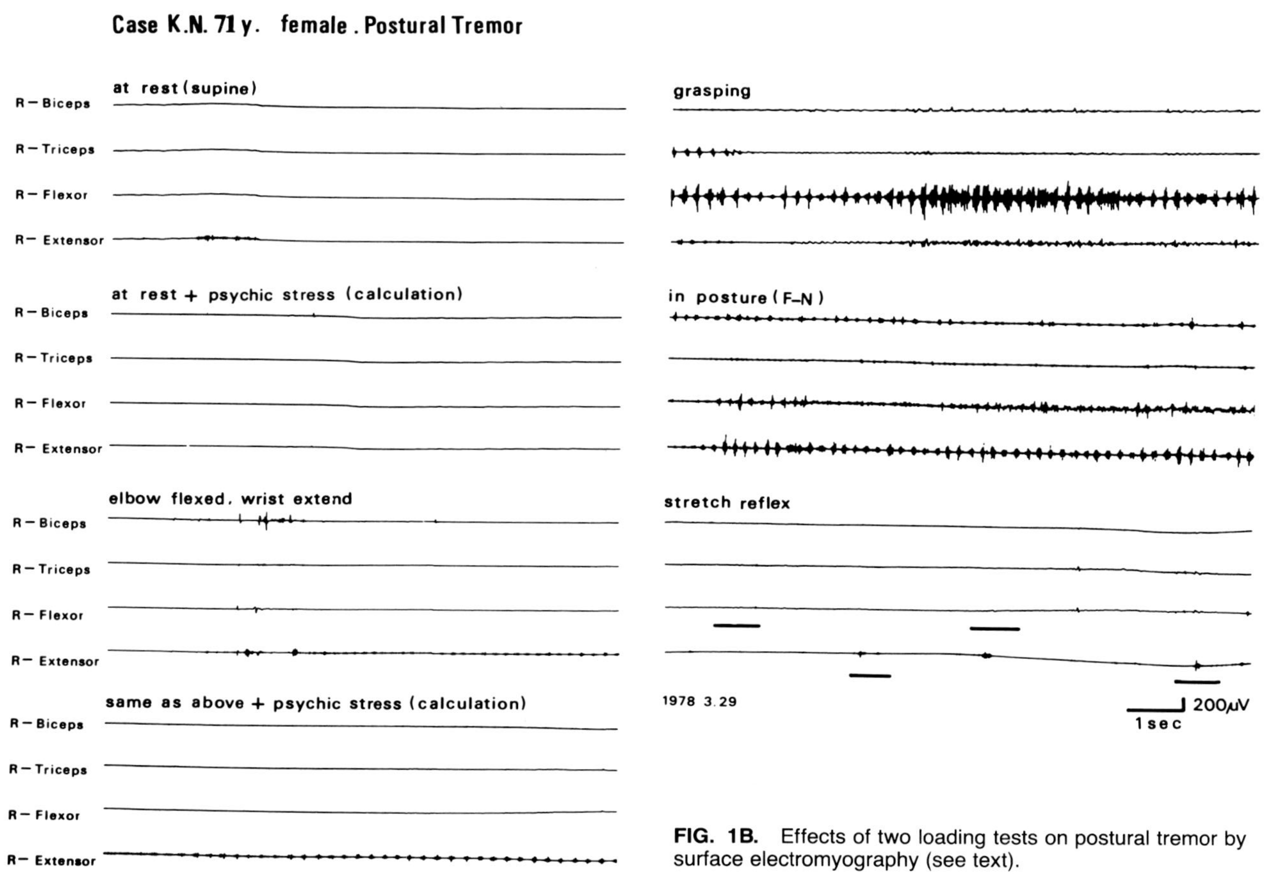

FIG. 1B. Effects of two loading tests on postural tremor by surface electromyography (see text).

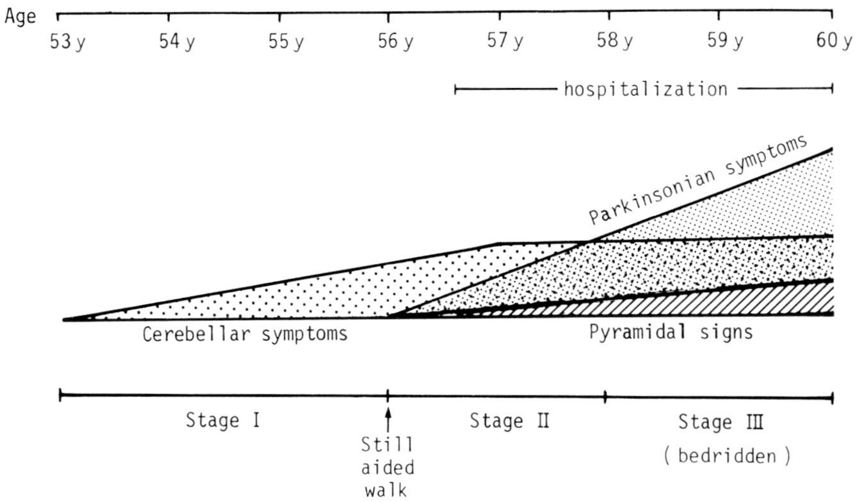

FIG. 2. Course of cerebellar and parkinsonian symptoms in OPCA (case M.O.)

second with beginning extrapyramidal symptoms, and the third with parkinsonian symptoms predominating.

In the first stage in this patient, cerebellar signs, such as horizontal nystagmus, ataxia of gait with a wide base, muscular hypotonia and hypermetria, which were more marked on the right, slight tremor in movement, and slowing in speech, had been slowly progressive for about 3 years since the onset of the disease at the age of 53. When he was admitted to our hospital in the second stage about 4 years after onset, the patient still could move and walk with assistance. Muscle tone was still generally hypotonic, except that the wrist joint presented the *signe de poignet figé* (Froment), a sign of slight rigidity. In several months, rigidity began to be added, first in the neck and proximal upper extremities, more marked on the right side than on the left. Within a year, this spread to other parts of the body. A slight, regular, rhythmic tremor was present in both arms. Progressive rigidity resulted with the patient immobile in bed in the third stage, which lasted for 2 years until his death.

In the last year, the clinical picture was much like that of advanced parkinsonism in the bedridden state, and it was almost impossible to think of the initial picture of cerebellar symptoms. Speech was soft and slurred, difficult to understand, and without scanning. The extremities were fixed in severe, rigid, semiflexed posture, with a moderate resting tremor of about 4 Hz in both arms and hands. The neck and truncal muscles were equally rigid, and the patient could not roll over. L-DOPA, anticholinergic drugs, and Symmetrel were relatively effective in lessening the muscular hypertonus, but the patient's truncal immobility and activities of daily living were not benefited. He died of pneumonia at the age of 60.

At autopsy, there was severe atrophy of the cerebellar hemispheres, the anterior vermis, and the pons. Brownish pigmentation in the putamen and depigmentation of the nigral region were prominent.

On microscopic examination, as shown in Table 1, loss of cortical neurons of the cerebellum, especially of the vermis, was marked, but degeneration of the dentate nucleus was moderate. The neurons of the pontine nuclei and the olivary nucleus had disappeared almost completely with marked gliosis. In the basal ganglia, there was severe nerve cell loss in the putamen with gliosis. The red nucleus and the nigra also showed moderate neuronal loss and depigmentation. There was degeneration of the pyramidal tract at the level of the pons. Clinical course, symptoms, and neuropathologic findings in this case are typical of OPCA.

Changes in the pattern of tremulous movement in each stage of the illness were carefully observed. In stage 1, when only cerebellar signs were found, tremor was slight and observable only on performing delicate voluntary movements of the hand, such as writing. Coarse tremor was not seen at any time during the course of the illness. At the time of admission in stage 2, i.e., about 4 years after onset, a regular, rhythmic tremor of the hands of small amplitude was occasionally seen on maintaining a posture and even at rest, although the muscle was slightly hypotonic;

TABLE 1. *Neuropathologic findings of OPCA*[a]

	Severity[b]			Severity[b]	
Site	Neuron	Glia	Site	Neuron	Glia
Cerebellum			Thalamus	—	—
cortex			Corpus luysi	(+)	1+
vermis	2+	1+	Substantia nigra	2+	1+[d]
hemisphere	1+	(+)	Nucleus ruber	2+	(+)
medulla	4+	3+	Locus ceruleus	1+	(+)[d]
nucleus dentatus	(+)	1+	Cerebral cortex	(+)	(+)
Brachium conjunctivum	(+)	(+)	Centrum semiovale	1+	1+
Brachium pontis	4+	3+	Tractus corticopontinus	3+	2+
Corpus restiforme	3+	2+	Tractus pyramidalis		
Nuclei pontis	4+	3+	cerebral peduncles	1+	1+
Nucleus olivaris	4+	3+	pons	2+	1+
Nucleus caudatus			medulla oblongata	1+	—
small cell	—	1+	medulla spinalis	1+	—
large cell	3+		Tractus spinocerebellaris	(+)	—
Putamen			Nucleus dorsalis (Clarke)	2+	1+
small cell	3+	4+[c]	Funiculus posterior	(+)	—
large cell	4+		Dorsal column	—	—
Globus pallidus			Lateral column	2+	—
pars lateralis	3+	1+[c]	Anterior column	(+)	—
pars medialis	2+	(+)[c]			

[a]Case M. O. (From ref. 4.)
[b]1+, least severe pathologic changes; 4+, most severe.
[c]Pigment granule deposit.
[d]Depigmentation.

only slight rigidity at the wrist was detectable. This small postural or rest tremor tended to become more marked when the patient was trying to write or to hold something; i.e., it was enhanced by movement.

In the last 2 years in the bedridden state of stage 3, the patient continuously presented a parkinsonian tremor in the supine or lateral recumbent position. The muscles were relatively rigid, even though cerebellar-type hypermetria and decomposition were still detectable on careful examination.

The gradual change in the phenotype of movement from a slight tremor during movement to a postural tremor enhanced by voluntary movement culminating in a parkinsonian tremor at rest paralleled the gradual change in the general neurologic picture from the cerebellar phase to the cerebellar plus extrapyramidal phase, which is described above. These changes in tremor pattern occurred as steps in a continuum.

The patient's speech was slowed and slurred at the onset. It progressively worsened to a scanning type of speech when the patient was admitted early in the second stage. In the third stage, however, the disturbance resembled that in severe parkinsonism. Protrusion of the tongue was not limited in the early stage but was poor in the third stage of the disease. No deviation was observed.

Other cerebellar signs such as gait, ataxia, hypermetria, or oscillation in the heel-to-knee test were obvious in the first and early second stages. With diminished mobility, these signs became more difficult to detect in later stages.

One of the main factors that may be responsible for these changes in clinical features, especially in tremor, is the gradual change of background muscle tone from hypotonia to its mixture with rigidity and finally to the highly rigid state.

The author (7) has previously pointed out that the frequency of tremor is changeable and determined to some extent by the grade of coexisting muscle hypertonus. In parkinsonism, an increase in tremor frequency within 1 Hz is observed in parallel with a gradual increase in passive muscle stretch, which may mean a gradual increase of muscle afferent discharge. In exceptional situations, e.g., in the borderline between parkinsonian and familial tremor, tremor is not observed at rest but can be elicited easily by passive muscle stretch without voluntary contraction. This may mean that the increase of muscle afferent discharge would be important in producing tremor and determining its frequency.

In the case of OPCA, the gradual change of tremor type from a slight action tremor in the earlier stages to a parkinsonian rest tremor seemed to parallel the slow increase of muscular hypertonus through the course of several years. In the third stage, L-DOPA and Symmetrel were administered to reduce the marked rigidity, with relatively good effect. When the rigidity was diminished, it became easier to identify the increase of intention tremor on voluntary movement.

These observations suggest the importance of muscle tone and thus of the role of muscle afferent activity in influencing tremor, which seems to reflect a peripheral mechanism.

DISCUSSION

The facilitatory influence of the cerebellothalamic inflow on involuntary movement of diencephalic origin was suggested as a working hypothesis. The distribution of the cerebellar projections to the thalamic subnuclei, the ventral anterior nucleus, the ventral lateral nucleus, and the VIM has been studied intensively, mostly in animals (3,6). The pattern of distribution is known to vary slightly in different species. In man, the VIM seems to be especially important, since the cerebellar and vestibular projections and the proprioceptive or kinesthetic afferents converge on this specific area. At the present stage of our knowledge, there is no detailed physiologic understanding of the integration of diencephalic and cerebellar functions to apply to pathologic symptoms.

The author has studied dyskinesia in the macaque induced by the administration of 10 to 20 mg of a peripheral dopa-decarboxylase inhibitor intraperitoneally and 100 to 200 mg L-DOPA intravenously. When dyskinesia of the neck and jaw appeared, it was continuously present for a period of about 1 hr. A previous cerebellectomy tended to abolish this symptom, and the animal sat quietly on his chair (8). Thus both clinical observation and these animal models suggest that the cerebellum exerts a facilitatory influence on involuntary movements produced at the diencephalic level. In the absence of cerebellar influence, involuntary movements become less apparent. However, cerebellar pathology seriously affects the peripheral motor mechanism by producing muscular hypotonia, which obviously is fed back promptly to the central nervous system as a change in the amount and modus of muscle afferent and kinesthetic input. The important role of muscle tone in modifying centrally produced abnormal movement was also discussed; this role may be interpreted in terms of the amount of muscle afferents. The simple motor loading test described seems to offer a useful tool for analyzing the role of muscle tone.

Two possible mechanisms of cerebellodiencephalic interrelation, one central and the other peripheral, are important in analyzing the clinical features of OPCA. These two mechanisms are considered to closely influence each other, as in an integrated circuit (1).

REFERENCES

1. Asanuma, H. (1984): Function role of sensory inputs to the motor cortex. *Prog. Neurobiol. (in press).*
2. Eccles, J. C., Ito, M., and Szentágothai, J. (1967): *The Cerebellum as a Neuronal Machine.* Springer-Verlag, New York.
3. Hassler, R. (1959): Anatomy of the thalamus. In: *Introduction to Stereotaxis with an Atlas of the Human Brain, Vol. 1*, edited by G. Schaltenbrand and P. Bailey, pp. 230–290. Thieme, Stuttgart.
4. Hirayama, K., Saito, M., Chida, T., Iizuka, R., and Murofushi, K. (1977): A clinicopathological study on extrapyramidal components in cerebellar degeneration with special reference to olivo-ponto-cerebellar atrophy. *Adv. Neurol. Sci.*, 21:37–54.
5. Hirayama, K. (1980): Analysis of clinical features in cerebello-extrapyramidal system degeneration. In: *Spinocerebellar Degenerations*, edited by Japan Medical Research Foundation, pp. 23–34. University of Tokyo Press, Tokyo.
6. Mehler, W. R. (1971): Idea of a new anatomy of the thalamus. *J. Psychiatr. Res.*, 8:203–217.

7. Narabayashi, H. (1973): Importance of muscle tone in production or modification of tremorous movements. In: *Parkinson's Disease, Vol. 2*, edited by J. Siegfried, pp. 27–36. Hans Huber, Bern.
8. Narabayashi, H., Goto, A., Miyazaki, S., and Kosaka, K. (1974): Importance of the cerebellar hemisphere in production of tremulous movement or choreodystonic movement in monkeys. *Acta Neurochir. [Suppl.]*, 21:35–38.
9. Narabayashi, H., and Ohye, C. (1978): Parkinsonian tremor and nucleus ventralis intermedius of the human thalamus. In: *Progress in Clinical Neurophysiology, Vol. 5*, edited by J. E. Desmedt, pp. 165–172. Karger, Basel.
10. Narabayashi, H. (1979): Involuntary movements and cerebellar pathology. In: *Cerebro-Cerebellar Interactions*, edited by J. Massion and K. Sasaki, pp. 231–248. Elsevier, Amsterdam.
11. Narabayashi, H., Chida, T., and Kondo, T. (1979): Analysis of two factors influencing involuntary movement: Psychological stress effect and motor effect. In: *Advances in Neurology, Vol. 24*, edited by L. J. Poirier, T. L. Sourkes, and P. J. Bedard, pp. 361–371. Raven Press, New York.
12. Narabayashi, H. (1982): Surgical approach to tremor. In: *Movement Disorders*, edited by C. D. Marsden and S. Fahn, pp. 293–299. Butterworth Scientific, London.
13. Narabayashi, H. (1982): Tremor mechanisms. In: *Stereotaxy of the Human Brain*, edited by G. Schaltenbrand and A. E. Walker, pp. 510–514. Thieme, Stuttgart.
14. Ohye, C., and Narabayashi, H. (1979): Physiological study of presumed ventralis intermedius neurons in the human thalamus. *J. Neurosurg.*, 50:290–297.

The Olivopontocerebellar Atrophies, edited by R. C. Duvoisin and A. Plaitakis. Raven Press, New York © 1984.

Disorders of Ocular Motility in the Olivopontocerebellar Atrophies

Frederick E. Lepore

Department of Neurology, University of Medicine and Dentistry of New Jersey, Rutgers Medical School, Academic Health Science Center, New Brunswick, New Jersey 08903

Wilson (39) attributed our knowledge of olivopontocerebellar atrophy (OPCA) to Dejerine and Thomas (11), who described "atrophy of cerebellar cortex, bulbar olives, and pontine grey matter, complete degeneration of middle peduncles and partial of restiform bodies, with relative integrity of the central nuclei." Although 40 years had elapsed since their original description in 1900, Wilson still conceded the clinician's dilemma of "a clearly outlined pathological picture . . . to which, it so happens, no distinct clinical syndrome corresponds; the symptoms are those of chronic progressive cerebellar atrophies in general" (39).

The diagnosis of OPCA during life remains a demanding exercise of clinical acumen. Over the years, however, a spectrum of disordered ocular motility has been noted, presumably reflecting dysfunction of the cerebellum and brainstem. Beginning with the original paper by Dejerine and Thomas (11) noting disturbances of ocular motility in both patients with OPCA, subsequent authors have estimated ocular motor dysfunction to be present in roughly one-quarter of 117 anatomically confirmed cases of familial and sporadic OPCA (3). This figure may substantially underestimate the prevalence of disordered motility, since older authors did not have the benefit of later refinements of the clinical neuroophthalmologic examination. Although a grouping of ocular motor deficits may not be specific for OPCA [such a specific grouping is claimed for other spinocerebellar disorders (15)], these findings can be of great utility and should receive the consideration accorded to the more well-known signs, such as disturbance of gait and balance, dysarthria, and extrapyramidal disturbance.

We reviewed the presence of disordered ocular motility in 108 cases of OPCA from the world literature. These cases included hereditary and sporadic OPCA as well as variant OPCA with retinal degeneration and/or optic atrophy. For this review, OPCA had to be documented on postmortem examination or by neuroradiologic studies. Family members of anatomically proven index cases of OPCA were included if they demonstrated similar clinical signs.

NUCLEAR AND INTERNUCLEAR DISORDERS OF EYE MOVEMENT

Involvement of nuclei III, IV, and VI is distinctly uncommon in the OPCAs. Third nerve paresis was accurately described in one member of the Schut family (22). Pathologic confirmation of combined involvement of the third and fourth nerves was made in an unusual case of unilateral OPCA (10) and in a case of severe external ophthalmoplegia (25). Internuclear ophthalmoplegia was found in three patients, all members of a kindred with OPCA and retinal degeneration (37). Dilated or sluggishly reactive pupils (19,26,28,37) and ptosis (28) were not found in the company of the typical motility deficits of an oculomotor nerve lesion. Clearly, nuclear or internuclear lesions are infrequent causes of disturbed ocular motility in the OPCAs (3). External ophthalmoplegia in OPCA is almost invariably of supranuclear origin, and to understand motility in OPCA we must consider the cerebellar and brainstem gaze systems.

SUPRANUCLEAR DISORDERS OF EYE MOVEMENT

Saccades are rapid eye movements with a peak velocity between 30 and 700°/sec. They enable the fovea to be rapidly trained on objects of visual interest. A marked slowing of velocity of this eye movement subsystem has been reported in hereditary, sporadic, glutamate dehydrogenase-deficient, and retinal degeneration-associated OPCA (2,7,12,19–21,24,29,30,35). Wadia and Swami (35,36) examined 24 members of 13 families with OPCA and found that all 24 had marked slowing of saccades. Quantitative electrooculography showed maximum saccadic velocity in several patients to be one-sixth to one-eighth that of controls. There was no nystagmus, diplopia, squint, ptosis, or pupillary abnormality. Limitation of ocular excursions did not occur until 8 to 10 years after onset of the progressive cerebellar and oculomotor signs that marked the authors' cases. Although defects of saccadic eye movements may be more common in OPCA than has heretofore been realized (20), they are not an invariable accompaniment of OPCA; neither are slow saccades specific to OPCA. They have been described in a variety of other diseases: Huntington's disease, Wilson's disease, ataxia telangiectasia, juvenile lipidosis, and progressive supranuclear palsy (PSP). Saccades in OPCA can be defective in amplitude as well as velocity. Multiple hypometric saccades may be required for target attainment by patients with OPCA (2), PSP, Parkinson's disease, status posthemispherectomy (34), and congenital ocular motor apraxia (COMA) (43).

Head thrusting is an associated finding reported in some OPCA patients with saccadic palsy (7,20,35). Typically, a patient suddenly turns the head, overshooting the desired point of fixation. The eyes, lagging behind the rate of head turn, eventually fixate on the desired target. With the target now placed on fovea, the head turns back and the eyes remain in primary position in the orbits. These head thrusts are a striking example of a gaze strategy employed to overcome a defect of saccadic velocity by using compensatory vestibular eye movements. Cogan et al (7) note similar head thrusts in children with the slow horizontal saccades of COMA, although the acquired motility disorder in OPCA involves both vertical and horizontal gaze. Zee et al. (43) have described a form of COMA characterized by delay of saccadic initiation and normal velocity saccades, in contradistinction to OPCA in which there is no increased latency of initiation and saccades may be slow (1). The pattern of head thrusts in COMA with normal velocity saccades differs from the more extreme head overshooting found in OPCA (7,20,35) and COMA with slow saccades (7). The coupling of saccades and head movements is typical of afoveate, less phylogenetically advanced animals (27); thus patients with OPCA and COMA may employ primitive eye-head synkineses to overcome defective saccadic initiation or velocity.

Any disorder of saccadic velocity must upset the sequence of a burst of 400 to 600 spikes per second emanating from ocular motoneurons. This is sufficient to overcome the viscous inertia of the globe in the orbit. The new eye position is maintained by a tonic ("step") discharge of the motoneurons (41). The immediate origins of the motoneuron bursts are the medium-lead burst cells, which are to be found in the paramedian pontine reticular formation (PPRF). Computer modeling of slow saccades is compatible with the premise of scaling down velocity commands by decreasing the number of burst neurons in the PPRF (40). Currently, there is no compelling neuropathologic evidence of loss of these neurons in OPCA (20,35). Saccades are preceded by neuronal discharge in many areas of the brain: frontal eye fields (18), thalamus, cerebellum, vestibular nuclei, superior colliculus, pontine reticular formation, and mesencephalic periaqueductal gray (40). The neural pathway for saccades is multisynaptic, and multiple lesions may be a requisite for slow saccades in OPCA. A single lesion of a discrete structure, such as the cerebellum (27,40), cannot account for slow saccades in OPCA.

Once the desired visual image has been placed on the fovea by the saccadic system, the pursuit system holds it in position by tracking at rates up to 130°/sec and accelerating slowly as compared to saccades (27). The pursuit system is flawed in OPCA; in their original cases, Dejerine and Thomas (11) noted that upward gaze was performed in jerky nystagmoid fashion. The abnormal jerkiness of the usually smooth pursuit movement may be due to (a) interposed "catch-up" saccades when the eyes lag too far behind the target, (b) square wave oscillations superimposed on pursuit, or (c) nystagmus interacting with pursuit movements (8).

Another aspect of the stabilization of image upon fovea of the pursuit system may be cancellation of the vestibuloocular reflex (VOR). This reflex would tend to keep the eyes fixed relative to the external world and would prevent a target from being followed by the eyes whenever the head turned. The pursuit system in effect "cancels" the VOR and permits the eyes to follow a target as the head turns (27). Faulty suppression of the VOR is indicated by the intrusion of saccades as the eyes follow a target moving at the same rate as the head turns. This defective cancellation has been observed in hereditary cerebellar ataxia (42) and OPCA (13).

Pursuit system abnormalities can be a nonspecific sign (8) and have been noted in fatigued normal subjects (2). Nevertheless, cerebellectomy abolishes pursuit in monkeys (38), and the Purkinje cells of the flocculus modulate their discharge rate in proportion to pursuit gaze velocity in space (23). The extensive and widespread loss of Purkinje cells in OPCA may provide a neuropathologic substrate for impaired smooth pursuit.

Fifteen per cent of sporadic and familial OPCA patients may have external ophthalmoplegia of supranuclear origin (3). One year before his first published report of two cases of OPCA (11), Thomas (32) documented a typical pattern of supranuclear ophthalmoplegia in a third case of OPCA. Later authors have noted a characteristic sequence of limitation of gaze in which there is first involvement of upward gaze and convergence, then slowing of lateral saccadic eye movements to the point of extinction, and finally loss of downward gaze. Typically, there is no ptosis (19). This contrasts with PSP, in which downward gaze usually is first affected (33). Despite marked limitation of volitional eye movements in OPCA, reflexive vestibular motility can persist until 10 years after clinical onset, when there may be paralysis of all reflex and voluntary eye movements (35). This pattern of ocular motility loss resembles the progression in PSP which has been attributed to degeneration of ocular motoneurons.

Despite the similarities of supranuclear ophthalmoplegia in OPCA and PSP, the neuropathologic findings are dissimilar. The degenerative changes of PSP are most prominent in the globus pallidus, subthalamic nucleus, red nucleus, substantia nigra, periaqueductal gray, deep tegmental gray, superior colliculus, and dentate nucleus (31). With such diffuse brainstem involvement, it is reasonable to assume that supranuclear gaze centers and, in more advanced cases, the ocular motor nuclei (4) are involved. In autopsied cases of OPCA with supranuclear limitation of gaze, the pontine and mesencephalic tegmentum, periaqueductal gray, and ocular motor nuclei are typically spared (19,20,35). As in the abnormally slowed saccades, a discrete lesion causing supranuclear ophthalmoplegia in OPCA remains elusive. There may be more than one anatomical locus that causes this gaze disturbance.

The biphasic ocular oscillation of nystagmus is the most common disturbance of ocular motility in Berciano's (3) combined series of familial and sporadic OPCA. Gaze-evoked nystagmus elicited by holding the eyes in an eccentric position is the most prevalent type of nystagmus in OPCA (2,7,9,16,22,26,28,32) and was described in Dejerine and Thomas' original paper (11). Downbeat nystagmus, classically associated with disease at the craniocervical junction (6), has been reported in two cases of OPCA (5,7). Rebound nystagmus, a type of gaze-evoked nystagmus that changes direction with sustained lateral gaze or return to primary position, has been noted in one case of OPCA (2) and in intrinsic cerebellar disease (42).

It has been suggested that the disappearance of nystagmus during the course of OPCA might reflect a more generalized disturbance of saccades (4). Although nystagmus is typically absent when slow saccades are found (20,30,35), Cogan et al. (7) and Baloh et al. (2) have observed that these signs are not mutually exclusive.

Gaze-evoked nystagmus has been attributed to "leakiness" of neural integrators, which match the firing pattern of ocular motoneurons to the requirements of maintaining a given position of gaze (17). Although this integrator has been tentatively localized to the PPRF at the level of the abducens nuclei (27,34), it is known that lesions of the cerebellum interfere with the neural integrator and disturb gaze-holding by having the eye slip back toward center after an eccentric saccade (27). Although clinicopathologic correlation must be proposed cautiously since gaze-evoked nystagmus can be elicited in normal individuals in the dark (17), cerebellar pathology would appear to be the most likely source of gaze-evoked nystagmus in OPCA.

The entire spectrum of cerebellar disorders of ocular motility (8,14,42) can be viewed in OPCA. This includes gaze-evoked nystagmus, downward beating nystagmus, defective smooth pursuit, rebound nystagmus, enhanced VOR, instability of gaze fixation (i.e., square wave jerks), ocular dysmetria, and ocular flutter. The last three signs illustrate the defective maintenance of fixation of the diseased cerebellum with intrusion of saccades spontaneously in flutter and square wave jerks or following a refixation movement in dysmetria. In OPCA, gaze-evoked nystagmus and/or defective smooth pursuit are seen more commonly than are downbeat or rebound nystagmus, fixation instability, flutter, and dysmetria (2). Additionally, "noncerebellar" or brainstem disorders of ocular motility (7,8) are prominent in OPCA. These include slowing of saccades, supranuclear ophthalmoplegia, internuclear ophthalmoplegia, and oculomotor nerve palsy. These ocular motor deficits are not specific for OPCA, and some can be found in other spinocerebellar degenerations, including parenchymal cerebellar atrophy and Friedreich's ataxia (2).

The full repertoire of ocular motor dysfunction is not found in each case of OPCA, and there may be distinct subgroups of OPCA as defined by defective ocular motility, e.g. Wadia's (35) patients with slow saccades. Alternatively, the phenotypic expression of defective ocular motility may vary considerably, despite an identical genotype in affected patients. The varied clinical expression of the same genetic defect was described in the Schut family, in which, clinically, one member had Friedreich's ataxia, two had hereditary spastic paraplegia, and 19 had cerebellar ataxia (28). Equally varied disturbances of ocular motility were observed in these family members. Despite the protean clinical pictures, autopsies demonstrated OPCA. Similarly, Cogan et al. (7) describe two brothers with OPCA: one has slowing of saccades with conspicuous head thrusts, while the other has marked jerk nystagmus and normal saccadic velocity. Finally, ocular motor dysfunction may appear much differently in the same patient at the clinical onset of OPCA than in later years; e.g., nystagmus may cease (3), or a gaze palsy may evolve into external ophthalmoplegia (35).

It would seem that there are no pathognomonic eye signs in OPCA. However, by virtue of the ability to break down ocular motility into subsystems (27), we may be able to discern more of the disordered cerebellar and brainstem physiology of OPCA as reflected by defective ocular movements.

REFERENCES

1. Baloh, R. W. (1979): Reply to "A-T and other cerebellar atrophy syndromes." *Neurology*, 29:757.
2. Baloh, R. W., Konrad, H. R. E., and Honrubia, V. (1975): Vestibulo-ocular function in patients with cerebellar atrophy. *Neurology*, 25:160–168.

3. Berciano, J. (1982): Olivopontocerebellar atrophy—a review of 117 cases. *J. Neurol. Sci.*, 53:253–272.
4. Blumenthal, H., and Miller, C. (1969): Motor nuclear involvement in progressive supranuclear palsy. *Arch. Neurol.*, 20:362–367.
5. Case Records of the Massachusetts General Hospital, Case 39–1980 (1980): *N. Engl. J. Med.*, 303:803–809.
6. Cogan, D. G. (1968): Down-beat nystagmus. *Arch. Ophthalmol.*, 80:757–768.
7. Cogan, D. G., Chu, F. C., Reingold, D., and Barranger, J. (1981): Ocular motor signs in some metabolic diseases. *Arch. Ophthalmol.*, 99:1802–1808.
8. Cogan, D. G., Chu, F. C., and Reingold, D. B. (1982): Ocular signs of cerebellar disease. *Arch. Ophthalmol.*, 100:755–760.
9. Critchley, M., and Greenfield, J. G. (1948): Olivo-ponto-cerebellar atrophy. *Brain*, 71:343–363.
10. Davison, C., and Wechsler, I. S. (1938): Olivopontocerebellar atrophy and unilateral involvement of cranial nerve nuclei. *J. Nerv Ment. Dis.*, 88:569–588.
11. Dejerine, J., and Thomas, A. (1900): L'atrophie olivo-ponto-cérébelleuse. *Nouv. Inconogr. Salpet.*, 13:330–370.
12. Duvisoin, R. C., Chokroverty, S., Lepore, F., and Nicklas W. (1982): The clinical expression of glutamate dehydrogenase deficiency. *Neurology*, 32:A82 (Abstr.).
13. Duvoisin, R. C., Chokroverty, S., Lepore, F., and Nicklas, W. *Unpublished data.*
14. Ellenberger, C., Keltner, J. L., and Stroud, M. H. (1972): Ocular dyskinesia in cerebellar disease. *Brain*, 95:685–692.
15. Furman, J., Perlman, S., and Baloh, R. W. (1982): Eye movements in Friedreich ataxia. *Neurology*, 32:A83 (Abstr.).
16. Geary, J. R., Earle, K. M., and Rose, A. S. (1956): Olivopontocerebellar atrophy. *Neurology*, 6:218–224.
17. Glaser, J. S. (1978): *Neuro-ophthalmology*. Harper and Row, Hagerstown, Maryland.
18. Goldberg, M. E., and Bushnell, M. C. (1981): Behavioral enhancement of visual responses in monkey cerebral cortex: II. Modulation in frontal eye fields specifically related to saccades. *J. Neurophysiol.*, 46:773–787.
19. Jampel, R. S., Okazaki. H. and Bernstein, H. (1961): Ophthalmoplegia and retinal degeneration associated with spinocerebellar ataxia. *Arch. Ophthalmol.*, 66:247–259.
20. Koeppen, A. H., and Hans, M. B. (1976): Supranuclear ophthalmoplegia in olivopontocerebellar degeneration. *Neurology*, 26:764–768.
21. Koeppen, A. H., Hans, M. B., Shepherd, D. I., and Best, P. V. (1977): Adult-onset hereditary ataxia in Scotland. *Arch. Neurol.*, 34:611–618.
22. Landis, D. M. Rosenberg, R. N. Landis, S. C., Schut, L., and Nyhan, W. L. (1974): Olivopontocerebellar degeneration. *Arch. Neurol.*, 31:295–307.
23. Lisberger, S. G., and Fuchs, A. F. (1978): Role of primate flocculus during rapid behavioral modification of the vestibuloocular reflex: I. Purkinje cell activity during visually guided horizontal smooth-pursuit eye movements and passive head rotation. *J. Neurophysiol.*, 41:733–763.
24. Maas, O., and Scherer, H. J. (1933): Zur Klinik und anatomie einiger seltener kleinhirnerkrankungen. *Z. Gesamte Neurol. Psychiatr.*, 145:420–444.
25. Pellegrini, G., and Scarlato, G. (1969): Contributo anatomo-clinico allo studio dell'atrofia olivo-ponto-cerebellare ereditaria. *Riv. Patol. Nerv. Ment.*, 90:252–279.
26. Perry, T. L., Currier, R. D., Hansen, S., and MacLean, J. (1977): Aspartate-taurine imbalance in dominantly inherited olivopontocerebellar atrophy. *Neurology*, 27:257–261.
27. Robinson, D. A. (1981): The control of eye movements. In: *Handbook of Physiology, Vol. II*, edited by V. B. Brooks, pp. 1275–1320. American Physiological Society, Bethesda.
28. Schut, J. W. (1950): Hereditary ataxia: Clinical study through six generations. *Arch. Neurol. Psychiatry*, 63:535–568.
29. Sears, E. S., Hammerberg, E. K., Norenberg, M. D., Wilson, B., and Nellhaus, G. (1975): Supranuclear ophthalmoplegia and dementia in olivopontocerebellar atrophy: A clinicopathologic study. *Neurology*, 25:395 (Abstr.).
30. Staal, A., Stefanko, S. Z., Busch, H. F. M., Jennekens, F. G. I., and DeBruijn, W. C. (1981): Autonomic nerve calcification and peripheral neuropathy in olivopontocerebellar atrophy. *J. Neurol. Sci.*, 51:383–394.
31. Steele, J. C., Richardson, J. C., and Olzewski, J. (1964): Progressive supranuclear palsy. *Arch. Neurol.*, 10:333–359.

32. Thomas, A. (1903): Atrophie du cervelet et sclérose en plaques. *Rev. Neurol. (Paris)*, 1:121–131.
33. Troost, B. T., and Daroff, R. B., (1977): The ocular motor defects in progressive supranuclear palsy. *Ann. Neurol.*, 2:397–403.
34. Troost, B. T., and Dell'Osso, L. F. (1979): Fast eye movements (saccades): Basic science and clinical correlations. In: *Topics in Neuro-Ophthalmology*, edited by H. S. Thompson, pp. 246–265. Williams & Wilkins, Baltimore.
35. Wadia, N. H. (1977): Heredo-familial spinocerebellar degeneration with slow eye movements—another variety of olivopontocerebellar degeneration. *Neurology (India)*, 25:147–160.
36. Wadia, N. H., and Swami, R. K. (1971): A new form of heredo-familial spinocerebellar degeneration with slow eye movements (nine families). *Brain*, 94:359–374.
37. Weiner, L. P., Konigsmark, B. W., Stoll, J., and Magladery, J. W. (1967): Hereditary olivopontocerebellar atrophy with retinal degeneration. *Arch. Neurol.*, 16:364–376.
38. Westheimer, G., and Blair, S. M. (1973): Oculomotor defects in cerebellectomized monkey. *Invest. Ophthalmol.*, 12:618–621.
39. Wilson, S. A. K. (1940): In: *Neurology*, edited by A. N. Bruce, Chap. LX, p. 965. Williams & Wilkins, Baltimore.
40. Zee, D. S., Optican, L. M., Cook, J. D., Robinson, D. A., and Engel, W. K. (1976): Slow saccades in spinocerebellar degeneration. *Arch. Neurol.*, 33:243–251.
41. Zee, D. S., and Robinson, D. A. (1979): Clinical applications of oculomotor models. In: *Topics in Neuro-Ophthalmology*, edited by H. S. Thompson, pp. 266–285. Williams & Wilkins, Baltimore.
42. Zee, D. S., Yee, R. D., Cogan, D. G., Robinson, D. A., and Engle, W. K. (1976): Ocular motor abnormalities in hereditary cerebellar ataxia. *Brain*, 99:207–234.
43. Zee, D. S., Yee, R. D., and Singer, H. S. (1977): Congenital ocular motor apraxia. *Brain*, 100:581–599.

The Olivopontocerebellar Atrophies, edited by R.C. Duvoisin and A. Plaitakis. Raven Press, New York © 1984.

Autonomic Dysfunction in Olivopontocerebellar Atrophy

Sudhansu Chokroverty

Department of Neurology, University of Medicine and Dentistry of New Jersey, Rutgers Medical School, Academic Health Science Center, New Brunswick, New Jersey 08903; and Neurology Service, Veterans Administration Medical Center, Lyons, New Jersey 07939

During the past two decades, there has been growing awareness of the presence of autonomic dysfunction causing severe disability in many neurologically afflicted patients. One such disorder, a multisystem neurodegenerative disease, which had generally come to be known as the Shy-Drager variant of the primary orthostatic hypotension syndrome, has attracted considerable attention. First alluded to by Piorry in 1826 (156) and later characterized by Bradbury and Eggleston in 1925 (29), this entity was more recently brought to the forefront by Shy and Drager in 1960 (186). There are certain similarities in the clinical features and pathoanatomical alterations of this disorder and olivopontocerebellar atrophy (OPCA), first described in detail by Dejerine and Thomas in 1900 (51). To better understand the effects of autonomic dysfunction, it is useful to outline briefly the anatomy, physiology, and pharmacology of the autonomic nervous system (ANS) and review some of the tests used to evaluate ANS function. For detailed treatment of the subject, the reader is referred to monographs by Mitchell (129), Pick (155), and Gabella (72).

ANATOMY OF THE ANS

The ANS consists of sympathetic and parasympathetic divisions, each with its central and peripheral components. Internal homeostasis is maintained by the two divisions, which are closely integrated and regulated in the hypothalamus, the head ganglion of the ANS (93,94,129,155). The cerebral cortex may also influence the ANS (102,103,153,155). From experimental observations in animals, it is concluded that the anterior hypothalamus is primarily concerned with the regulation of the parasympathetic division, whereas the posterior and lateral hypothalamic areas regulate sympathetic responses (22). According to Ingram (93,94), however, it is not possible to demarcate sharply between parasympathetic and sympathetic areas. The course of the descending sympathetic pathways is not well delineated (32), but the fibers probably traverse the brainstem tegmentum in the region of the lateral reticular formation and descend to the intermediolateral neurons of the spinal cord at T_1 through L_1 segments. The dorsal longitudinal bundle of Shütz probably plays a role in the hypothalamic control of the parasympathetic neurons of the brainstem (94,129,155). Recently, Saper et al. (172) demonstrated direct fiber connections from the hypothalamus to the preganglionic autonomic efferent neurons. The brainstem autonomic neurons are connected with the autonomic centers in the diencephalon and forebrain by suprasegmental pathways which travel in the reticular formation. According to Brodal (32), the functional significance of reciprocal connections between the hypothalamus and the medullary autonomic nuclei is little known.

Figure 1 schematically outlines the central autonomic neurons. The efferent autonomic pathway consists of two neurons: one preganglionic and one postganglionic. Preganglionic neurons originate in the central nervous system (CNS) and are myelinated; postganglionic fibers usually are unmyelinated and terminate at their effectors, such as smooth muscles, glands, and the heart. Preganglionic parasympathetic neurons have long fibers; postganglionic parasympathetic cell bodies are close to or even in the organ they supply, and their axons are short.

Parasympathetic Efferent Organization

The parasympathetic efferent nervous system is represented in the cranial and sacral subdivisions. The preganglionic neurons of the cranial portion are located in the nuclei of the third, seventh, ninth, and tenth cranial nerves. The tectal outflow consists of the preganglionic parasympathetic fibers originating in the Edinger-Westphal nucleus of the third cranial nerve; these travel along the oculomotor nerve. Postganglionic fibers from the ciliary ganglion supply the sphincter pupillae and the ciliary muscles for pupilloconstriction and accommodation. The secretomotor

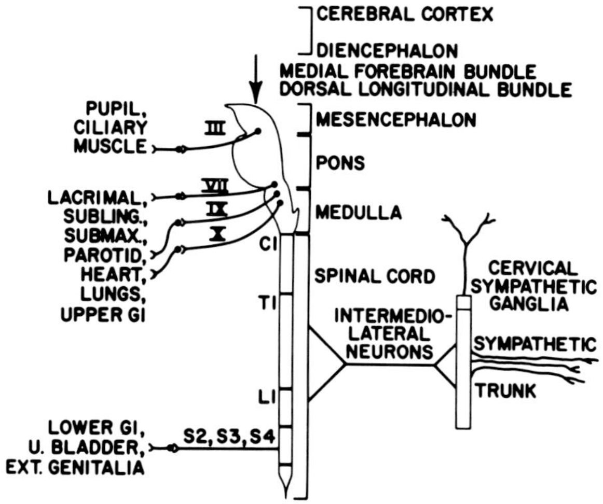

FIG. 1. Central autonomic neurons.

and vasodilator fibers from the superior salivatory nucleus in the pontomedullary junction travel along the seventh cranial nerve to innervate the lacrimal, sublingual, submandibular, and mucosal glands in the nasal cavity and palate. The preganglionic parasympathetic fibers from the inferior salivatory nucleus in the medulla leave by way of the ninth cranial nerve and synapse with cells of the otic ganglion. The postganglionic fibers from the otic ganglion join the auriculotemporal nerve to innervate the parotid gland. Preganglionic fibers from the dorsal motor nucleus and the nucleus ambiguus of the vagus nerve travel along the main trunk of the nerve to innervate the larynx, pharynx, esophagus, heart, lungs, and alimentary canal down to the descending colon. The preganglionic neurons of the sacral division of the parasympathetic system are located in the gray matter lateral to the central canal of the second, third, and fourth sacral segments and travel in the ventral spinal roots. These fibers then continue as the nervi erigantes to the postganglionic cell bodies in the pelvic plexus and the walls of the urinary bladder and rectum. The postganglionic fibers terminate in the lower segment of the colon, rectum, urinary bladder, and reproductive system.

Sympathetic Efferent Organization

The preganglionic sympathetic nerve fibers forming the thoracolumbar outflow arise from the intermediolateral neurons of the spinal cord from segments T_1 to L_1. The suprasegmental projections to these neurons derive from the cell bodies in the posterior and lateral hypothalamic regions (22,32,155) as well as brainstem catecholaminergic neurons (48,108) via the reticulospinal projections (32). The preganglionic axons emerge from the spinal cord as the white rami communicantes in each ventral root and join the paravertebral sympathetic ganglia. Some fibers synapse with postganglionic neurons in the paravertebral sympathetic ganglia on each side of the vertebral column. Other preganglionic fibers do not synapse with the paravertebral sympathetic chain but pass peripherally as the splanchnic nerves to synapse with the prevertebral ganglia (celiac and superior and inferior mesenteric) from which the postganglionic neurons arise to supply the smooth muscles of the viscera and the visceral blood vessels.

The postganglionic unmyelinated fibers from the paravertebral sympathetic ganglia join the spinal nerves as the gray rami communicantes. The fibers then travel along the spinal nerves to the blood vessels (vasomotor), sweat glands (sudomotor), and erector pilorum muscles of the skin (pilomotor), and to the blood vessels of the striated muscles and bone. The superior cervical ganglion contains the neurons of the postganglionic sympathetic fibers to the head and neck. The middle and inferior cervical sympathetic ganglia and the ganglia from T_1 to T_4 provide postganglionic sympathetic innervation to the heart and upper limbs.

Autonomic Afferent Fibers

There are afferent fibers in both the sympathetic and parasympathetic nerves, but the exact anatomical distribution and the physiologic significance of most of these fibers are unknown (32,72,129,155). Some important parasympathetic afferents include the sinus nerve of Hering, a branch of the glossopharyngeal nerve, and the aortic nerve of Cyon and Ludwig, a branch of the vagus nerve (128), which carry afferent impulses from the baroreceptors and chemoreceptors in the walls of the carotid artery, heart, and aorta to the CNS (85,184). These fibers are important for the reflex control of the circulation and respiration. The baroreceptor fibers terminate in the nucleus tractus solitarius of the medulla (192). The efferent arc of the baroreceptor reflex for the control of circulation consists of the sympathetic fibers via the reticulospinal projection to the intermediolateral columns of the thoracic spinal cord and parasympathetic fibers from the dorsal motor nucleus and the nucleus ambiguus of the vagus nerve (197). Recently, Ricardo and Koh (165) demonstrated direct projections from the nucleus tractus solitarius to the hypothalamic nuclei. This nucleus also gives off fibers to other regions in the brainstem and cerebellum (46,142,189).

Some sympathetic afferent fibers from the viscera travel along the splanchnic nerves, while others join the somatic nerves on their way to the dorsal root ganglia. These autonomic afferent fibers probably subserve visceral sensation and various autonomic reflexes, such as vasomotor, respiratory, viscerosomatic, and baroreceptor reflexes.

Noradrenergic and Cholinergic Pathways

The central noradrenergic neuronal cell bodies are located in the locus ceruleus and the neighboring brainstem reticular formation (7,45,47,48,67,71,108,146). Peripheral noradrenergic neuronal cell bodies are located in the sympathetic ganglia. The peripheral organs are depleted of norepinephrine following postganglionic, but not preganglionic, sympathectomy.

Biochemical and histochemical mapping in the rat brain have demonstrated ascending and descending noradrenergic pathways from the central noradrenergic neurons in the brainstem (7,45,47,48,67,71,108,146). The descending axons terminate in the intermediolateral neurons of the spinal cord at various levels. The ascending noradrenergic pathways form two major bundles: dorsal and ventral. The dorsal bundle arises from the locus ceruleus and terminates in the cerebellum, hippocampus, and cerebral cortex ipsilaterally. The ventral bundle arises from other cell groups in the reticular formation and ends primarily in the ipsilateral hypothalamus and in some limbic structures.

The central cholinergic neurons in the rat brainstem are located by measuring the distribution of choline acetyltransferase (107). The highest concentration is found in the cranial motor nuclei (III, VII, IX, X, and XII), salivatory nucleus, nucleus of the tractus solitarius, and caudate putamen. These are the major cholinergic structures in the rat brain. The lowest levels are found in the cerebellum, and low levels are found in the reticular formation, raphe nuclei, and sensory nuclei. Tracer studies in monkeys and rats have demonstrated cholinergic neurons also in the basal forebrain (75,101,105,126) in the regions of the medial septum, diagonal band of Broca, and nucleus basalis of Meynert supplying a diffuse projection to the neocortex, hippocampus, and amygdala.

PHYSIOLOGY AND PHARMACOLOGY OF THE ANS

The physiologic responses of the two divisions of the ANS are basically opposite in nature (4,8,33,99). Activation of the sympathetic nervous system causes mydriasis, vasoconstriction, acceleration of cardiac rate, bronchodilatation, inhibition of intestinal peristalsis, constriction of intestinal sphincters, release of renin and norepinephrine, secretion of the adrenal medulla, and ejaculation. Parasympathetic stimulation produces pupilloconstriction, bradycardia, bronchconstriction, increased peristalsis, increased gland secretion, sweating, and penile erection.

Acetylcholine is the neural transmitter for all preganglionic and postganglionic parasympathetic fibers and postganglionic sympathetic innervation to the sweat glands. Postganglionic sympathetic fibers release norepinephrine at their terminals. The sympathetic effects are determined by two types of receptors: alpha and beta (4,5). The alpha receptors, in general, are excitatory; the beta receptors are inhibitory, except for those in the heart, which are excitatory. Some of the sympathetic vasodilator fibers (in skeletal muscle and possibly coronary blood vessels) are cholinergic.

CEREBELLAR CONTROL OF THE ANS

Recent studies based on stimulation and ablation experiments have confirmed previous observations of a cerebellar role in autonomic function (55,92,93,128). The evidence is based on physiologic findings; no anatomical pathways from the cerebellum are known. Mitchell (129) and Ingram (93,94) summarized past observations on the role of the cerebellum in autonomic function. Willis (210) in 1664 had considered the cerebellum a center of autonomic activity. The cerebellar influence of the ANS was known to 19th century physiologists (124). Eckhard (63) in 1872 noted an increase in heart rate and blood pressure following stimulation of the posterior vermal regions in dogs. Experimental studies by Ferrier (68) in 1876 and Spencer (190) in 1894 suggested a role for the cerebellum in the regulation of pupillary motion (68) and respiration, but Pick (155) cautioned that the medulla probably was excited by a spread of the current in those experiments. Most of the pioneering studies of the present century were done by Moruzzi (134), Hare et al. (84), Zanchetti and Zoccolini (213), and Dow and Moruzzi (55). Many of these studies showing influence of cerebellar cortical stimulation on the cardiovascular system, however, have been variable and contradictory (124). In most of these investigations, the circulatory influences were induced from the cerebellar cortex, especially from the vermal part.

Recently, Miura and Reis (131) and Achari and Downman (1) elicited pressor responses induced by electrical stimulation of the rostral fastigial nucleus. They suggested that fastigial pressor responses resulted from widespread sympathetic activation. In 1972, Doba and Reis (53) found that stimulation of the rostral fastigial nucleus in cats caused elevation of blood pressure, tachycardia, and an increase of peripheral vascular resistance. These vascular responses were neurogenic and mediated by alpha-adrenergic receptors, since the responses were abolished by phentolamine. The authors also noted an increase in myocardial contractility mediated by beta receptors. The responses observed by Doba and Reis (53) closely approximated the cardiovascular reflex responses evoked by assumption of the upright posture. The investigators noted that bilateral rostral fastigial electrolytic lesions impaired the compensatory reflex response to tilting in cats. Lesions in the nucleus interpositus, however, did not impair these responses. These findings suggest that the cerebellum actively participates in the regulation of orthostatic cardiovascular responses, probably acting in concert with systemic baroreceptors.

Several investigators have reported cerebellar modulation of gastrointestinal and urinary bladder functions, but the results have been inconsistent. Martner (124) noted that the role of the cerebellum in the regulation of the ANS was obvious, but the pathways and precise mechanisms were not known. He found pressor and other autonomic responses as well as behavioral changes after stimulation of the rostral fastigial nucleus in the cat. The author concluded that a restricted fastigial area in the cerebellum linked the parasympathetic and sympathetic systems and affected virtually all types of autonomic mechanisms, including reflexes concerned with bulbospinal and homeostatic mechanisms. All these result in cardiovascular, gastrointestinal, or urinary bladder adjustments. These influences probably take place mainly at spinal and bulbar levels, but the cerebellar interactions may also occur at higher levels via fastigial projections to the hypothalamus and limbic structures. In summary, substantial evidence now points to cerebellar participation in the ANS. Hence one might expect to find autonomic dysfunction in patients with cerebellar degeneration who have lesions of the fastigial nucleus or the fastigiobulbar projections.

CLINICAL MANIFESTATIONS OF AUTONOMIC DYSFUNCTION

The four most important manifestations in autonomic neuropathy are postural hypotension, urinary bladder dysfunction, hypohidrosis or anhidrosis, and impotence in men. Most autonomic disorders manifest at least two of these. The most severe and often disabling feature is orthostatic hypotension (8,99). Its symptoms include dizziness, blurring of vision, unsteadiness, faintness or even frank unconsciousness, and generalized seizures, depending on the degree and rapidity of the fall of systemic blood pressure. There is no generally accepted normal range of postural variation of blood pressure. Thomas et al. (200) defined significant orthostatic hypotension as a consistent and persistent fall of 30 mm Hg or more in systolic and 15 mm Hg or more in diastolic pressure accompanied by clinical symptoms. Others believe that any postural fall of blood pressure, if accompanied by postural symptoms as described above, should be diagnostic of postural hypotension.

The maintenance of blood pressure in the erect posture involves a complex interplay of circulatory, neural, humeral, and physical factors (25,34,171,183). It has been aptly stated that "when man became a biped and assumed the upright position, he immediately made an enemy of gravity, and he has been fighting this relentless foe ever since" (100). When an individual assumes the upright position, the hydrostatic force resulting from the weight of the intravascular column of blood exerts an unusual degree of stress on the circulation (34,128,171). A shift of blood results from the upper to the lower parts of the body, causing a decrease in central blood volume and an excess accumulation of blood in the peripheral venous reservoir. With the pooling of blood in the periphery, venous return to the heart is diminished, and cardiac output falls by 20 to 25% (26,34,171). Transient postural hypotension (usually a fall of 5–15 mm Hg systolic blood pressure) occurs within 10 sec of assuming the erect position. All these changes cause a decrease in blood flow to various tissues and organs in the body, including heart and brain (99).

The human organism is extremely sensitive to even slight falls in blood pressure, and striking compensatory mechanisms are immediately mobilized to counteract the deleterious effects of gravity (24,25,34,85,171,183,184). The immediate compensation is neural and is mediated through the carotid sinus-aortic arc baroreceptor reflex mechanism (85,184). The delayed compensation consists of humoral and physical factors (34,182). Carotid hypotension in the upright position stimulates immediately the pressure-sensitive stretch receptors of the carotid sinus and aortic arc, resulting in sympathetic stimulation and vagal inhibition (173). Peripheral resistance, venous return, and cardiac output all increase; within 30 to 45 sec, blood pressure returns to its previous level. The primary baroreceptor mechanism is aided by secondary factors, such as increase in the levels of plasma catecholamine, renin, and aldosterone and the physical factors of accumulation of tissue fluid in the legs, "muscle pump," and respiratory mechanisms. If compensatory regulatory responses fail as a result of disease of the afferent, central, or efferent pathways, the physiologic postural hypotension becomes prolonged, and pathologic orthostatic hypotension results.

The parasympathetic innervation of the urinary bladder is of major importance in the physiology of micturition. It is responsible for the contraction of the detrusor muscles and relaxation of the sphincter. The symptoms resulting from autonomic dysfunction may consist of urgency, hesitancy, and frequency of micturition, nocturia, dribbling, incontinence, and retention of urine (8,99).

An important manifestation in many patients with autonomic neuropathy is hypohidrosis or anhidrosis affecting first the lower limb (8,99). There may also be patchy involvement of the trunk and face. In severe cases, the entire body may be affected.

Dysfunction of the sacral parasympathetic innervation may cause impotence, which is often an early manifestation of autonomic neuropathy (8,99). Retrograde ejaculation of semen into the urinary bladder or failure of ejaculation may occur in sympathetic neuropathy affecting the urogenital system.

Additional clinical manifestations of dysautonomia (8,99) include Horner's syndrome, impairment of pupillary responses to light and accommodation, gustatory facial sweating, diminished lacrimation, sialorrhea, dryness of the mouth, persistent tachycardia, difficulty in swallowing and vomiting due to achalasia of the cardia or gastric atony, constipation, intermittent and often nocturnal diarrhea, and fecal incontinence.

DIAGNOSTIC EVALUATION OF AUTONOMIC DYSFUNCTION

A number of tests are available for evaluation of the function of the ANS (4,8,54,92,98,135). One can localize the sites of lesions to the sympathetic or parasympathetic division of the ANS. To further localize the lesions to preganglionic or postganglionic sites to assess the integrity of the entire ANS, one must perform a combination of tests. Hemodynamic, pharmacologic, biochemical, morphologic, and radiologic techniques are available.

TESTS OF BARORECEPTOR FUNCTION

Tilt-Table Study

Blood pressure, heart rate (electrocardiogram), and electroencephalogram may be recorded simultaneously in the supine position and at different degrees of upright tilt on a tilt-table, preferably an electrically powered table. One can simply measure the supine and standing pulse and blood pressure at intervals of 1 to 2 min for 10 min if tolerated, as suggested by Thomas et al. (200); however, the physical factors of compensation are not eliminated, and, therefore, mild degrees of orthostatic hypotension may be missed. In patients with autonomic neuropathy, there may be orthostatic hypotension accompanied by postural symptoms.

Right Heart Catheterization

Cardiac catheterization is an invasive test by which one can determine the cardiac output and the peripheral vascular resistance in the supine and erect positions. A marked decrease of cardiac output (more than 25%) and lack of rise of peripheral resistance would indicate autonomic insufficiency (26,86,99).

Valsalva Maneuver

The Valsalva maneuver consists of forced expiration for 10 to 15 sec with an intraoral pressure of approximately 40 mm Hg while continuously recording the brachial arterial pressure and electrocardiogram before, during, and immediately after release of the expiratory pressure (8,99,174). Blood pressure and heart rate changes (83) go through four phases (Fig. 2). During phase 1, or the onset of expiratory strain, there is an initial rise of blood pressure due to expulsion of pulmonary blood into the left atrium, thereby increasing cardiac output, and to transmittal of the increased intrathoracic pressure to all the vessels within the thorax, producing an abrupt rise of systolic and diastolic blood pressure. During phase 2, or the period of sustained strain, raised intrathoracic pressure obstructs

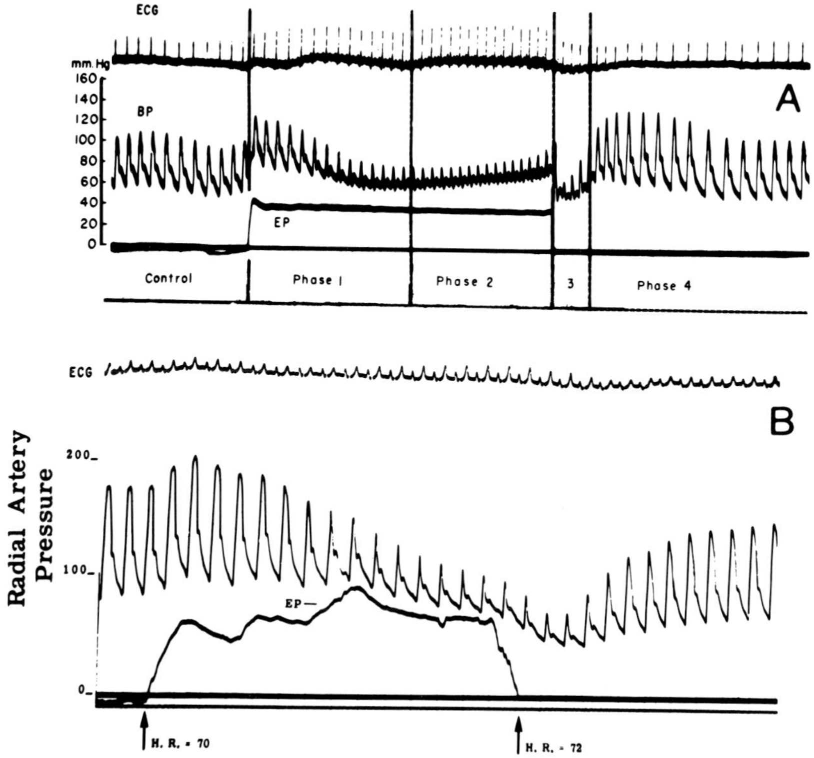

FIG. 2. Valsalva response in a normal adult male **(A)** and in a case of the Shy-Drager syndrome **(B)**. EP, intraoral expiratory pressure; ECG; electrocardiogram; HR, heart rate. **B** is reproduced from *Brain*, 92:743–768, 1969, with permission from the publisher.

venous return; therefore, cardiac output falls rapidly. Phase 3 is the period of release of intrathoracic pressure lasting from 1 to 2 sec. There is an abrupt fall in arterial blood pressure, presumably due to transient pooling of the right ventricular output in the expanding pulmonary vascular bed. Phase 4 is the stage of recovery and "overshoot," with subsequent increase of blood pressure above the pre-Valsalva level due to a combination of increased cardiac output and persistence of reflex peripheral arterial constriction. Following release, the maximum rise in blood pressure usually occurs within 3 to 4 sec. The rise in blood pressure is followed within 15 sec by bradycardia. The rising pulse pressure reflexly stimulates vagal innervation to the heart, which causes bradycardia. The baroreceptor reflex mechanism is stimulated in phases 2, 3, and 4. Lack of post-Valsalva overshoot and reflex bradycardia would indicate autonomic dysfunction due to interruption of the baroreceptor reflex arc (Fig. 2).

Levin (116) devised a simple, noninvasive test of cardiac autonomic function, the Valsalva ratio, based on the heart rate change induced by the maneuver. This is the ratio of the longest to the shortest R-R interval, excluding premature beats.

The mean value of three tests is taken as the Valsalva ratio. The author defined a value of 1.50 or higher as normal; however, Ewing et al. (64) considered a ratio of 1.10 or less as abnormal, 1.1 to 1.20 as borderline, and 1.21 or better as a normal response. My own data *(unpublished observations)* suggest a ratio of 1.20 to 1.30 as borderline, less than 1.20 as abnormal, and more than 1.30 as a normal response.

TESTS OF SYMPATHETIC EFFERENT PATHWAYS

Cold Pressor Test

Immersing the hand in ice-cold water (4°C) for 1 to 3 min in normal subjects produces a slight rise of blood pressure and pulse rate. A normal cold pressor test demonstrates the integrity of the efferent sympathetic pathways (164).

Mental Arithmetic Test

The stress of mental concentration in simple arithmetic stimulates the efferent sympathetic pathways in many normal individuals to increase blood pressure and pulse rate transiently.

Tests of Sudomotor Function

Anatomically, the fibers to the sweat glands are sympathetic; pharmacologically, however, they are cholinergic. Sweating in response to increasing body temperature by 1°C with an electric blanket or a heat cradle tests the integrity of the efferent sympathetic fibers (4,8,99,135). Sweat can be detected by topical application of quinizarin (1,4-dihydroxyanthraquinone) powder, which turns purple in sweated areas (99). The density of functioning sweat glands may be counted by application of silicone elastic impression material (104) or graph paper containing starch and iodine, which will turn blue when wet. The number of dark spots per unit area may then be counted. The amount of sweating also can be estimated by weighing small squares of filter papers applied to different parts of the body. An additional method is noting the lowering of skin resistance in response to sweating; this method, the psychogalvanic or electrodermal reflex (99), is not reliable. Sweating induced by the subcutaneous injection of 10 mg pilocarpine demonstrates the integrity of the sweat glands and the peripheral sudomotor fibers. Axon reflex sweating may be used to test the integrity of the postganglionic sympathetic fibers to the sweat glands. Hence impairment of thermal and axon reflex sweating but presence of sweating after pilocarpine injection would suggest central or postganglionic sympathetic fiber lesions but intact sweat glands (99).

Norepinephrine Infusion

The intravenous infusion of norepinephrine in normal individuals causes an increase in blood pressure and a reflex bradycardia resulting from baroreceptor stimulation. In postganglionic sympathetic denervation following Cannon's law of denervation (35), there is a supersensitive response to the intravenous infusion of norepinephrine. The increased blood pressure is accompanied by bradycardia, if the afferent baroreceptor reflex arc and efferent vagal innervation to the heart are intact. There may be a moderate increase in blood pressure response after a central lesion, called "decentralization hypersensitivity" (14,160,172), resulting from reduced sympathetic impulse traffic, but this response is much less than that noted after postganglionic denervation. Therefore, the norepinephrine infusion test may be helpful in determining the site of the lesion (14,38,99,160). When blood pressure is stablized, an infusion of norepinephrine (2.5 mg dissolved in 500 ml of 5% dextrose) is started at a rate of 89.9 ng/kg/min. In normal individuals during this infusion, the diastolic pressure should rise 20 mm Hg, according to Roguska et al. (168).

Intravenous Tyramine Infusion Test

In normal individuals, tyramine increases blood pressure by releasing norepinephrine from stores at the sympathetic nerve terminals. Therefore, the intravenous infusion of 1 to 3 mg tyramine may be used to test the integrity of the postganglionic sympathetic nerve endings (14,92,135).

Plasma Norepinephrine Levels in Supine and Erect Positions

Plasma levels of norepinephrine may be determined in the supine and erect positions to test the integrity of the efferent sympathetic fibers (17,113,136,214). The plasma concentration of catecholamines is directly portional to the activity of the sympathetic nerve terminals. In normal individuals, as a result of gravitational stress in the upright posture, there is increased sympathetic stimulation through the baroreceptor mechanism, and an increased amount of catecholamine is liberated at the sympathetic nerve endings. According to Lake et al. (113), the plasma level of norepinephrine increases to twice the resting value after standing for 5 min. Norepinephrine in plasma may be measured by the radioenzymatic assay method (113). If there is postganglionic sympathetic denervation, then the resting plasma level of norepinephrine should be low, and norepinephrine will not rise appreciably in the upright position. If the lesion is preganglionic, the resting level may remain normal but will fail to increase in the upright position because of inadequate impulse traffic at the nerve endings.

Serum Dopamine-Beta-Hydroxylase Activity

In addition to the release of norepinephrine at the sympathetic nerve endings in the upright position, the enzyme dopamine-beta-hydroxylase, which converts dopamine to norepinephrine, is also released. Its blood level reflects sympathetic nerve activity over hours to days (212). This test may supplement the plasma norepinephrine level in the supine and erect positions. However, low serum dopamine-beta-hydroxylase activity may not help distinguish preganglionic from postganglionic sympathetic nerve dysfunction.

Catecholamine Fluorescence in Muscle Biopsy Specimen

Marked decrease or absence of catecholamine fluorescence in the perivascular nerve plexus in muscle biopsy samples may indicate depletion of norepinephrine in the sympathetic vasomotor nerve endings (10,13,65,111).

Plasma Renin Activity in Supine and Erect Positions

Renin, an enzyme synthesized in the kidney, acts on angiotensinogen to form angiotensin I, which is then converted to angiotensin II. Angiotensin II is a potent vasoconstrictor and increases blood pressure significantly. It also acts directly on the zona glomerulosa of the adrenal cortex to stimulate aldosterone secretion (138). Renin release depends on a complex interplay of a variety of stimuli, such as changes in blood volume, renal perfusion pressure, systolic blood pressure, renal blood flow, fluid osmolality, renal nerve activity, and catecholamine release (50,147,152,188,203,204). An intrarenal mechanism for the control of renin release probably acts synergistically with the sympathetic nervous system and other complex extrarenal reflex and CNS pathways. In normotensive healthy subjects on *ad libitum* sodium intake, renin activity always increases upon changing from the supine to the upright position (43). The postural changes in plasma renin activity in normal subjects result from hemodynamic changes, such as a shift in blood volume and renal vasoconstriction. The integrity of the ANS is essential to the stimulation of the renin-angiotensin system (43,74,148). Thus the activity of the renal sympathetic nerves can be tested by determining plasma renin activity by the radioimmunoassay method (82) in the supine and erect positions and also after norepinephrine infusion. During this study, urine should be collected for 24 hr to determine its sodium content. Absence of a rise in plasma renin activity in the erect position and after intravenous norepinephrine infusion in the presence of normal urinary sodium excretion suggests dysfunction of the renal sympathetic nerves.

Sural Nerve Biopsy

The sural nerve contains unmyelinated sympathetic fibers. Morphometry of sural nerve biopsy samples revealing reduction in the unmyelinated fibers may provide morphologic evidence of peripheral sympathetic nerve involvement (59,145).

Sympathetic Reflex Response (Sympathetic C-Fiber Recording)

Recently, an attempt has been made to obtain sympathetic C-fiber recording in the clinical electromyographic laboratory immediately after a deep breath and after nerve stimulation (28). The usefulness of this test must be documented by recording in a large number of controls and patients with various types of autonomic neuropathies, correlating the results with microneurographic recordings.

Pharmacologic Tests of Pupillary Function

Intraocular instillation of 1:1,000 epinephrine in normal eyes produces no response. If sympathetic postganglionic denervation is present, however, there will be pupillary dilatation due to denervation supersensitivity (99).

Intraocular instillation of 1% paredrine (hydroxyamphetamine), an indirect sympathomimetic amine that acts by releasing norepinephrine from endogenous stores in sympathetic nerve terminals, causes pupillary dilatation in a normally innervated eye (201,202). In patients with postganglionic sympathetic denervation of the pupils, the nerve terminals will be degenerated, the stores of norepinephrine will be reduced or absent, and instillation of paredrine will cause the pupils to dilate incompletely or not at all.

Cocaine acts presynaptically, blocking the reuptake and inactivation of norepinephrine from nerve endings. The instillation of a 4% solution normally causes pupillary dilatation; as with paredrine, however, there is no response in the presence of postganglionic sympathetic denervation (99,201). This test is not reliable in differentiating preganglionic from postganglionic sympathetic denervation.

TESTS TO DETERMINE THE INTEGRITY OF PARASYMPATHETIC EFFERENT PATHWAYS

Atropine Tests

Following intravenous (1–3 mg) or intramuscular (0.8 mg) atropine injections, the heart rate normally increases due to paralysis of the vagal action and unopposed sympathetic activity (92,99). Lack of tachycardia after atropine injection may indicate either vagal or sympathetic cardiac denervation.

Neostigmine Test

Intramuscular injection of neostigmine (1 mg), a parasympathomimetic agent, will cause bradycardia if the cardiac parasympathetic innervation is intact (99).

Beat-to-Beat Variation of Heart Rate

Absence of beat-to-beat variation in heart rate on deep inspiration (sinus arrhythmia) indicates cardiac vagal denervation (209).

Insulin Test for Gastric Acidity

Insulin-induced (0.1 U insulin/kg body weight) hypoglycemia may be used to test the integrity of vagal activity in the stomach (89). Hypoglycemia causes secretion of gastric acidity if the vagal innervation to the stomach is intact. In vagal denervation, gastric acidity fails to increase.

Radiologic Study

Cineradiography and barium studies may be used to detect abnormalities of gastrointestinal motility, such as esophageal and gastric atony and abnormal peristaltic waves, indicating parasympathetic dysfunction (99).

Cystometrogram

Cystometric study of urinary bladder function with manometric recording of detrusor muscle contractions in relation to the intravesicular pressure increment may be useful (31). An important observation in autonomic neuropathy is the cystometric finding of detrusor areflexia.

Pupillary Function

Conjunctival instillation of a freshly prepared solution of methacholine (mecholyl) 2.5% (99) or pilocarpine 0.062% (44) does not show any significant response in normal pupils. Postganglionic parasympathetic denervation supersensitivity, however, will be manifested by pupillary constriction. Pilocarpine is preferable to methacholine because of its stronger miotic action.

DETERMINING THE INTEGRITY OF THE AFFERENT LIMB OF THE BARORECEPTOR REFLEX ARC

There is no single test to determine the integrity of the afferent limb of the baroreceptor reflex arc (99). However, imparied function of the total reflex arc in the presence of normal tests of the efferent limb would suggest afferent limb dysfunction. If there is reflex bradycardia after the Valsalva maneuver and intravenous norepinephrine infusion, then the afferent limb of the reflex arc must be intact.

AUTONOMIC DYSFUNCTION IN OPCA

Clinically, OPCA may be defined as a chronic, slowly progressive neurologic disorder, occurring with or without a positive family history, presenting initially with either a predominantly cerebellar or extrapyramidal syndrome (atypical parkinsonism) or a mixed cerebellar-parkinsonian syndrome but always associated with some evidence of cerebellar dysfunction on clinical examination or cerebellar atrophy on computerized tomography brain scan. Involvement of the ANS has rarely been mentioned in the literature on spinocerebellar degeneration, including OPCA. In those subgroups with peripheral nerve involvement (36,95), disturbances of the ANS have been mentioned sporadically. Vasomotor disturbances resulting from preferential involvement of the postganglionic sympathetic nerve fibers have been described in some patients with Charcot-Marie-Tooth disease (95).

Miyazaki (133) evaluated 45 patients with cerebellar degeneration for the presence of orthostatic hypotension. His subjects included patients with parenchymatous cerebellar degeneration, OPCA, and the Shy-Drager syndrome. He found orthostatic hypotension in 20 patients, four of whom had the Shy-Drager syndrome. A high percentage of those showing orthostatic hypotension also had urinary incontinence (85%), pyramidal signs (40%), extrapyramidal symptoms (35%), and dementia (35%). Patients without orthostatic hypotension had no urinary incontinence or extrapyramidal symptoms, but some had pyramidal signs. The Valsalva maneuver was abnormal in four of nine subjects, two of whom had the Shy-Drager syndrome. Three of these four patients had no supersensitivity to the intravenous infusion of norepinephrine. The author concluded that there was no merit in separating the Shy-Drager syndrome from OPCA, and he used the inclusive term "multiple system atrophy" for these two conditions, in agreement with other authors (15,16,76,148,149). It is notable, however, that in his Table 2, Miyazaki (133) listed autonomic symptoms preceding cerebellar and other somatic neurologic features in the Shy-Drager syndrome by 1 to 5 years, while the sequence was reversed in other patients with cerebellar degeneration.

In the description of the pathologic findings, adequate emphasis has not been placed on the status of autonomic neurons in OPCA. Structural lesions in the locus ceruleus (catecholaminergic neurons), nucleus ambiguus (114), and dorsal motor nucleus of the vagus (parasympathetic neurons) have been described (23,61,78, 79,148). Neuropathologic examination in three siblings in one generation of five patients with an unusual form of dominant OPCA by Staal et al. (193) disclosed a unique observation of abundant intrafascicular calcification in the sympathetic nerve fibers and their ganglia, in addition to abnormalities of the peripheral nerves, atrophy of the spinal cord, and the typical findings of OPCA. Clinically, the patients did not have any symptoms attributable to autonomic nerve dysfunction. Whether there are lesions in the intermediolateral neurons of the spinal cord and the sympathetic ganglia or other autonomic structures in classic OPCA cannot be stated with certainty.

Because of the close proximity of the central autonomic and somatic neurons, which are known to degenerate in OPCA (23,60,78,79), and because of morphologic evidence of degeneration of some central autonomic neurons, it is logical to expect degeneration of the autonomic and somatic structures in parallel fashion. Furthermore, as noted above, recent physiologic studies have suggested that the cerebellum participates in autonomic control mechanisms. How commonly or severely the ANS is involved in the various types of OPCA is not known, because a systematic study of the ANS has not been undertaken in a large number of OPCA patients. Urinary and rectal spincter dysfunction, which may be a manifestation of autonomic neuropathy, was noted by Dejerine and Thomas (51). Bakker (12) later emphasized urinary sphincter dysfunction in OPCA. Urinary incontinence has been mentioned in some cases of dominant (Menzel) OPCA (61,125), and urinary sphincter dysfunction has been reported frequently although later in the course of Holmes' cerebelloolivary atrophy (90).

The pathogenesis of urinary incontinence in OPCA is not clear. It is probably multifactorial in origin. Various hypotheses have been postulated. Bakker (12) suggested a loss of control of the cerebellum over the sympathetic nervous system. In light of the recent evidence of a cerebellar influence on the ANS, this suggestion remains a possibility. Another hypothesis is that urinary bladder dysfunction is secondary to degeneration of Clarke's column cells (77). Eadie (60) suggested that the urinary sphincter dysfunction was a consequence of dementia; this is unlikely, however, since dementia is not prominent in most cases of OPCA. Clinical expression of the dysautonomia may be mild and evident only on formal tests of autonomic function. In the author's personal experience, autonomic function tests demonstrate deficits in only some (40,41) OPCA patients (Tables 1 and 2). Neuropathologic examination at necropsy in one patient confirmed the clinical diagnosis of OPCA and showed marked neuronal loss and gliosis in the substantia nigra, pons, cerebellum, locus ceruleus, inferior olives, and lateral reticular nucleus of the medulla. There was widespread loss of Purkinje cells in the cerebellum, along with severe degeneration of the fastigial nucleus. The nucleus tractus solitarius did not show significant morphologic changes. Examination of the spinal cord revealed loss of neurons in the anterior horns and in Clarke's column and demyelination of the posterior columns. There were no significant qualitative changes in the intermediolateral columns, but a quantitative assessment of the neuronal population of the lateral horns was not made.

TABLE 1. *Comparison of clinical data in the Shy-Drager syndrome and OPCA*

Parameter	Shy-Drager syndrome ($N = 12$)[a]	OPCA ($N = 10$)[a]
Ages (years)	49–68 (mean, 57)	32–64 (mean, 53)
Family history	None	Dominant, 2; recessive, 1; sporadic, 7
Initial presentation	Dysautonomic symptoms (orthostatic syncope, urinary dysfunction, impotence, and impaired sweating)	Somatic symptoms (predominantly cerebellar in all)
Later presentation	Predominantly cerebellar in 9 and extrapyramidal in 3	Urinary dysfunction (? autonomic) in 4, and dysautonomic symptoms (orthostatic, syncope, impotence, and impaired sweating) in 1
Duration of illness	2–12 yr	2–20 yr
Course of illness	10 died, 2 lost to follow-up	2 died, 2 alive, 6 lost to follow-up
Necropsy study	Performed in 3 patients: features of OPCA in 1, striatonigral degeneration in 1, and mixed in 1	Performed in 1 patient: typical features of OPCA

[a]All subjects were men.

TABLE 2. *Comparison of autonomic function data in the Shy-Drager syndrome and OPCA*

Parameter	Shy-Drager syndrome (N = 12)	OPCA (N = 10)
Orthostatic hypotension	Severe in all	Mild in 4; severe in 1
Valsalva response	Abnormal in all	Abnormal in 1
Cold pressor test	Impaired in all	Impaired in 4
Mental arithmetic test	Impaired in all	Impaired in 4
Plasma renin activity (supine and erect)	Impaired in 5 of 5 patients tested	Impaired in 5 of 8 patients tested
Norepinephrine infusion test	Supersensitive response in 5 of 5 patients tested	Normal in 1 patient tested
Plasma norepinephrine	Abnormal in 1 patient tested	Abnormal in 1 of 2 patients tested
Atropine test	Abnormal in 5 of 5 patients tested	Not performed
Neostigmine test	Abnormal in 5 of 5 patients tested	Not performed
Sweat test	Abnormal in 5 of 5 patients tested	Not performed
Cardiac catheterization data	Abnormal in 4 of 4 patients tested	Not performed
Cystometrogram	Abnormal in 5 of 5 patients tested	Not performed
Barium swallow and cineradiography	Normal in 4 of 4 patients tested	Not performed

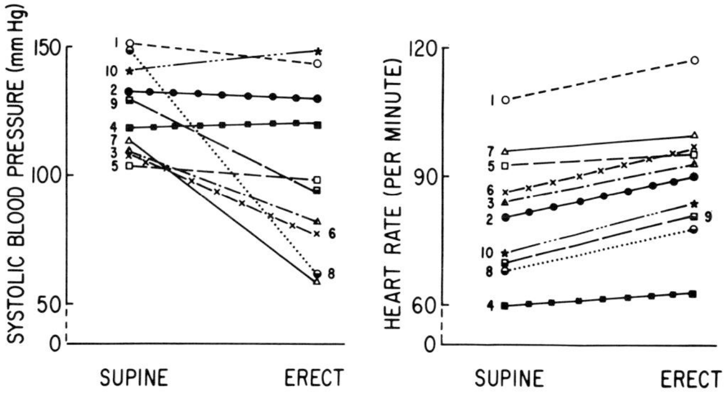

FIG. 3. Response to tilting in 10 OPCA patients.

Study of autonomic function in 10 OPCA patients (Table 2) demonstrated a fall of 20 to 50 mm Hg systolic blood pressure in the erect position (Fig. 3), accompanied by postural symptoms of dizziness, faintness, or sweating in five patients and fixed heart rate in two. These findings indirectly suggested a critical reduction of cerebral blood flow and impaired circulatory homeostasis (99) in the erect posture. One patient had a low Valsalva ratio and absence of post-Valsalva reflex bradycardia, indicating interruption of the baroreceptor reflex arc. Postural hypotension without impairment of the Valsalva response in four patients may be consistent with a central defect above the level of medulla, as suggested by Gross et al. (81) in their studies of patients with Parkinson's disease. Impaired cold pressor (Fig. 4) and mental arithmetic tests and fixed heart rate in the erect position in two patients indicated efferent sympathetic dysfunction. Normal cold pressor and mental arithmetic tests and tachycardia on tilting in the remaining patients (Table 2), however, implied intact efferent cardiac sympathetic pathways.

Low supine plasma renin or its failure to rise adequately in the upright position (Fig. 5) in five patients with normal urinary sodium suggested reduction of impulse traffic from supraspinal centers to the sympathetic nerve terminals. A normal supine level of plasma norepinephrine and its failure to rise adequately in the erect position in one patient (Table 2; Fig. 6) without postural hypotension may also indicate reduced impulse traffic at the sympathetic nerve endings due to reduced descending impulses from supraspinal centers, which were not directly concerned with mediation of circulatory reflexes. Aminoff and Wilcox (6) made a similar suggestion in explanation of norepinephrine supersensitivity without postural hypotension in cases of paralysis agitans. Therefore, the autonomic dysfunction in some patients with OPCA as manifested by orthostatic hypotension, impaired Valsalva response, cold pressor and mental arithmetic tests, and less than normal rise of plasma renin and norepinephrine in the erect posture suggested a sympathetic defect.

The exact site of the responsible central lesion remains speculative. Lesions in the nucleus tractus solitarius, where the central baroreceptor neurons are presumed to be located (192), supramedullary controlling pathways to the nucleus tractus solitarius (32), fastigial nucleus of the cerebellum (131,132), fastigiobulbar fibers, and intermediolateral columns of the spinal cord may all be implicated. As described above, at least in one patient, the nucleus tractus solitarius and the intermediolateral columns were not involved. In this patient, however, there was severe

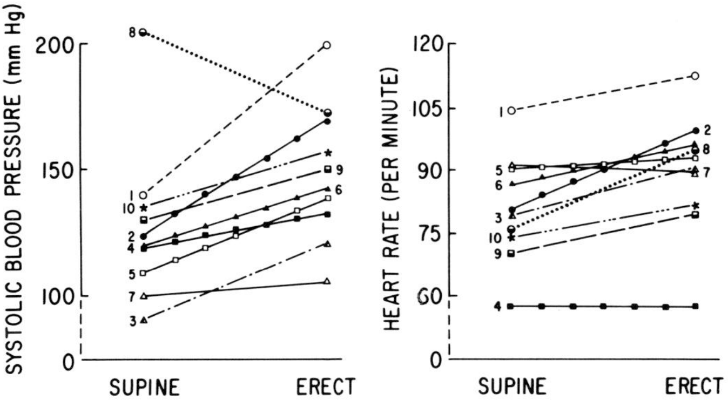

FIG. 4. Cold pressor test in 10 OPCA patients.

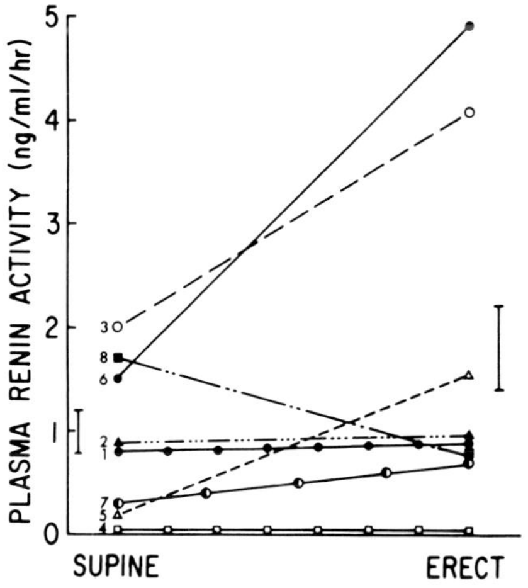

FIG. 5. Plasma renin activity in eight OPCA patients. Vertical bars indicate normal range.

degeneration of the fastigial nucleus, making this the most likely site of the lesion responsible for the autonomic deficit. Few data are available on the extent and frequency of involvement of the parasympathetic nervous system in OPCA.

In summary, patients with classic OPCA (familial or sporadic) may manifest mild to moderate dysautonomia. It is often subclinical but may be elicited by special tests of autonomic function.

THE SHY-DRAGER SYNDROME AND PURE PRIMARY DYSAUTONOMIA

There are striking similarities in the clinical and morphologic findings (148) of the Shy-Drager syndrome and classic OPCA, Parkinson's disease, and striatonigral degeneration (Table 3).

Bradbury and Eggleston (29) in 1925 gave a complete clinical description of three patients with orthostatic hypotension. Two years later (30), they reported the postmortem findings in one of these patients. Unfortunately, the brain and the spinal cord were not examined. The authors found no morphologic evidence of peripheral sympathetic nervous system involvement or suprarenal disease. Between 1925 and 1960, more cases with orthostatic hypotension were reported (11,19, 20,23,80,86,87,96,112,115,122,142,169,187,194,207,208). Diffuse CNS signs, although present in many of these cases, were not emphasized (19,169); indeed, in some reports, they were thought to be incidental (19). Wagner (207) in 1959 described a classic case of what we now call the Shy-Drager syndrome.

Shy and Drager (186) in 1960 first suggested that some cases of idiopathic orthostatic hypotension may be due to a primary degenerative disease of the nervous system. Their conclusion was based on the clinical features in two patients and a careful autopsy study in one of them. The full syndrome comprised orthostatic hypotension, urinary and rectal incontinence, impotence in men, atonic urinary bladder, loss of rectal sphincter tone, anhidrosis, iris atrophy, external ocular palsy,

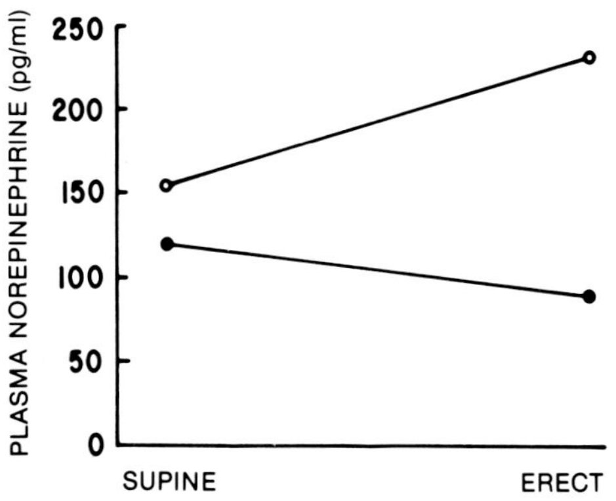

FIG. 6. Plasma norepinephrine levels in two patients with OPCA.

rigidity, tremor, loss of associated movements, fasciculation, and amyotrophy with evidence of a neuropathic lesion on electromyograph and on muscle biopsy. The relevant autopsy findings consisted of alterations and loss of neurons in the autonomic ganglia, ventral, intermediolateral, and Clarke's columns of the spinal cord, inferior olives, dorsal vagal nucleus, nucleus ambiguus, Purkinje cells in the cerebellum, locus ceruleus, substantia nigra, oculomotor nucleus, periaqueductal gray matter, caudate nucleus, and putamen. Although cerebellar and pyramidal tract signs were present in their cases, Shy and Drager did not list these in the clinical definition offered in their paper. Their first case clearly had cerebellar signs: "rapid alterating movements and the finger-to-nose and heel-to-knee-to-tibia tests were performed poorly. The dysmetria was more marked on the right" (186). The second patient had an unsteady and wide-based gait and impaired coordination bilaterally.

Neuropathologic findings in the second patient included degenerative changes in the cerebellum and inferior olives and minor changes in the pons. Thus the clinical and morphologic findings in the original cases of Shy and Drager resemble those noted in OPCA.

Later reports (15,17,21,38,42,69,76,79,91,98,117,123,140,148,166,167,176–178, 196,198–200,205) confirmed those original findings of Shy and Drager and strengthened the idea that the Shy-Drager variant of primary orthostatic hypotension is a multisystem neurodegenerative disease resembling OPCA, Parkinson's disease, or striatonigral degeneration but with prominent dysautonomia. Oppenheimer and others (16,76,148,149,195) have suggested that the term multiple system atrophy be used to include cases showing the combination of degenerative lesions in the striatum, pons, pigmented nuclei, cerebellar cortex, and inferior olives, such as may be seen in the Shy-Drager syndrome, OPCA, and striatonigral degeneration. However, the temporal sequence of clinical features with manifestations of autonomic dysfunction, presenting initially before somatic neurologic deficits, differentiates the Shy-Drager syndrome from the other entities. Rarely, autonomic and somatic features present simultaneously at the onset. Although there are occasional reports of patients with Shy-Drager syndrome presenting initially with somatic

TABLE 3. *Neuronal sites of degeneration in four groups of neurodegenerative diseases*[a]

Site of degeneration	OPCA	Shy-Drager syndrome	Parkinson's disease	Striatonigral degeneration
Cerebral cortex	±	±	±	±
Basal ganglia	+	+	+ +	+ +
Substantia nigra	+	+	+ +	+ +
Locus ceruleus	+	+	+	?
Pontine nuclei	+ +	+	—	±
Nucleus ambiguus	+	+	—	—
Dorsal vagal nucleus	+	+	?	—
Inferior olives	+ +	+	—	±
Cerebellum	+ +	+	—	±
Motor nuclei	±	±	—	—
Pyramidal tracts	+	+	—	—
Intermediolateral columns	?	+ +	±	±
Sympathetic ganglia	?	+	±	?

[a]Modified from ref. 148; ±, occasional, mild; +, common; + +, always or almost always; —, not affected.

neurologic manifestations before dysautonomic symptoms (199), it is difficult to decide whether these patients do in fact have the Shy-Drager syndrome.

Clinical and autonomic function data in 12 patients with the Shy-Drager syndrome studied in detail by the author are summarized in Tables 1 and 2. Reports of seven of these patients have been published previously (38,42). These data and the information gleaned from the literature suggest that the clinical manifestations of the Shy-Drager syndrome pass through three successive stages. The first is characterized by a tetrad of urinary bladder dysfunction, impotence, impairment of sweating, and symptoms related to orthostatic hypotension. Some patients may present with other dysautonomic features described above. Both the sympathetic and parasympathetic divisions (38,105) are affected, although sympathetic dysfunction has been emphasized in the literature. In the second stage, somatic neurologic manifestations are added to the dysautonomia, e.g., dysfunction of extrapyramidal, cerebellar, and corticospinal pathways and the lower motoneuron and oculomotor systems. The motor systems are predominantly affected. Sensory and mental functions are spared, except in the last stage, when some patients may have mild dementia perhaps secondary to repeated episodes of cerebral hypoxia experienced in the erect position. The third stage is characterized by inexorable progression of the features described above, despite partial correction of the postural hypotension, extreme generalized muscle weakness, and inability to stand or walk. The course is slowly progressive over a period of years but is accelerated after the onset of stage 2. The patients usually die of respiratory or urinary tract infection 2 to 6 years after the onset of somatic neurologic features.

Some authors (111,160,214) think idiopathic orthostatic hypotension (pure primary dysautonomia) and Shy-Drager syndrome are separate entities, whereas others do not make a clear distinction. One of the author's previously published cases (case 1 in ref. 38) developed somatic neurologic features 3½ years after the onset of pure dysautonomia (37) and, at autopsy, had classic pathologic findings of the Shy-Drager syndrome *(unpublished data)*.

Plasma norepinephrine levels may differentiate between peripheral and central sympathetic lesions and may separate pure autonomic failure from cases of the Shy-Drager syndrome (214). Low supine plasma norepinephrine levels and an insufficient rise in the erect posture suggest postganglionic (peripheral) sympathetic dysfunction, whereas a normal supine plasma norepinephrine level and its failure to rise adequately in the erect posture suggest a preganglionic (central) lesion. However, the findings may depend on the extent and duration of the illness. Patients with the Shy-Drager syndrome may develop lesions in the sympathetic ganglia (27,154,186) and manifest postganglionic sympathetic dysfunction. In Fig. 7 are data on a patient with the Shy-Drager syndrome who initially had a normal supine plasma norepinephrine level; later, however, the supine plasma norepinephrine level was found to be low, indicating progression of the disease. Bannister et al. (17) also subscribe to this view. Bannister and Oppenheimer (16) stated that the autonomic deficits were the first to appear in many cases of the Shy-Drager syndrome; hence, at an early stage, cases of the Shy-Drager syndrome were similar to cases of pure autonomic failure.

PARKINSON'S DISEASE AND AUTONOMIC DYSFUNCTION

Prominent dysautonomia is not typical of Parkinson's disease. Later in the course of their illness, however, some patients with classic Parkinson's disease may develop autonomic deficits, which are often mild and uncovered by autonomic function tests. James Parkinson (151) in 1817 described manifestations of autonomic dysfunction in Parkinson's disease, including excessive sweating, urinary incontinence, and loss of bowel control. Orthostatic hypotension, although less common, has also been noted (81,163). Some of the reports of autonomic deficits have been

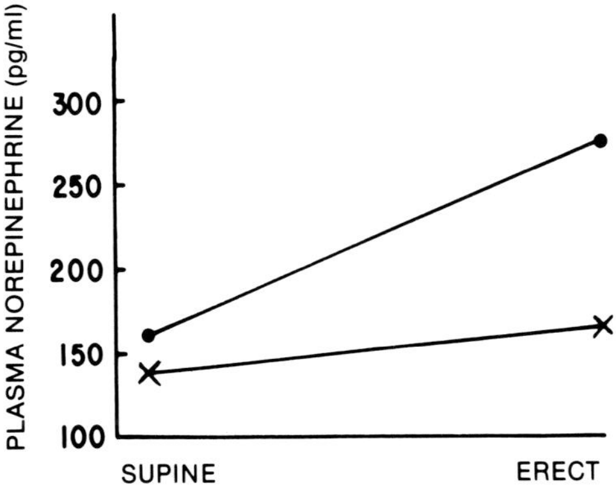

FIG. 7. Plasma norepinephrine levels on two separate occasions in a patient with the Shy-Drager syndrome: (x) levels obtained 6 months after (●) levels.

contradictory. Circulatory studies by Gross et al. (81) demonstrated postural hypotension but normal Valsalva responses. The authors suggested that these findings may be due to a lesion at a higher level of the nervous system above the medulla. Reid et al. (163) found impairment of Valsalva responses and orthostatic hypotension in their study of 30 patients with Parkinson's disease, but the authors correlated these abnormalities with advancing age. On the other hand, Appenzeller and Goss (9) demonstrated impaired thermoregulatory sweating and marked deficits in the post-Valsalva overshoot but no significant postural hypotension in 25 Parkinson's patients. The authors concluded that there was a profound failure in baroreceptor and thermoregulatory functions in Parkinson's disease, and these deficits may have resulted from a central failure of autonomic control due to lesions of the hypothalamus, perhaps aggravated by peripheral degenerative changes in the autonomic ganglia. Barbeau et al. (18) observed reduced supine plasma renin activity in patients with Parkinson's disease. Similarly Michelakis and Robertson (127) found suppressed plasma renin activity in the supine and upright positions in approximately half of 35 patients. Aminoff and Wilcox (6) found no significant postural hypotension but an increased sensitivity to infused norepinephrine, a patchy impairment of thermoregulatory sweating, and a disturbance of urinary bladder function. These authors postulated that the hypersensitive norepinephrine infusion response indicated reduced impulse traffic at the sympathetic nerve terminals due to reduced descending impulses from supraspinal centers which were not directly concerned with mediation of circulatory reflexes. This explanation could also account for the low resting blood pressure and reduced renin activity reported by Barbeau and others (18,127).

Rajput and Rozdilsky (162) studied six patients with Parkinson's disease at necropsy. They found Lewy bodies in the sympathetic ganglia in five cases, three of whom had orthostatic hypotension. The authors concluded that the lesions in the sympathetic ganglia played a major role in the production of orthostatic hypotension.

STRIATONIGRAL DEGENERATION AND AUTONOMIC DEFICITS

Adams and Victor (4) noted that a prominent orthostatic hypotension may be a feature of striatonigral degeneration, but they did not give details about these findings and other autonomic dysfunctions. They further stated that in some of these patients, intermediolateral cells of the spinal cord were depleted. The pathologic findings in the cases described by Adams et al. (2,3) under the heading of striatonigral degeneration consisted of a striking striatonigral lesion resembling that noted in Huntington's chorea, but the lesions were more marked in the putamen than in the caudate. There were no Lewy bodies or neurofibrillary tangles. Their fourth case had, in addition, pathologic findings of OPCA. These authors (4) stated that since the original cases, they have seen several cases showing a combination of OPCA and striatonigral degeneration and clinical signs of both cerebellar ataxia and extrapyramidal dysfunction. It is difficult to be certain whether some of these cases are OPCA rather than striatonigral degeneration. These difficulties led Oppenheimer (148,149) and Takei and Mirra (195) to include striatonigral degeneration and OPCA under the general category of multiple system atrophy.

CEREBELLAR AND EXTRAPYRAMIDAL DEGENERATIVE DISORDERS WITH DYSAUTONOMIA AND THEIR INTERRELATIONSHIP

"Social and scientific observations of Homo sapiens (Var. medicus) have shown that he tends to function as a 'splitter' or as a 'lumper'" (211). The degenerations of the nervous system have been a happy ground for "splitters" or "lumpers." One could lump Parkinson's disease, OPCA, striatonigral degeneration, the Shy-Drager syndrome, and progressive supranuclear palsy under the general heading of multiple system atrophy. Such excessive lumping will not improve our understanding, however, and clearly lumps together disorders of different etiologies. On the other hand, our knowledge of OPCA will not be increased by excessive splitting. One can split OPCA into multitudinous and almost meaningless entities based on clinical "pattern" recognition, such as variants with dementia and retinal degeneration (62,110), peripheral neuropathy, extrapyramidal manifestations (110), slow eye movements (205), those with dysautonomia, and so on. Some of these may represent separate morbid entities. Until a specific primary biochemical deficiency or gene defect is consistently associated with a characteristic clinical pattern, e.g., OPCA with glutamate dehydrogenase deficiency (56–58,157,158), classifications of OPCA will remain uncertain and provisional.

Autonomic (adrenergic or cholinergic, or both) dysfunction for which no obvious cause is found should simply be called primary dysautonomia (adult onset and nonfamilial) rather than idiopathic orthostatic hypotension; the patients invariably have dysautonomic features other than orthostatic hypotension. If a patient initially presents with dysautonomia and later in the course of the illness develops somatic neurologic manifestations (cerebellar, parkinsonian, or other features), then the disease may be labeled multiple system atrophy with dysautonomia (Shy-Drager syndrome).

There are certain differences between those patients with Parkinson's disease, OPCA, and striatonigral degeneration who may later develop evidence of dysautonomia and those presenting initially with dysautonomia who later show somatic neurologic manifestations (cerebellar or parkinsonian, or both). The course of the illness, the biochemical findings in general, and the response to various therapeutic modalities appear to be different. Generally, the course is relentlessly progressive and shorter in multiple system atrophy with dysautonomia (Shy-Drager syndrome) than in the other degenerative diseases.

The characteristic biochemical deficits of Parkinson's disease are not noted in many patients with the Shy-Drager syndrome, probably because these frequently have not been sought. Some reports show similar biochemical findings. Spokes et al. (191) found reduced levels of dopamine and norepinephrine in the brains of four patients with autopsy-proven multiple system atrophy and autonomic failure, particularly in the striatum, substantia nigra, nucleus accumbens, and locus ceruleus. These authors found that the levels of dopamine in the substantia nigra and striatum were comparable to the low levels found in Parkinson's disease (119), but norepinephrine levels were lower than in patients with Parkinson's disease (66). The hypothalamus and anterior perforated substance had marked loss of the enzyme tyrosine hydroxylase; this was not found in Parkinson's disease. Quik et al. (161) estimated dopamine receptor sites in the striatum, substantia nigra, and frontal cortex by measuring (^{3}H)-spiperone binding in four cases of the Shy-Drager syndrome, eight cases of Parkinson's disease, and 18 normal controls. They found loss of dopamine receptors in the substantia nigra in Parkinson's disease and in the Shy-Drager syndrome. Spokes et al. (191) also estimated the enzymes choline acetyltransferase and glutamic acid decarboxylase in the brains of four patients with multiple system atrophy and autonomic failure; but the results have been inconclusive.

Patients with the Shy-Drager syndrome may also have specific catecholamine enzyme deficits in the brain and sympathetic ganglia. Black and Petito (27,154) found depressed activity of the enzyme tyrosine hydroxylase in the adrenergic neurons of the locus ceruleus and reduced level of the enzyme dopamine-beta-hydroxylase in the sympathetic ganglia. However, Bannister and Oppenheimer (16) disagreed with their diagnosis of the Shy-Drager syndrome in their four cases.

A new dimension has been added to the neurochemistry of the Shy-Drager syndrome by the finding of abnormalities of substance P, a putative peptide neurotransmitter (143). Substance P-containing neurons have been found anatomically to be intimately related to the autonomic neurons of the brainstem (catecholaminergic cell groups), spinal cord (intermediolateral columns), and peripheral nervous system (sympathetic ganglia). In the lumbar cerebrospinal fluid of seven patients with the Shy-Drager syndrome, the mean concentration of substance P-like immunoreactivity was reduced; in 22 parkinsonian patients, however, the mean concentration did not differ significantly from control values.

Bannister and Oppenheimer (16) suggested that in order to understand the significance of neurochemical findings, careful investigations should be carried out in patients with pure autonomic failure, Parkinson's disease with progressive autonomic failure, and multiple system atrophy without evidence of autonomic failure. According to these authors, there are no reports of chemical observations in patients with autonomic failure associated with Parkinson's disease. In one case of striatonigral degeneration with severe parkinsonism but without overt autonomic dysfunction, Sharpe et al. (182) found a virtual absence of dopamine and homovanillic acid from the striatum and pallidum. This writer agrees with Bannister and Oppenheimer (16) that without further neurochemical studies, including observations on the lateral horns and the autonomic ganglia, suggestions about specific neurochemical deficits in primary autonomic failure, OPCA, and striatonigral degeneration are highly speculative.

The Shy-Drager syndrome is characteristically associated with loss of intermediolateral neurons of the spinal cord. Oppenheimer (150) found a mean loss of 70% of these sympathetic preganglionic cells in 21 cases of progressive autonomic failure, two of whom had presented clinically as pure autonomic failure. He did not find reduction of these neurons on quantitative study as compared with controls in three cases of Parkinson's disease without autonomic dysfunction. Furthermore, he found a loss of 50% of the lateral horn cells in three cases of multiple system atrophy without clinical dysautonomia. Although intermediolateral nerve cell loss has been described in patients with Parkinson's disease (148), the significance of this loss and its relationship to clinical autonomic deficits cannot be determined without careful study. Low et al. (121), after a quantitative study of the cells of the intermediolateral columns of the seventh thoracic spinal cord segment, stated that there was a general tendency for these neurons to decay with advancing years. These authors found a significant reduction of the preganglionic autonomic neurons in patients with the Shy-Drager syndrome in addition to a reduction of the B fibers in the corresponding ventral spinal roots, suggesting involvement beyond the central autonomic neurons in this condition. Low et al. (121) further stated that a loss of less than 50% of these neurons may not be clinically significant.

It appears, then, that the data presently available distinguish the Shy-Drager syndrome from classic Parkinson's disease, striatonigral degeneration, and OPCA, all of which share some common clinical and morphologic findings. The most important features separating the Shy-Drager syndrome from the other entities are the initial presentation with severe dysautonomic manifestations, the shorter duration of the illness, and the finding of severe loss of neurons of the intermediolateral cell column of the thoracic spinal cord. The latter abnormality has occurred in most of the cases studied thus far. Finally, patients with the Shy-Drager syndrome and patients with striatonigral degeneration and OPCA do not respond as well to levodopa treatment as do patients with Parkinson's disease. The Shy-Drager syndrome appears to be a distinct entity rather than simply representing one end of a spectrum of neurodegenerative disease. Future research should be directed toward detailed correlated physiologic, pharmacologic, biochemical, and morphologic investigations, including quantitative studies of the intermediolateral column cells of the thoracic spinal cord in patients with classic OPCA, Parkinson's disease, striatonigral degeneration, and the Shy-Drager syndrome.

THERAPEUTIC CONSIDERATION

Treatment of the autonomic deficits in OPCA and other neurodegenerative diseases is unsatisfactory. The etiologic mechanisms in these disorders have remained largely unresolved. In many, there is a tendency to hereditary transmission. Recent discovery of a reduction of the enzyme glutamate dehydrogenase in the leukocytes and skin fibroblasts of some patients with OPCA (58,157) offers the promise of improving our understanding of the neurodegenerative diseases. This also opens up the possibility for pharmacologic manipulation to normalize glutamate dehydrogenase activity in patients with a deficiency of this enzyme. The patients might benefit from a high leucine diet and oral supplementation (39,159) with branched chain amino acids (leucine, isoleucine, and valine).

In the absence of a specific treatment, one must rely on a comprehensive symptomatic treatment program. One should approach patients with a positive point of view rather than an attitude of therapeutic nihilism. The most disabling and serious dysautonomic manifestation in OPCA and other neurodegenerative diseases is orthostatic hypotension. Therefore, this section deals exclusively with the treatment of postural hypotension. It is important to remember that asymptomatic patients do not require treatment. The symptoms of postural hypotension depend on a critical reduction of cerebral blood flow, which is again dependent on the level of the systolic blood pressure and cerebral autoregulation in the upright position.

Mechanical Measures

Stead and Ebert (194) in 1941 first noted improvement in orthostatic blood pressure after immersion of two patients in water up to the level of the heart in order to neutralize the effects of hydrostatic pressure. Since then, beneficial effects from counter-pressure garments have been observed by several authors (26,91, 117,178,185,187,200). Other physical measures include elastic stockings and abdominal binders, in addition to the antigravity suit (19,20,177,185). All these reduce the amount of blood pooled in the lower extremities during standing and prevent orthostatic hypotension. MacLean and Allen (122) first advocated, and others (177,200) later recommended, the use of a head-up bed position in orthostatic hypotension, but not all patients benefit from this treatment (26). The head-up tilt reduces renal arterial pressure and increases renin release and blood volume, thereby improving postural hypotension.

Mineralocorticoids

Desoxycorticosterone acetate was first used with benefit by Gregory (80). Wagner (207) in 1959 used 2-methyl-9-alpha-fluorohydrocortisone in one patient; subsequently, several reports (16,21,38,70,87,88,123,175–177,200) have appeared in the literature describing the efficacy of 9-alpha-fluorohydrocortisone for the treatment of orthostatic hypotension in the Shy-Drager syndrome. Dosage ranged from 0.1 to 0.4 mg up to a maximum of 1 mg/day. The undesirable side effects include supine hypertension, congestive cardiac failure, edema of the legs, and hypokalemia. Fluorohydrocortisone is often supplemented with high sodium (150 mEq/day). Several mechanisms of action of fluorohydrocortisone for the control of orthostatic hypotension have been postulated and summarized by Hohl et al. (88) as follows: (a) hypervolemia, (b) sensitization of the peripheral arterioles which, therefore, respond to a diminished norepinephrine pool in the vessel walls, (c) "water-logging" of the peripheral arteriolar walls, thereby increasing the peripheral vascular resistance and thus raising systemic blood pressure, and (d) an altered peripheral reflex venoconstriction.

Vasoconstrictive Agents

Vasoconstrictive drugs have been used with partial success in many patients with orthostatic hypotension; Ghrist and Brown (73) in 1928 first successfully used ephedrine tablets. Subsequently, ephedrine (11,96,176,178,196,207) and other drugs, such as neosynephrine (20,96), paredrine (112), epinephrine (144), metaraminol (26), benzedrine (11,96,112), and vasopressin (208), have been used with varying degrees of success.

Indirect sympathomimetic drugs with or without monoamine oxidase (MAO) inhibitors have been used with success in many patients with orthostatic hypotension (21,49,52,118,139,166,167,179,180,200). It should be noted that the response of these agents will depend on whether the lesion is preganglionic or postganglionic. This can be decided on the basis of basal supine plasma norepinephrine levels and from the degree of supersensitivity following intravenous norepinephrine infusion (214). In postganglionic degeneration of the sympathetic nerves, the supine plasma norepinephrine level will be very low and will show a subnormal response in the erect position. In these lesions, intravenous norepinephrine infusion will show denervation supersensitivity. In the preganglionic lesions, the supine plasma norepinephrine level may be normal but also will show a subnormal response in the erect position; the intravenous norepinephrine infusion test will show a "decentralization" response, in which the degree of rise of blood pressure will be much less than that noted after postganglionic denervation supersensitivity (14,170). In postganglionic degeneration of the sympathetic nerve terminals, indirect sympathomimetic agents, such as hydroxyamphetamine (paredrine) and tyramine with or without MAO inhibitors, e.g., tranylcypromine (parnate), will be ineffective. These agents should first be tried in patients in whom the lesion is thought to be in the preganglionic regions. In both groups of patients, the drug that could be used with benefit is 9-alpha-fluorohydrocortisone, as described above.

Seller (179,180) first used a combination of hydroxyamphetamine and tyramine with success; subsequently, others (49,52,118,139) used MAO inhibitors and tyramine in the form of cheese or a chemical preparation of tyramine with benefit in some patients with the Shy-Drager syndrome and primary dysautonomia. Some authors have used a combination of MAO inhibitor and L-DOPA (181).

In severe cases of orthostatic hypotension, Thomas et al. (200) used a new drug, midodrine, with encouraging results. This is a peripheral alpha agonist and causes constriction of both resistance and capacitance vessels.

Jennings et al. (97) treated four patients with autonomic failure and orthostatic hypotension with oral dihydroergotamine; improvement was shown in all. When combined with fluorohydrocortisone, there was further improvement. The mode of action of this agent seems to be due to constriction of the capacitance vessels, thereby increasing venomotor tone and venous drainage; hence it prevents venous pooling in the upright position (141).

Other Modes of Therapy

Kochar and Itskovitz (109) used indomethacin in the treatment of four patients with the Shy-Drager syndrome. All patients improved. The authors suggested that indomethacin acted by inhibiting prostaglandin synthesis, thereby preventing accumulation of vasodilator prostaglandin in the peripheral vessels. In another report (16), however, there was no improvement in orthostatic hypotension after this treatment. Propranolol has recently been advocated as a therapy for orthostatic hypotension (36). This beta receptor inhibitor reduces the vasodilatation and thus improves orthostatic hypotension. Moss and co-workers (137) treated a patient with primary orthostatic hypotension with atrial tachypacing, resulting in marked improvement.

In conclusion, effective treatment of the most dramatic manifestation of dysautonomia, namely, orthostatic hypotension, and its accompanying symptoms continues to elude us. The best therapeutic measure appears to be a combination of a physical mode of treatment using elastic stockings and an abdominal binder with 9-alpha-fluorohydrocortisone. Despite these measures and initial success in the maintenance of blood pressure in the upright position and improvement of postural disability, the nervous system degeneration continues to progress (37,198) in an inexorable fashion, indicating that cerebral ischemia and hypoxia do not play significant roles in causing these degenerations. The search for an effective measure to prevent and halt disease progression must continue.

ACKNOWLEDGMENTS

The author thanks Dr. Roger C. Duvoisin and Dr. Kevin D. Barron for their valuable suggestions, and Lena DiMauro for typing the manuscript. This work was supported in part by the Veterans Administration Medical Research Service.

REFERENCES

1. Achari, N. K., and Downman, C. B. B. (1970): Autonomic effector responses to stimulation of nucleus fastigius. *J. Physiol.*, 210:637–659.
2. Adams, R. D. (1968): Striatonigral degenerations: In: *Handbook of Clinical Neurology*, edited by P. J. Vinken and J. W. Bruyn, pp. 694–702. North Holland, Amsterdam.
3. Adams, R. D., Van Bogaert, L., and Van der Ecken, H. (1964): Striatonigral degeneration. *J. Neuropathol. Exp. Neurol.*, 23:584–608.
4. Adams, R. D., and Victor, M. (1981): *Principles of Neurology*, McGraw-Hill, New York.
5. Ahlquist, R. P. (1948): A study of adrenotropic receptors. *Am. J. Physiol.*, 153:586–600.
6. Aminoff, M. J., and Wilcox, C. S. (1971): Assessment of autonomic function in patients with a Parkinsonian syndrome. *Br. Med. J.*, 4:80–84.
7. Andén, N. E., Dahlstrom, A., Fuxe, K., Larsson, K., Olson, L., and Understedt, V. (1966): Ascending monoamine neurons to the telencephalon and diencephalon. *Acta Physiol. Scand.*, 67:313–326.
8. Appenzeller, O. (1970): *The Autonomic Nervous System*. North Holland, London.
9. Appenzeller, O., and Goss, J. E. (1971): Autonomic deficits in Parkinson's syndrome. *Arch. Neurol.*, 24:50–57.
10. Axelsson, S., Bjorklund, A., Falck, B., Lindvall, O., and Svensson, L-A. (1973): Glyoxylic acid condensation: A new fluoroscence method for the histochemical demonstration of biogenic monoamines. *Acta Physiol. Scand.*, 87:57–62.

11. Baker, T. W. (1938): Recognition of orthostatic hypotension. *Proc. Staff Meeting Mayo Clinic*, 13:169–174.
12. Bakker, S. P. (1924): Atrophia olivo-pontocerebellaris. *Z. Gesamte Neurol. Psychiatr.*, 89:213–246.
13. Bannister, R., Crowe, R., Eames, R., and Burnstock, G. (1981): Adrenergic innervation in autonomic failure. *Neurology*, 31:1501–1506.
14. Bannister, R., Davis, B., Holly, E., Rosenthal, T., and Sever, P. (1979): Defective cardiovascular reflexes and supersensitivity to sympathomimetic drugs in autonomic failure. *Brain*, 102:163–176.
15. Bannister, R., and Oppenheimer, D. R. (1972): Degenerative disease of the nervous system associated with autonomic failure. *Brain*, 95:457–474.
16. Bannister, R., and Oppenheimer, D. (1982): Parkinsonism, system degenerations and autonomic failure. In: *Movement Disorders*, edited by C. D. Marsden and S. Fahn, pp. 174–190. Butterworth, Boston.
17. Bannister, R., Sever, P., and Gross, M. (1977): Cardiovascular reflexes and biochemical responses in progressive autonomic failure. *Brain*, 100:327–344.
18. Barbeau, A., Gillo-Joffroy, L., Boucher, R., Nowsczynski, W., and Genest, J. (1969): Renin-alderstone system in Parkinson's disease. *Science*, 165:291–292.
19. Barker, N. W. (1933): Postural hypotension: A report of a case and review of the literature. *Med. Clin. North Am.*, 16:1301–1312.
20. Barnett, A. J., Hamilton, M. D., and Kay, H. B. (1955): Severe orthostatic hypotension. *Aust. Ann. Med.*, 4:183–194.
21. Barr, A. N. (1979): The Shy-Drager syndrome. In: *Handbook of Clinical Neurology*, edited by P. J. Vinken and J. W. Bruyn, pp. 233–256. North-Holland, Amsterdam.
22. Beattie, J., Brown, G. R., and Long, C. N. H. (1930): The hypothalamus and the sympathetic nervous system. *Assoc. Res. Nerv. Ment. Dis. Proc.*, 9:249.
23. Berciano, J. (1982): Olivopontocerebellar atrophy: A review of 117 cases. *J. Neurol. Sci.*, 53:253–272.
24. Berne, R. M., and Levy, M. N. (1967): *Cardiovascular Physiology*, C. V. Mosby, St. Louis.
25. Best, C. H., and Taylor, N. B. T. (1966): Regulation of the circulation under states of stress. In: *Physiological Basis of Medical Practice*, edited by J. R. Brobeck, Chap. 48, pp. 883–914. Williams & Wilkins, Baltimore.
26. Bickelmann, A. G., Lippschutz, E. J., and Brunjes, C. F. (1961): Hemodynamics of idiopathic orthostatic hypotension. *Am. J. Med.*, 30:26–38.
27. Black, I. B., and Petito, C. K. (1976): Catecholamine enzymes in the degenerative neurological disease idiopathic orthostatic hypotension. *Science*, 192:910–912.
28. Boulu, P., Cohen, J. A., and Shahani, B. T. (1982): Autonomic dysfunction in peripheral neuropathies investigated with sympathetic reflex response. *Muscle Nerve*, 5:564.
29. Bradbury, S., and Eggleston, C. (1925): Postural hypotension. A report of 3 cases. *Am. Heart J.*, 1:73–86.
30. Bradbury, S., and Eggleston, C. (1927): Postural hypotension: Autopsy on a case. *Am. Heart J.*, 3:105–106.
31. Bradley, W. E. (1980): Diagnosis of urinary bladder dysfunction in diabetes mellitus. *Ann. Intern. Med.*, 92:323–326.
32. Brodal, A. (1981): *Neurological Anatomy: In Relation to Clinical Medicine*, Oxford University Press, New York.
33. Burn, J. H. (1971): *The Autonomic Nervous System for Students of Physiology and Pharmacology*, Blackwell Scientific, Oxford.
34. Burton, A. C. (1965): *Physiology and Biophysics of the Circulation*. Year Book, Chicago.
35. Cannon, W. B., and Rosenblueth, A. (1949): *The Supersensitivity of Denervated Structures: A Law of Denervation*. Macmillan, New York.
36. Chobanian, V. A., Volicer, L., Liang, C. S., Kershaw, G., and Tifft, C. (1977): Use of propranolol in the treatment of idiopathic orthostatic hypotension. *Clin. Res.*, 25:513A.
37. Chokroverty, S., Barron, K. D., Arieff, A. F., and Rovner, R. N. (1967): A case of severe orthostatic hypotension. *Trans. Am. Neurol. Assoc.*, 92:216–219.
38. Chokroverty, S., Barron, K. D., Katz, F. H., Del Greco, F., and Sharp, J. T. (1969): The syndrome of primary orthostatic hypotension. *Brain*, 92:743–768.
39. Chokroverty, S., Duvoisin, R. C., Sage, J., Sachdeo, R., and Nicklas, W. (1983): Neurophysio-

logical study in olivopontocerebellar atrophy with and without glutamate dehydrogenase deficiency. *Ann. Neurol.*, 14:148.
40. Chokroverty, S., and Sachdeo, R. (1978): Autonomic deficits in spinocerebellar degeneration. *Neurology*, 28:403.
41. Chokroverty, S., Sachdeo, R., and Masdeu, J. (1984): Autonomic dysfunction and sleep apnea in olivopontocerebellar degeneration. *Arch. Neurol. (In press.)*
42. Chokroverty, S., Sharp, J. T., and Barron, K. D. (1978): Periodic respiration in erect posture in Shy-Drager syndrome. *J. Neurol. Neurosurg. Psychiatry*, 41:980–986.
43. Cohen, E. L., Conn, J. W., and Rovner, D. R. (1967): Postural augmentation of plasma renin activity and aldosterne excretion in normal people. *J. Clin. Invest.*, 46:418–428.
44. Cohen, D., and Zakov, N. (1975): The diagnosis of Adie's pupil using 0.062% pilocarpine solution. *Am. J. Ophthalmol.*, 23:883–885.
45. Cooper, J., Bloom, A., and Roth, R. H. (1974): *The Biochemical Basis of Neuropharmacology*, Oxford University Press, New York.
46. Cottle, M. K. W., and Calaresu, F. R. (1975): Projections from the nucleus and tractus solitarius in the cat. *J. Comp. Neurol.*, 161:143–158.
47. Dahlstrom, A., and Fuxe, K. (1964): Evidence for the existence of monoamine-containing neurons in the central nervous system. I. Demonstration of monoamines in the cell bodies of brain stem neurons. *Acta Physiol. Scand. [Suppl. 62]*, 232:1–55.
48. Dahlstrom, A., and Fuxe, K. (1965): Evidence for the existence of monoamine neurons in the central nervous system. *Acta Physiol. Scand. [Suppl. 64]*, 247:1–36.
49. Davies, B., Bannister, R., and Sever, P. (1978): Pressor amines and monoamine-oxidase inhibitors for treatment of postural hypotension in autonomic failure. *Lancet*, 1:172–175.
50. Davis, J. O. (1971): What signals the kidney to release renin? Review. *Circ. Res.*, 28:301–306.
51. Dejerine, J., and Thomas, A. (1900): L-atrophic olivopontocerebelleuse. *Nouv. Iconogr. Salpet.*, 13:330–370.
52. Diamond, M. A., Murray, R. H., and Schmid, P. G. (1970): Idiopathic postural hypotension: Physiologic observations and report of a new mode of therapy. *J. Clin. Invest.*, 49:1341–1348.
53. Doba, N., and Reis, D. J. (1972): Cerebellum: Role in reflex cardiovascular adjustment to posture. *Brain Res.*, 13:495–500.
54. Dobken, B. H., and Rosenthal, N. P. (1975): Clinical assessment of autonomic dysfunction: An approach to the Shy-Drager syndrome. *Bull. Los Angeles Neurol. Soc.*, 40:101–110.
55. Dow, R. S., and Moruzzi, G. (1958): *The Physiology and Pathology of the Cerebellum*. University of Minnesota Press, Minneapolis.
56. Duvoisin, R. C., and Chokroverty, S. (1983): *This volume*.
57. Duvoisin, R. C., Chokroverty, S., Lepore, F., and Nicklas, W. (1982): The clinical spectrum of glutamate deyhydrogenase deficiency. *Neurology*, 32:A82.
58. Duvoisin, R. C., Chokroverty, S., Lepore, F., and Nicklas, W. (1984): Glutamate dehydrogenase deficiency in patients with olivopontocerebellar atrophy. *Neurology*, 33:1322–1326.
59. Dyck, P. J. (1975): Inherited neuronal degeneration and atrophy affecting peripheral motor, sensory and autonomic neurons. In: *Peripheral Neuropathy*, edited by P. J. Dyck, P. K. Thomas, and E. H. Lambert, pp. 825–867. Saunders, Philadelphia.
60. Eadie, M. J. (1975): Olivo-ponto-cerebellar atrophy (Dejerine-Thomas type). In: *Handbook of Clinical Neurology*, edited by P. J. Vinken and G. W. Bruyn, pp. 415–431. North-Holland, Amsterdam.
61. Eadie, M. J. (1975): Olivo-ponto-cerebellar atrophy (Menzel type). In: *Handbook of Clinical Neurology*, edited by P. J. Vinken and G. W. Bruyn, pp. 433–449. North-Holland, Amsterdam.
62. Eadie, M. J. (1975): Olivo-ponto-cerebellar atrophy (variants). In: *Handbook of Clinical Neurology*, edited by P. J. Vinken and G. W. Bruyn, pp. 451–457. North-Holland, Amsterdam.
63. Eckhard, C. (1872): Beitrage Anat. und physiol. (Giessen). 6:IV Abhandl., 51–94; VII Abhandl., 177–192. [Cited by Wiggers, K. (1943): The influence of the cerebellum on the vegetative functions. 1. A review. *Arch. Néerl. Physiol.*, 27:286–300.]
64. Ewing, D. J., Campbell, I. W., Burt, A. A., and Clarke, B. F. (1973): Vascular reflexes in diabetic autonomic neuropathy. *Lancet*, 2:1354–1356.
65. Falck, B., Hillarp, N. A., Thieme, G., and Torp, A. (1962): Fluoroscence of catecholamines and related compounds condensed with formaldehyde. *J. Histochem. Cytochem.*, 10:348–354.
66. Farley, I. J., and Hornykiewicz, O. (1977): Noradrenaline in subcortical brain regions of patients with Parkinson's disease and control subjects. In: *Advances of Parkinsonism—Biochemistry, Phys-*

iology, Treatment, edited by W. Birkmayer and O. Hornykiewicz, pp. 178–185. Editions Roche, Basel.
67. Farley, I. J., and Hornykiewicz, O. (1977): Noradrenaline distribution in subcortical areas of the human brain. *Brain Res.*, 126:53–62.
68. Ferrier, D. (1876): *The Functions of the Brain.* Smith, Elder and Company, London.
69. Fischefet, J. P., Sternon, J. E., Franken, Demanet, J. C., and Vanderhaeghen, J. J. (1965): Etude anatomo-clinique d'un cas d'hypotension orthostatique "idiopathique:" Considerations pathogeniques. *Acta Cardiol.*, 20:332–348.
70. Frick, M. H. (1966): 9-Alpha-fluorohydrocortisone in the treatment of postural hypotension. *Acta Med. Scand.*, 179:293–299.
71. Fuxe, K., Hokfelt, T., and Ungerstedt, U. (1970): Morphological and functional aspects of central monoamine neurons. In: *International Review of Neurobiology, Vol. 13*, edited by C. C. Pfeiffer and J. R. Smythies, pp. 93–126. Academic Press, New York.
72. Gabella, G. (1968): *Structure of the Autonomic Nervous System.* Wiley, New York.
73. Ghrist, D. G., and Brown, G. E. (1928): Postural hypotension with syncope: Its successful treatment with ephedrine. *Am. J. Med. Sci.*, 175:336–349.
74. Gordon, R. D., Kuchel, O., Liddle, G. W., and Island, D. P. (1967): Role of the sympathetic nervous system in regulating renin and aldosterone production in man. *J. Clin. Invest.*, 46:599–605.
75. Gorry, J. R. (1963): Studies on the comparative anatomy of the ganglion basale of Meynert. *Acta Anat. (Basel)*, 55:51–104.
76. Graham, J. G., and Oppenheimer, D. R. (1969): Orthostatic hypotension and nicotine sensitivity in a case of multiple system atrophy. *J. Neurol. Neurosurg. Psychiatry.*, 32:28–34.
77. Gray, R. C., and Oliver, C. P. (1941): Marie's hereditary cerebellar ataxia (olivopontocerebellar atrophy). *Minn. Med.*, 24:327–335.
78. Greenfield, J. G. (1954): The spino-cerebellar degenerations. Blackwells, Oxford.
79. Greenfield, J. G. (1958): System degenerations of the cerebellum, brain stem and spinal cord. In: *Neuropathology*, edited by J. G. Greenfield, W. Blackwood, A. Meyer, W. H. McMenemy, and R. M. Norman, pp. 529–549. Edward Arnold, London.
80. Gregory, R. (1945): The treatment of orthostatic hypotension with particular reference to the use of desoxycorticosterone. *Am. Heart J.*, 29:246–252.
81. Gross, M., Bannister, R., and Godwin-Austen, R. (1972): Orthostatic hypotension in Parkinson's disease. *Lancet*, 1:174–176.
82. Haber, E., Koerner, T., Page, L. B., Kliman, B., and Purnode, A. (1969): Application of a radioimmunoassay for angiotensin I to the physiologic measurements of plasma renin activity in normal human subjects. *J. Clin. Endocrinol.*, 29:1349–1355.
83. Hamilton, W. F., Woodbury, R. A., and Harper, H. T., Jr. (1936): Physiological relationships between intrathoracic, intraspinal and arterial pressures. *JAMA*, 107:853–856.
84. Hare, W. K., Magoun, H. W., and Ranson, S. W. (1937): Localization within the cerebellum of reactions to faradic cerebellar stimulation. *J. Comp. Neurol.*, 67:145–182.
85. Heymans, C., and Neil, E. (1958): *Reflexogenic Areas of the Cardiovascular System.* Little, Brown, Boston.
86. Hickam, J. B., and Pryor, W. W. (1951): Cardiac output in postural hypotension. *J. Clin. Invest.*, 30:401–405.
87. Hickler, R. B., Thompson, G. R., Fox, L. M., and Hamlin, J. T. (1959): Successful treatment of orthostatic hypotension with 9-alpha-fluorohydrocortisone. *N. Engl. J. Med.*, 261:788–791.
88. Hohl, R. T., Frame, B., and Schatz, I. J. (1965): The Shy-Drager variant of idiopathic orthostatic hypotension. *Am. J. Med.*, 39:134–141.
89. Hollander, F. (1964): Insulin test for presence for intact nerve fibers after vagal operation for peptic ulcer. *Gastroenterology*, 7:607–614.
90. Holmes, G. (1907): A form of familial degeneration of the cerebellum. *Brain*, 30:466–489.
91. Hughes, R. C., Cartlidge, N. E. F., and Miller, P. (1970): Primary neurogenetic orthostatic hypotension. *J. Neurol. Neurosurg. Psychiatry*, 33:363–371.
92. Ibrahim, M. M. (1975): Localization of lesion in patients with idopathic orthostatic hypotension. *Br. Heart J.*, 37:868–872.
93. Ingram, W. R. (1940): Nuclear organization and chief connections of the primate hypothalamus. *Res. Publ. Assoc. Nerv. Ment. Dis.*, 20:195–244.

94. Ingram, W. R. (1960): Central autonomic mechanisms. In: *Handbook of Physiology, Section 1, Neurophysiology, Vol. 2*, p. 951. American Physiology Society, Washington, D.C.
95. Jammes, J. L. (1972): The autonomic nervous system in peroneal muscular atrophy. *Arch. Neurol.*, 27:218–220.
96. Jeffers, W. A., Montgomery, H., and Burton, A. C. (1941): Types of orthostatic hypotension and their treatment. *Am. J. Med. Sci.*, 202:1–14.
97. Jennings, G., Esler, M., and Holmes, R. (1979): Treatment of orthostatic hypotension with dihydroergotamine. *Br. Med. J.*, 1:307.
98. Johnson, R. H., Lee, G., De, J., Oppenheimer, D. R., and Spalding, J. M. K. (1966): Autonomic failure with orthostatic hypotension due to intermediolateral column degeneration. *Q. J. Med.*, 35:276–292.
99. Johnson, R. H., and Spalding, J. M. K. (1974): *Disorders of the Autonomic Nervous System*. F. A. Davis, Philadelphia.
100. Jones, J. A. (1933): Effect of posture work on the health of children. *Am. J. Dis. Child.*, 46:148–154.
101. Jones, E. G., Burton, H., Saper, C. B., and Swanson, L. W. (1976): Midbrain, diencephalic and cortical relationships of the basal nucleus of Meynert and associated structures in primates. *J. Comp. Neurol.*, 167:385–420.
102. Kaada, B. R. (1960): Cingullate, posterior orbital, anterior insular and temporal pole cortex. In: *Handbook of Physiology, Section 1, Neurophysiology, Vol. 2*, p. 1345. American Physiological Society, Washington, D.C.
103. Kennard, M. A. (1945): Focal autonomic representation in the cortex and its relationship to sham rage. *J. Neuropathol. Exp. Neurol.*, 4:295–304.
104. Kennedy, W. R., and Sakuta, M. (1982): Sweat gland dysfunction in diabetic neuropathy. *Ann. Neurol.*, 12:106.
105. Khurana, R. K., Nelson, E., Azzarelli, B., and Garcia, J. H. (1980): Shy-Drager syndrome: Diagnosis and treatment of cholinergic dysfunction. *Neurology*, 30:805–809.
106. Kimura, H., McGeer, P. L., Peng, J. H., and McGeer, E. G. (1981): The central cholinergic system studies by choline acetyltransferase immunohistochemistry in the cat. *J. Comp. Neurol.*, 200:151–201.
107. Kobayashi, R. D. M., Brownstein, M., Saavedra, J. M., and Palkovits, M. (1975): Choline acetyltransferase content in discrete regions of the rat brain stem. *J. Neurochem.*, 24:637–640.
108. Kobayashi, R. D. M., Palkovits, M., Jacobowitz, D. M., and Kopin, I. J. (1975): Biochemical mapping of the noradrenergic projection from the locus coeruleus. *Neurology*, 25:223–233.
109. Kochar, M. S., and Itskovitz, H. D. (1978): Treatment of idiopathic orthostatic hypotension (Shy-Drager syndrome) with indomethacin. *Lancet*, 1:1011–1014.
110. Konigsmark, B. W., and Weiner, L. P. (1970): The olivo-ponto-cerebellar atrophies: A review. *Medicine*, 49:227–241.
111. Kontos, H. A., Richards, D. W., and Narvell, J. E., (1975): Norepinephrine depletion in idiopathic orthostatic hypotension. *Ann. Intern. Med.*, 82:336–341.
112. Korns, H. M., and Randall, W. L. (1937): Orthostatic hypotension treated with benzedrine. *Am. Heart J.*, 13:114–118.
113. Lake, C. R., Ziegler, M. G., and Kopin, I. J. (1976): Use of plasma norepinephrine for evaluation of sympathetic neuronal function in man. *Life Sci.*, 18:1315–1326.
114. Lapresle, J., and Annabi, A. (1979): Olivopontocerebellar atrophy with velopharyngolaryngeal paralysis—A contribution to the somatotopy of the nucleus ambiguus. *J. Neuropathol. Exp. Neurol.*, 38:401–406.
115. Laubry, C., and Doumer, E. (1932): L-hypotension orthostatique. *Presse Med.*, 1:17–20.
116. Levin, A. B. (1966): A simple test of cardiac function based upon the heart rate changes induced by the Valsalva maneuver. *Amr. J. Cardiol.*, 18:90–99.
117. Lewis, H. D., Jr., and Dunn, M. (1967): Orthostatic hypotension syndrome. *Am. Heart J.*, 74:396–401.
118. Lewis, R. K., Hazelrig, C. G., Fricke, F. J., and Russell, R. O., Jr. (1972): Therapy of idiopathic postural hypotension. *Arch. Intern. Med.*, 129:943–949.
119. Lloyd, K. G., Davidson, L., and Hornkiewicz, O. (1975): The neurochemistry of Parkinson's disease—effect of L-dopa therapy. *J. Pharmacol. Exp. Ther.*, 195:453–464.
120. Loewy, A. D., and Burton, H. (1978): Nuclei of the solitary tract: Efferent projections to the lower brain stem and spinal cord of the cat. *J. Comp. Neurol.*, 181:421–450.

121. Low, P. A., Thomas, J. E., and Dyck, P. J. (1978): The splanchnic autonomic outflow in Shy-Drager syndrome and idiopathic orthostatic hypotension. *Ann. Neurol.*, 4:511–514.
122. MacLean, A. R., and Allen, E. V. (1940): Orthostatic hypotension and orthostatic tachycardia: Treatment with the "head-up" bed. *JAMA*, 115:2162–2167.
123. Martin, J. B., Travers, R. H., and Van Den Noort, S. (1968): Centrally mediated orthostatic hypotension. *Arch. Neurol.*, 19:163–173.
124. Martner, J. (1975): Cerebellar influence on autonomic mechanisms. *Acta Physiol. Scand. [Suppl.]*, 425:8–35.
125. Menzel, P. (1891): Beitrag zur Kenntnis der Hereditarn ataxic und kleinhirnatrophie. *Arch. Psychiatr. Nervenkr.*, 22:160–190.
126. Mesulam, M. M., and Van Hoesen, G. W. (1976): Acetylcholinesterase-rich projections from the basal forebrain of the rhesus monkey to neocortex. *Brain Res.*, 109:152–157.
127. Michelakis, A. M., and Robertson, D. (1970): Plasma renin activity and levodopa in Parkinson's disease. *JAMA*, 213:83–85.
128. Milnor, W. R. (1980): *The circulation*. In: *Medical Physiology*, edited by V. B. Mountcastle, pp. 951–1146. C.V. Mosby, St. Louis.
129. Mitchell, G. A. G. (1953): *Anatomy of the Autonomic Nervous System*. Livingstone, Edinburgh.
130. Miura, M. (1975): Postsynaptic potentials recorded from nucleus of the solitary tract and its subjacent reticular formation elicited by stimulation of the carotid sinus nerve. *Brain Res.*, 100:437–440.
131. Miura, M., and Reis, D. J. (1970): A pressor response from fastigial nucleus and its related pathway in brain stem. *Am. J. Physiol.*, 219:1330–1336.
132. Miura, M., and Reis, D. J. (1972): The role of the solitary and paramedian reticular nuclei in mediating cardiovascular reflex responses from carotid baro- and chemo-receptors. *J. Physiol.*, 223:525–548.
133. Miyazaki, M. (1980): Shy-Drager syndrome: A nosological entity? The problem of orthostatic hypotension. In: *Spinocerebellar Degeneration*, edited by I. Sobue, pp. 35–43. University Park Press, Baltimore.
134. Moruzzi, G. (1950): *Problems in Cerebellar Physiology*. Charles C Thomas, Springfield, Illinois.
135. Moskowitz, M. A. (1977): Diseases of the autonomic nervous system. In: *Clinics in Endocrinology and Metabolism*, 6:745–768.
136. Moskowitz, M. A., and Wurtman, R. J. (1975): Catecholamines and neurologic disease. *N. Engl. J. Med.*, 293:274–280; 332–338.
137. Moss, A. J., Glasser, W., and Topol, E. (1980): Atrial tachypacing in the treatment of a patient with primary orthostatic hypotension. *N. Engl. J. Med.*, 302:1456–1457.
138. Mulrow, P. G. (1966): Neural and other mechanisms regulating aldosterone secretion. In: *Neuroendocrinology*, edited by L. Martini and W. F. Ganong, pp. 407–444. Academic Press, New York.
139. Nanda, R. N., Johnson, R. H., and Keogh, H. J. (1976): Treatment of neurogenic orthostatic hypotension with a monoamine oxidase inhibitor and tyramine. *Lancet*, 2:1164–1167.
140. Nick, J., Contamin, F., Escourolle, R., Guillard, A., and Marcantoni, J. (1967): Hypotension orthostatique idiopathique avec syndrome neurologique complexe a predominance extrapyrmidale: E'tude anatomo-clinique d'un cas. *Rev. Neurol.*, 116:213–227.
141. Nordenfeldt, I., and Mellander, S. (1972): Central hemodynamic effects of dihydroergotamine in patients with orthostatic hypotension. *Acta Med. Scand.*, 191:115–120.
142. Norgren, R. (1978): Projections from the nucleus of the solitary tract in the rat. *Neuroscience*, 3:207–218.
143. Nutt, J. G., Morz, E. A., Leman, S. E., Williams, A. C., King Engel, W., and Chase, T. N. (1980): Substance P in human cerebral spinal fluid: Reductions in peripheral neuropathy and autonomic dysfunction. *Neurology*, 30:1280–1285.
144. Nylin, G., and Levander, M. (1948): Studies on the circulation with the aid of tagged erythrocytes in a case of orthostatic hypotension. *Ann. Intern. Med.*, 28:723–746.
145. Ochoa, J., and Maier, W. G. (1969): The normal sural nerve in man. *Acta Neuropathol.*, 13:197–216.
146. Olson, L., and Fuxe, F. (1972): Further mapping out of central noradrenaline neuron systems: Projections of the "subcoeruleus" area. *Brain Res.*, 43:283–295.
147. Oparil, S., and Haber, E. (1974): The renin-angiotensin system. *N. Engl. J. Med.*, 291:389–401.
148. Oppenheimer, D. R. (1976): Diseases of the basal ganglia, cerebellum and motor neurons. In:

Greenfield's Neuropathology, edited by W. Blackwood and J. A. N. Corsellis, pp. 608–651. Year Book Medical, Chicago.
149. Oppenheimer, D. R. (1980): Multiple system atrophy and the Shy-Drager syndrome. In: *Spinocerebellar Degeneration*, edited by I. Sobue, pp. 165–170. University Park Press, Baltimore.
150. Oppenheimer, D. R. (1980): Lateral horn cells in progressive autonomic failure. *J. Neurol. Sci.*, 46:393–404.
151. Parkinson, J. (1817): *Essay on the Shaking Palsy*. London. Reprinted in: James Parkinson (1755–1824), edited by M. Critchley, pp. 145–218, 1955. MacMillan, London.
152. Peart, W. S. (1965): The renin-angiotensin system. *Pharmacol. Rev.*, 17:143–182.
153. Penfield, W., and Jasper, H. (1954): Epilepsy and the functional anatomy of the human brain. *Little, Brown*, Boston.
154. Petito, C. K., and Black, I. B. (1978): Ultrastructure and biochemistry of sympathetic ganglia in idiopathic orthostatic hypotension. *Ann. Neurol.*, 4:6–17.
155. Pick, J. (1970): *The Autonomic Nervous System. Morphological, Comparative, Clinical and Surgical Aspects*. J. B. Lippincott, Philadelphia.
156. Piorry, P. A. (1826): Recherches sur l'influence de la pesanteur sur le cours du sang: diagnostic de la syncope et de l'apoplexie; cause et traitement de la syncope. *Arch. Gen. Med.*, 12:527–544.
157. Plaitakis, A., Nicklas, W. J., and Desnick, R. J. (1980): Glutamate dehydrogenase deficiency in 3 patients with spinocerebellar syndrome. *Ann. Neurol.*, 7:297–303.
158. Plaitakis, A., Berl, S., and Yahr, M. D. (1982): Abnormal glutamate metabolism in an adult-onset degenerative neurological disorder. *Science*, 216:193–196.
159. Plaitakis, A., Berl, S., and Yahr, M. D. (1983): The treatment of GDH-deficient olivopontocerebellar atrophy with branched chain amino acids. *Neurology [Suppl. 2]*, 33:78.
160. Polinsky, R. P., Kopin, I. J., Ebert, M. H., and Weiss, V. (1981): Pharmacologic distinction of different orthostatic hypotension syndromes. *Neurology*, 31:1–7.
161. Quik, M., Spokes, E. G., Mackay, A. V. P., and Bannister, R. (1979): Alterations in (3H) spiperone binding in human caudate nucleus, substantia nigra and frontal cortex in the Shy-Drager syndrome and Parkinson's disease. *J. Neurol. Sci.*, 43:429–437.
162. Rajput, A. H., and Rozdilsky, B. (1976): Dysautonomia in Parkinsonism: A clinical-pathological study. *J. Neurol. Neurosurg. Psychiatry*, 39:1092–1100.
163. Reid, J. L., Calne, D. B., George, C. F., Pallis, C., and Vakil, S. D. (1971): Cardiovascular reflexes in Parkinsonism. *Clin. Sci.*, 41:63–67.
164. Reiser, M. F., and Ferris, E. B., Jr. (1948): The nature of the cold pressor test and its significance in relation to neurogenic and humoral mechanisms in hypertension. *J. Clin. Invest.*, 27:156–163.
165. Ricardo, J. A., and Koh, E. T. (1978): Anatomical evidence of direct projections from the nucleus of the solitary tract to the hypothalamus, amygdala and other forebrain structures in the rat. *Brain Res.*, 153:1–26.
166. Roessmann, U. (1975): Primary orthostatic hypotension. In: *Handbook of Clinical Neurology*, edited by P. J. Vinken and G. W. Bruyn, pp. 231–242. North Holland, Amsterdam.
167. Roessmann, U., Van den Noort, S., and McFarland, D. E. (1971): Idiopathic orthostatic hypotension. *Arch. Neurol.*, 24:503–510.
168. Roguska, J., Simon, N. M., and Del Greco, F. (1968): Pressor response to antiotensin II in hypertension: Correlation with plasma renin activity and response to norepinephrine and metaraminol. *Am. J. Cardiol.*, 21:705–713.
169. Rosecan, M., Glasser, R. J., and Goldmen, M. L. (1952): Orthostatic hypotension, anhidrosis and impotence. *Circulation*, 6:30–40.
170. Rubensten, A. E., Yahr, M. D., and Mytilineou, C. (1978): Peripheral adrenergic hypersensitivity in orthostatic hypotension: The effects of denervation versus decentralization. *Neurology*, 28:376.
171. Rushmer, R. F. (1976): *Structure and Function of the Cardiovascular System*. Saunders, Philadelphia.
172. Saper, C. B., Loewy, A. D., Swanson, L. W., and Cowan, W. M. (1976): Direct hypothalamo-autonomic connections. *Brain Res.*, 117:305–312.
173. Sarnoff, S. J., Gilmore, J. P., Brockman, S. K., Mitchell, J. H., and Linden, R. J. (1960): Regulation of ventricular contraction by the carotid sinus: Its effect on atrial and ventricular dynamics. *Circ. Res.*, 8:1123–1136.
174. Sarnoff, S. J., Hardenbergh, E., and Whittenberger, J. L. (1948): Mechanism of the arterial

pressure response to the Valsalva test. The basis for its use as an indicator of the sympathetic outflow. *Am. J. Physiol.*, 154:316–327.
175. Schatz, I. J., Miller, M. L., and Frame, B. (1976): Corticosteriods in the management of orthostatic hypotension. *Cardiology [Suppl. 1]*, 61:280–289.
176. Schatz, I. J., Podolsky, S., and Frame, B. (1963): Idiopathic orthostatic hypotension. *JAMA*, 186:537–540.
177. Schirger, A., Hines, E. A., Jr., Molnar, G. D., and Thomas, J. E. (1962): Idiopathic orthostatic hypotension. *JAMA*, 181:822–826.
178. Schwarz, J. A. (1967): The orthostatic hypotension syndrome of Shy-Drager. *Arch. Neurol.*, 16:123–139.
179. Seller, R. H. (1968): Idiopathetic orthostatic hypotension (I.O.H.): Report of successful treatment with a new form of therapy. *Circulation [Suppl. 6]*, 38:175.
180. Seller, R. H., (1969): Idiopathic orthostatic hypotension. Report of successful treatment with a new form of therapy. *Am. J. Cardiol.*, 23:838–844.
181. Sharpe, I., Marquez-Julio, A., and Ashby, P. (1972): Idiopathic orthostatic hypotension treated with levodopa and MAO inhibitor: A preliminary report. *Can. Med. Assoc. J.*, 107:296–300.
182. Sharpe, J. A., Rewcastle, N. B., Lloyd, K. G., Hornykiewicz, O., Hill, M., and Tasker, R. R. (1973): Striatonigral degeneration: Response to levodopa therapy with pathological and neurochemical correlation. *J. Neurol. Sci.*, 19:275–286.
183. Shepherd, J. T. (1963): *Physiology of the Circulation in Human Limbs in Health and Disease*. Saunders, Philadelphia.
184. Shepherd, J. T. (1973): Intrathoracic baroreflexes. *Proc. Mayo Clin.*, 48:426–437.
185. Sheps, S. G. (1976): Use of an elastic garment in the treatment of orthostatic hypotension. *Cardiology [Suppl. 1]*, 61:271–279.
186. Shy, G. M., and Drager, G. A. (1960): A neurological syndrome associated with orthostatic hypotension. *Arch. Neurol.*, 2:511–527.
187. Sieker, H. O., Burnum, J. F., Hickam, J. B., and Penrod, K. E. (1956): Treatment of postural hypotension with a counter pressure garment. *JAMA*, 161:132–135.
188. Skinner, S. L., McCubbin, J. W., and Page, I. H. (1964): Control of renin secretion. *Circ. Res.*, 15:522–531.
189. Somana, R., and Walberg, F. (1979): Cerebellar afferents from the nucleus of the solitary tract. *Neurosci. Lett.*, 11:41–47.
190. Spencer, W. G. (1894): The effect produced upon respiration by faradic excitation of the cerebrum in the monkey, dog, cat and rabbit. *Philos. Trans. R. Soc. Lond. [Biol.]*, 185:609–657.
191. Spokes, E. G., Bannister, R., and Oppenheimer, D. R. (1979): Multiple system atrophy with autonomic failure; clinical, histological and neurochemical observations on 4 cases. *J. Neurol. Sci.*, 43:59–82.
192. Spyer, K. M. (1975): Organization of baroreceptor pathways in the brain. *Brain Res.*, 87:221–226.
193. Staal, A., Stefanko, S. Z., Busch, H. F. M., Jennekens, F. G. I., and DeBruijn, W. C. (1981): Autonomic nerve calcification and peripheral neuropathy in olivopontocerebellar atrophy. *J. Neurol. Sci.*, 51:383–394.
194. Stead, E. A., Jr., and Ebert, R. V. (1941): Postural hypotension, a disease of the sympathetic nervous sytem. *Arch. Intern. Med.*, 67:546–562.
195. Takei, Y., and Mirra, S. S. (1973): Striatonigral degeneration: A form of multiple system atrophy with clinical Parkinsonism. In: *Progress in Neurolopathology*, edited by H. M. Zimmerman, pp. 217–251. Grune & Stratton, New York.
196. Thapedi, I. M., Ashenhurst, E. M., and Rozdilsky, B. (1971): Shy-Drager syndrome. *Neurology*, 21:26–32.
197. Thomas, M. R., and Calaresu, F. R. (1974): Localization and function of medullary sites mediating vagal bradycardia in the cat. *Am. J. Physiol.*, 226:1344–1349.
198. Thomas, J. E., and Schirger, A. (1963): Neurologic manifestations in idiopathic orthostatic hypotension. *Arch. Neurol.*, 8:204–208.
199. Thomas, J. E., and Schirger, A. (1970): Idiopathic orthostatic hypotension: A study of its natural history in 57 neurologically affected patients. *Arch. Neurol.*, 22:289–293.
200. Thomas, J. E., Schirger, A., Fealey, R. D., and Sheps, S. G. (1981): Orthostatic hypotension. *Mayo Clin. Proc.*, 56:117–125.

droxyamphetamine tests for diagnosis of postganglionic defects. *Am. J. Ophthalmol.*, 72:472–480.
202. Thompson, H. S., Newsome, D. A., and Loewenfeld, I. E. (1971): The fixed dilated pupil: Sudden iridoplegia or mydriatic drops? A simple diagnostic test. *Arch. Ophthalmol.*, 86:21–27.
203. Tobian, L. (1960): Physiology of the juxtaglomerull cells. *Ann. Intern. Med.*, 52:395–410.
204. Vander, A. J. (1967): Control of renin release. *Physiol. Rev.*, 47:359–382.
205. Vanderhaeghen, J. J., Perier, O., and Sternon, J. E. (1970): Pathological findings in idiopathic orthostatic hypotension. *Arch. Neurol.*, 22:207–214.
206. Wadia, N. H., and Swami, R. K. (1971): A new form of heredo-familial spinocerebellar degeneration with slow eye movements (nine families). *Brain*, 94:359–374.
207. Wagner, H. N., Jr. (1959): Orthostatic hypotension. *Bull. Johns Hopkins Hosp.*, 105:322–359.
208. Wagner, H. N., Jr., and Braunwald, E. (1956): The pressor effect of the antidiuretic principle of the posterior pituitary in orthostatic hypotension. *J. Clin. Invest.*, 35:1412–1418.
209. Wheeler, T., and Watkins, P. J. (1973): Cardiac denervation in diabetes. *Br. Med. J.*, 4:584–586.
210. Willis, T. (1664): *Cerebri anatome, cui accessit nervorum descriptio et usus.* Flesher, Londini.
211. Woodworth, J. A., Beckett, R. S., and Netsky, M. G. (1959): A composite of hereditary ataxias. *Arch. Intern. Med.*, 104:594–606.
212. Wooten, G. F., and Cardon, P. V. (1973): Plasma dopamine-beta-hydroxylase activity: Elevation in man during cold pressor test and exercise. *Arch. Neurol.*, 28:103–106.
213. Zanchetti, A., and Zoccolini, A. (1954): Autonomic hypothalamic outbursts elicited by cerebellar stimulation. *J. Neurophysiol.*, 17:475–483.
214. Ziegler, M. G., Lake, C. R., and Kopin, I. J. (1977): The sympathetic nervous system defect in primary orthostatic hypotension. *N. Engl. J. Med.*, 296:293–297.

The Olivopontocerebellar Atrophies, edited by R. C. Duvoisin and A. Plaitakis. Raven Press, New York © 1984.

The Pharmacology of Olivopontocerebellar Atrophy

Christopher G. Goetz, Caroline M. Tanner, and Harold L. Klawans

Department of Neurological Sciences, Rush Presbyterian St. Luke's Medical Center, Chicago, Illinois 60612

The pharmacology of olivopontocerebellar atrophy (OPCA) has not been extensively or systematically studied. Klawans and Zeitlin (6) reported a levodopa response in two patients with a clinical diagnosis of OPCA. Levodopa ameliorated parkinsonian bradykinesia, resting tremor, rigidity, and postural reflex compromise but had no marked effect on cerebellar intention tremor, titubation, and broad-based gait.

Since this early report, many investigators have studied pharmacologic characteristics of various groups of patients with cerebellar dysfunction but have not selectively focused on OPCA. In this chapter, we present a retrospective analysis of 24 patients with clinical OPCA (one with proven autopsy) from our patient population, with attention to differential drug effects on parkinsonian, cerebellar, and other motor features of OPCA.

PATIENTS AND METHODS

Fifteen men and nine women with a diagnosis of OPCA identified from the data base of the movement-disorder outpatient clinic of Rush Presbyterian St. Luke's Medical Center were studied. Patients who had the clinical features of parkinsonism and cerebellar or corticospinal dysfunction with or without other neurologic deficit or associated family histories were included in the study. Any patient with another identifiable etiology or with exposure to carbon monoxide, hypoxia, toxins, or drugs causing extrapyramidal or cerebellar syndromes was excluded.

The average age of symptom onset was 56 years, with a range of 40 to 64 years. Fourteen patients had a definite or suspected family history of similar neurologic disorders; seven reported families without neurologic disease; and three did not know their families well. The predominant clinical feature at disease onset was parkinsonian disability in 11 patients, cerebellar disability in 6, and a clinically mixed presentation in 7. Only two patients had prominent spasticity at the time of data collection. The mean disease duration was 10 years, with a range of 5 to 20 years; the mean duration of drug therapy was 9.8 years, with a range of 6 to 18 years.

TABLE 1. *Pharmacologic data on 22 patients with OPCA*

Drug	No. of patients	Global effect[a]	Specific feature helped[b]	Comment
Levodopa or levodopa–carbidopa	19	16++, 3n	B, R, P: 16/17 RT: 2/6	RT in 4 patients not helped; cerebellar features not helped
Amantadine	10	9+, 1n	B: 8/10 R: 6/10 P: 9/10 RT: 2/10	Cerebellar features not helped
Bromocriptine	5	1++, 3+, 1n	B, R, P, RT: 4/5	Cerebellar features not helped
Lergotrile	1	1+	B, R, P, RT: 1/1	Cerebellar features not helped
Central anticholinergic agents	2	2n	None	RT prominent in both patients not helped
Lecithin	6	6n	None	All patients found lecithin difficult to ingest
Propranolol	12	9++, 3n	IT: 9/12 A: 2/12	No change in parkinsonian features, including resting tremor
Baclofen	5	5n	None	Complaints of nonspecific global weakness

[a] ++, Marked improvement; +, improvement; n, no change.
[b] B, bradykinesia; R, rigidity; P, postural reflex compromise; RT, resting tremor; IT, intention tremor; A, ataxia; D, dysarthria; S, spasticity.

The entire medical record of each patient was reviewed. Disease progression and drug therapy were recorded with attention to the relative efficacy of any therapeutic regimen. Differential effects of each agent on parkinsonian, cerebellar, or other neurologic signs and symptoms were noted. Retrospective analyses were supplemented with patient interviews and neurologic examinations.

RESULTS

Dopaminergic Agents

Levodopa or levodopa/carbidopa combination had been used in 19 of the 24 patients, all of whom demonstrated parkinsonian features. These patients included all those whose earliest disability was extrapyramidal, plus eight patients with prominent cerebellar and/or corticospinal features who had accompanying parkinsonian signs. Sixteen patients showed definite improvement in regidity, akinesia, and postural reflex compromise with levodopa. Resting tremor improved in two patients; but in the remaining four, all with intention tremor as well, levodopa induced no change. Three patients showed minimal or no improvement on levodopa even when the dose reached 3 g/day or its equivalent in levodopa/carbidopa combination.

Amantadine (100–300 mg/day) was used alone in two patients and in combination with levodopa in eight. As in idiopathic Parkinson's disease, this agent was of mild to moderate benefit in 9 of 10 patients, specifically in the control of postural reflex problems. Direct-acting agonists, including bromocriptine (5 patients; dose range, 10–80 mg/day) and lergotrile (1 patient; 20 mg/day), were used as supplements to levodopa therapy. In all but one patient, the response to other dopaminergic agents was similar to that seen with levodopa. Hence those who responded to levodopa responded to amantadine and direct-acting agonists, whereas those with a poor levodopa response proved poor responders to the latter drugs. One prominent exception was a man who improved dramatically when bromocriptine (22.5 mg/day) was added to levodopa after he failed to show significant improvement on levodopa/carbidopa combination or amantadine in the past. This improvement in his parkinsonian disability was maintained for 2.5 years.

Cerebellar features, including slurred speech, intention tremor, dyssynergia, and broad-based ataxic gait, were not altered with dopaminergic therapy. Thirteen patients treated with dopaminergic agents suffered with gradually progressive signs of central dopaminergic side effects. These included chorea (10 patients), sleep disruption (7 patients), and hallucinations (5 patients). The onset of first signs of central dopaminergic toxicity averaged 2.3 years.

Other Agents

Various agents were used in an attempt to control other symptoms in these patients. Propranolol (20–140 mg/day), a beta-adrenergic antagonist, was used successfully in nine of 12 patients with prominent intention tremor. The gait and speech difficulties in these patients were not altered. Lecithin (phosphatidylcholine), a presumed dietary precursor of central acetylcholine, was tried in six patients (10 to 25 g/day pure phosphatidylcholine in the form of lethicon) with no significant benefit after 2 months. Anticholinergic drugs were used in two patients with prominent extrapyramidal signs but did not markedly change their disability. Baclofen, a γ-aminobutyric acid (GABA) analog, was tried in five patients, four with cerebellar features and one with spasticity; in all of them, there were complaints of global weakness and more difficulty walking. The drug was discontinued after a maximum trial of 2 months (30–40 mg/day).

DISCUSSION

Although OPCA appears to be a single neurodegenerative process, the correlative anatomy and pharmacology of the different clinical features could be distinct. Parkinsonism is thought to relate to underactivity of the dopaminergic system of the nigrostriatal pathway. In Parkinson's disease, there is selective degeneration of the substantia nigra, where dopamine is synthesized. Levodopa, the amino acid precursor of dopamine, is the standard therapy for Parkinson's disease. Similar nigral degeneration has been documented in some cases of OPCA (2,3). With this background, it is reasonable to attempt dopaminergic augmentation therapy in OPCA patients with significant parkinsonian signs. Nineteen patients in our series showed improvement when treated with either levodopa or other dopaminergic drugs. This included the one patient for whom autopsied material was available; in this case, there was clear depigmentation of the substantia nigra and associated atrophy of the cerebellar cortex, inferior olivary and dentate nuclei, and basis pontis. Also in this group were three patients who received pretreatment lumbar punctures for analysis of homovanillic acid (HVA), the central metabolite of dopamine. In all three, the HVA level was low and similar to that seen in traditional idiopathic Parkinson's disease, indicating that dopamine metabolism was reduced in these patients. Since cerebrospinal fluid HVA levels reflect predominantly the function of the nigrostriatal dopaminergic pathway, these pharmacologic data suggest that in at least some patients with OPCA, there is markedly reduced activity of this system (5).

All patients, however, did not improve on dopaminergic therapy. Resistance to medication can be seen late in idiopathic Parkinson's disease. When poor response initially is seen to levodopa, however, an alternative diagnosis, primary striatal degeneration or "postsynaptic" parkinsonism, is suggested (5). In such cases, where the nigrostriatal dopaminergic path is intact, additional dopaminergic augmentation therapy would not be expected to induce marked improvement. Three patients in our series showed little or no response to dopaminergic drugs, suggesting that their parkinsonian features did not significantly relate to presynaptic nigrostriatal dopaminergic underactivity. Lesions of the striatum itself and the pallium have been reported in OPCA. Such postsynaptic lesions similar to those of striatonigral degenerative parkinsonism could underlie the clinical features of parkinsonism in some OPCA patients.

Central dopaminergic side effects seen in this patient population were identical to those seen in Parkinson's disease patients treated with the same agents. The mean duration of levodopa therapy at the first sign of established chorea, sleep disruption, or hallucinations compares well with previous reports for parkinsonian patients (10). This finding suggests that such side effects are not selective for patients with isolated nigrostriatal degeneration and that the complications can be seen after dopaminergic drug therapy in a variety of degenerative conditions.

The only other report of pharmacologic manipulation of the dopaminergic system is the early report of patients treated with levodopa by Klawans and Zeitlin (5,6). These patients are included in the present series.

Propranolol was moderately successful in the control of intention tremor in our series. This agent has not been previously studied in OPCA but has been used to treat essential tremor and is thought to have both central and peripheral effects (11). We found ataxia and titubation to be poorly controlled by propranolol, a finding that parallels our clinical experience with essential tremor when it is associated with titubation or gait dysfunction. The neurotransmitter pharmacology controlling midline cerebellar function may differ from that affecting extremity coordination.

Shimamoto et al. (9) attempted to alter cerebellar noradrenergic activity in patients with OPCA by using phthalazinol, an agent reported to increase cyclic AMP by inhibiting its phosphodiesterase. Their drug trial of four patients with clinical OPCA was based on the early identification by Hoffer et al. (4) of noradrenergic-containing afferent axons that synapse with and normally inhibit Purkinje cells. The authors hypothesized that cerebellar ataxia could result from primary cell death and/or lack of sufficient production of intracellular cyclic AMP in the cerebellum; thus they attempted to augment cyclic AMP. Phthalazinol improved speech, coordination, and ataxia in all patients; in addition, it improved rigidity in one, spastic bladder in another, and excessive salivation in the remaining two. This study has not been expanded but was the first to report an improvement in cerebellar, extrapyramidal, and other motor features with a single drug.

Cholinergic cerebellar pathways have been identified and appear to involve at least the mossy fibers (7). Barbeau (1) used lecithin in treating patients with established spinocerebellar disease and found improvement in speech and coordination in those with Friedreich's ataxia. Our small series of six OPCA patients with prominent cerebellar features receiving lecithin showed no clinical change with this therapy. The unpleasant weight gain associated with the therapy and the lack of improvement prompted us to abandon this medication.

Perry et al. (8) studied neurochemical alterations in autopsied brain from two patients with dominantly inherited OPCA. Aspartate and GABA levels in the cerebellar cortex and dentate nucleus were reduced, whereas the taurine content was elevated. Treatment with the GABA analog baclofen did not benefit our patients, two of whom showed evidence of dominant inheritance. Other experience with drugs altering GABA systems had not been reported. The possibility that dietary aspartate supplementation might ameliorate symptoms in these patients has not yet been investigated.

ACKNOWLEDGMENTS

This work was supported in part by grants from the United Parkinson Foundation and the Boothroyd Foundation, Chicago, Illinois. CGG is the recipient of a NINCDS Teacher/Investigator Award.

REFERENCES

1. Barbeau, A. (1979): Lecithin in movement disorders. In: *Nutrition and the Brain, Vol. 5*, edited by A. Barbeau, J. H. Growon, and R. J. Wurtman, pp. 263–272. Raven Press, New York.
2. Critchley, M., and Greenfield, J. G. (1948): Olivopontocerebellar atrophy. *Brain*, 71:343–363.
3. Greenfield, J. G., and Bosanquet, F. D. (1953): The brainstem lesions in parkinsonism. *J. Neurol. Neurosurg. Psychiatry*, 16:213–226.
4. Hoffer, B. J., Siggins, G. R., Oliver, A. P., and Bloom, F. E. (1972): Cyclic AMP-mediated adrenergic synapses to cerebellar Purkinje cells. In: *Advances in Cyclic Nucleotide Research, Vol. 1*, edited by P. Greengard and G. A. Robison, p. 411. Raven Press, New York.
5. Klawans, H. L. (1973): *Pharmacology of Extrapyramidal Movement Disorders*. Karger, Basel.

6. Klawans, H. L., and Zeitlin, E. (1971): Levodopa in parkinsonism associated with cerebellar dysfunction (probable olivoponto cerebellar degeneration). *J. Neurol. Nerurosurg. Psychiatry*, 34:14–19.
7. McGeer, P. L., Eccles, J. C., and McGeer, E. G. (1980): *Molecular Neurology of the Mammalian Brain*. Plenum, New York.
8. Perry, T. L., Currier, R. D., Hansen, S., and MacLean, J. (1977): Aspartate-taurine imbalance in dominantly inherited olivopontocerebellar atrophy. *Neurology*, 27:257–261.
9. Shimamoto, T., Murase, H., and Numans, F. (1976): Treatment of senile dementia and cerebellar disorders with phthalazinol. *Mech. Ageing Dev.*, 5:241–250.
10. Weiner, W. J., and Bergen, D. (1977): Prevention of side effects of levodopa. In: *Clinical Neuropharmacology, Vol. 2*, edited by H. L., Klawans, pp. 1–24. Raven Press, New York.
11. Young, R. R., and Shahani, B. T. (1979): Pharmacology of tremor. In: *Clinical Neuropharmacology, Vol. 4*, edited by H. L. Klawans, pp. 139–156. Raven Press, New York.

The Olivopontocerebellar Atrophies, edited by
R.C. Duvoisin and A. Plaitakis. Raven Press,
New York © 1984.

A Variety of Olivopontocerebellar Atrophy Distinguished by Slow Eye Movements and Peripheral Neuropathy

N. H. Wadia

J. J. Group of Hospitals and Grant Medical College, Byculla, Bombay 400 008; and Jaslok Hospital and Research Centre, Bombay 400 026, India

Although in 1933, Mass and Scherer (24) described an autopsy-proven sporadic case of olivopontocerebellar atrophy (OPCA) with progressive ataxia and slow voluntary eye movements without limitation in their range, it was Wadia and Swami (41) in 1971 who first drew attention to the type-specificity, hereditary nature, and frequency of this disease. They described 9 Indian families and reported that it appeared to be the most common heredofamilial spinocerebellar degeneration in India. Autosomal dominant heredity was clearly established in the majority of the 9 families; autopsy later demonstrated OPCA (43), and electromyography and sural nerve biopsy showed degeneration also in the peripheral nervous system (41–46). Although, in the earlier cases, it was not always clinically possible to distinguish that the slowing was restricted to the saccadic movements, electrooculographic recording later clearly demonstrated this feature (21). Sigwald et al. (36,37), Garcin and Man (10), and Kini and Venugopal (16) mention a similar oculomotor disorder in familial cerebellar ataxia, but oculometric examinations were not done. Autopsy of 1 of the 3 affected sisters in the family studied by Sigwald et al. showed OPCA. These and subsequent studies attest to the global prevalence of this disorder and its increasing recognition in India. The account here concerns the data gathered since the first family, still under review, was seen in 1962. Some of the findings have been previously published (21,41–45).

CLINICAL FEATURES

The clinical features at initial examination of 37 patients from 23 Indian families are summarized in Fig. 1. Twenty-seven patients have been seen on follow-up examination—some over a decade. The onset of the disease was most often in the third decade (average 27 years); the earliest occurring at 7 years and the latest at 51 years of age (Fig. 2). Cerebellar and oculomotor disorders were seen in every patient.

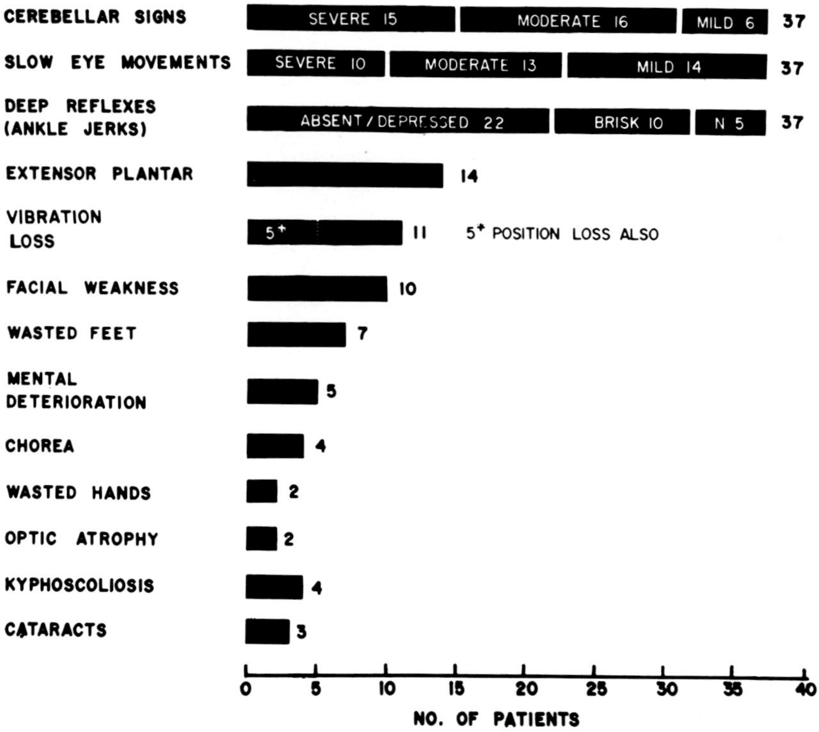

FIG. 1. Clinical features at initial examination.

Cerebellar Disorder

The symptoms were exclusively related to cerebellar disorders. Ataxia followed by an essentially symmetrical incoordination of limbs, intention tremor, titubation, and dysarthria were seen. There was no nystagmus. The disability worsened causing invalidism on an average of 8 years, with some patients mildly affected after 10 years and others disabled in 2 years. Ten died within a span of 7 to 23 years (average 13 years). The severity of disability was unrelated to the age of onset.

Ocular Disorder

There were no ocular symptoms even at the advanced stages of the disease. However, head jerking was occasionally noticed, and this helped to identify affected individuals. The disorder began with slowing of the horizontal, random, and command eye movements (saccades) through their full range, which was subtle enough to be missed by an uninformed examiner. A staring expression, owing to the loss of the small fixation saccades, and a slight compensatory jerk of the head appeared. Gradually the slowing became more obvious in all directions and reached a stage, often after years, of some limitation in their terminal range, which in combination

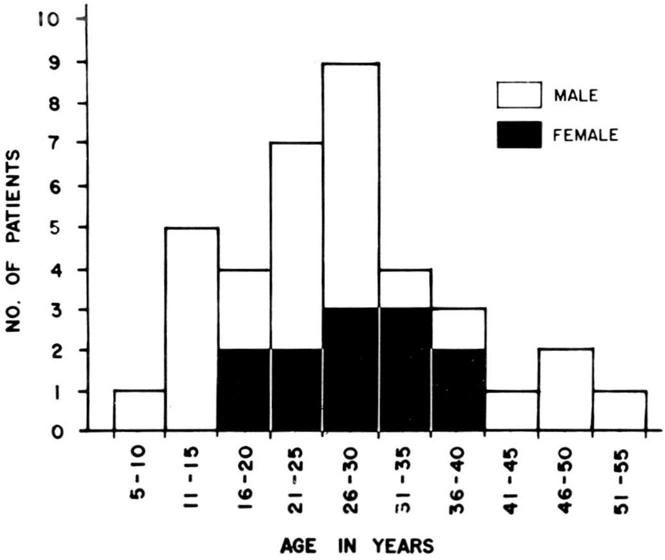

FIG. 2. Age at onset of OPCA with slow eye movements.

with a fixed expression gave the appearance of peripheral ophthalmoplegia. Yet the eyes could be moved fully by the doll's eye maneuvre, rapid rotation, and caloric stimulation. By contrast, there was no slowing of pursuit movements until the advanced stages of the disease, and no ptosis, squint, or pupillary abnormality was seen. Caloric stimulation early on caused horizontal gaze deviation with a slow saccade, but this later disappeared. Similarly, optokinetic nystagmus was either abnormal or absent.

The patient used compensatory head movements for looking at objects. The earliest movement was a sudden jerk of the head with blinking. As the eyes slowed further, the head and neck quickly turned toward the object, and the eyes were then seen to lock slowly on the target. As the eyes became more fixed, the patient was seen to jerk the neck adversely and tilt the face away from the object of gaze, in order to reflexly turn the eyes to the object. The ataxia and the ophthalmoplegia worsened simultaneously, but generally the severity of the ocular disorder trailed behind the cerebellar ataxia.

Other signs were less constant. Changes in deep reflexes, either depressed or exaggerated, were not related to the severity or the duration of the disease. The general tendency was for the reflexes to become depressed in time. Except in 6 patients, the knee and ankle jerks showed the same response; in 5, the ankle jerk was more depressed than the knee. Extensor plantar responses and impairment of vibration and postural sensibility appeared at all stages of the disease. Slight distal wasting and weakness appeared only in the severely affected patients. Mild bilateral facial weakness was occasionally observed. Chorea was seen in 4 severely affected patients, 2 of whom belonged to 1 family. Mild mental deterioration came late and was often mixed with depression. It was difficult to date the asymptomatic optic atrophy in the 2 severely affected patients. Kyphoscoliosis and cataracts were rarely found.

Genetic Data

Sixty members (38 males and 22 females) of 23 families were considered to be affected; 37 of these (25 males and 12 females) were examined. Ten patients died; 4 members of 3 families were autopsied. Of the 23 not examined by us, 17 were already deceased. Twenty-four members of these families were found to be normal. Twelve pedigrees published earlier are representative of these data (41,42).

More than 1 member was affected in 13 families. Ten families showed autosomal dominant inheritance (Figs. 3a,3c). The disease could be traced for 2 generations in 7 families, 3 generations in 2 families, and 4 generations in 1 family. Either parent of the propositus was affected, in equal numbers, in these families. Nearly 50% of members above the age of 10 years in the affected sibships were diseased.

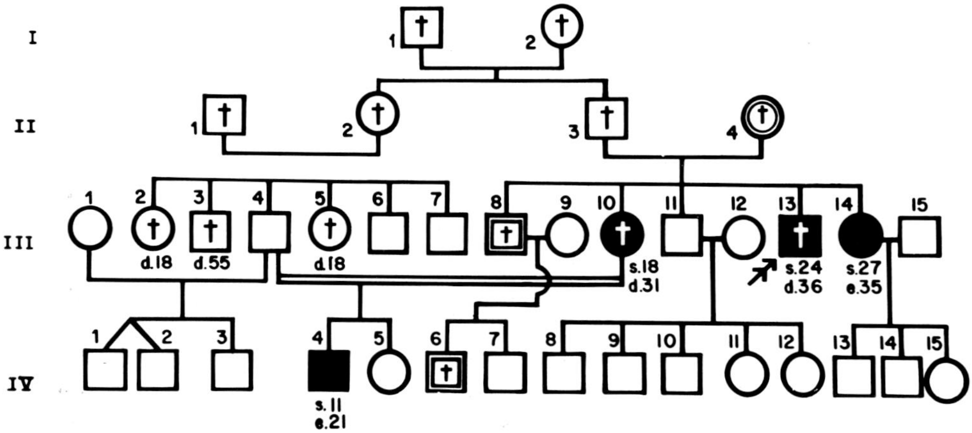

Fig. 3a. Pedigree of P.S.J. family with autopsied propositus.

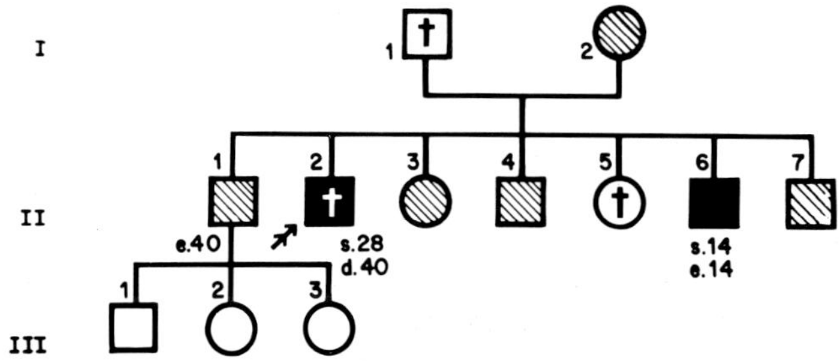

Fig. 3b. Pedigree of S.D.H. family with autopsied propositus.

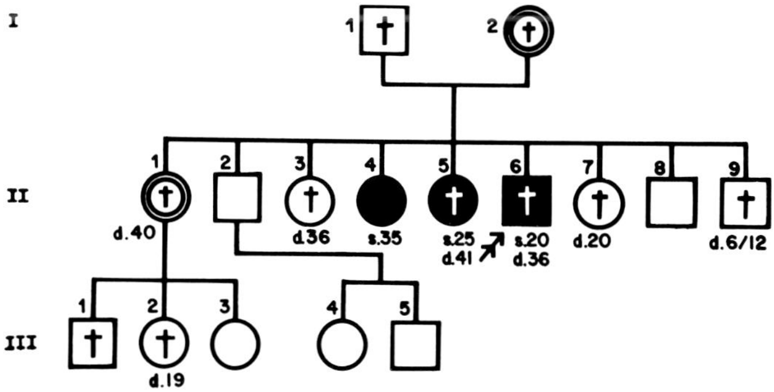

Fig. 3c. Pedigree of A.B. family with autopsied propositus.

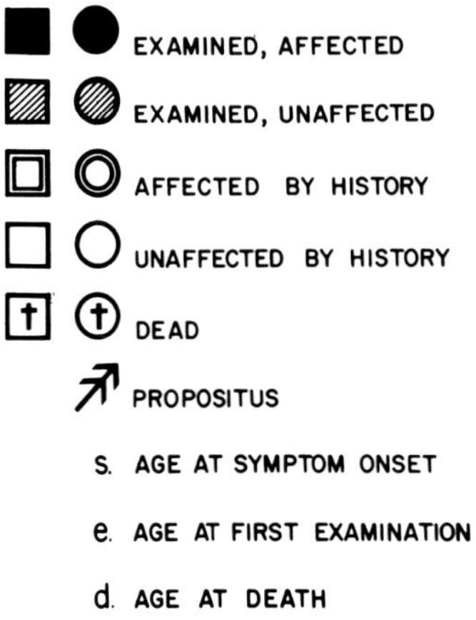

Fig. 3d. Key to symbols used in Figs. 3a to 3c.

In each of the other 3 families of nonconsanguineous parents, 2 siblings were affected.

In 2 of these families there were 4 and 7 unaffected sibs, and so far as could be ascertained, the parents had either remained unaffected or died at an age beyond the maximum age of onset (51 years) reported here. An autosomal recessive mode of inheritance cannot be excluded, despite absence of parental consanguinity (Fig. 3b), especially since we have not so far observed formes frustes of this disease, even in our clearly autosomal dominant families. To determine the pattern of inheritance will require greater follow-up of the next generation of these families. The pattern of inheritance was uncertain in the third family, since the parents were not examined and their ages were unknown.

In the remaining 10 families only the propositus was known to be affected. In many of these families, there were several younger siblings, and the parental age or cause of death could not be ascertained. Though new mutation is suggested, we cannot be certain of this. It thus appears that autosomal dominance is the common mode of inheritance, and genetic heterogeneity is not clearly established for the whole group.

Geographic and Ethnic Distribution

Among our patients were those whose origin was from several different states of India and Sindh (now in Pakistan). Eighteen Hindu, 3 Muslim, and 2 Catholic families were seen. These communities form the bulk of the population of India.

INVESTIGATIONS

Electroencephalography, electrocardiography, urinary amino acid testing, and electromyography (EMG) and biopsy of ocular muscles have revealed no significant abnormality. Pneumoencephalography has shown some generalized ventricular dilatation, a large cisterna magna, cerebellar atrophy, and slight cerebral cortical atrophy (41–43).

Electrooculographic examination has confirmed the reduced velocity of the saccade to a varying degree, in keeping with the clinical state (21,43); in the advanced cases it was reduced to 5°/sec. The fastest saccade in the patients was still only 30°/sec, as opposed to 150°/sec in normal controls for similar magnitude of step input. The smooth pursuit movement was at the same velocity as in controls, at least up to a target speed of 20°/sec (Fig. 4). Electromyographic studies of limb muscles showed evidence of denervation in 11 of 14 patients examined. The distal muscles were more affected. Giant motor units were recorded in 8 patients. Motor conduction velocities were normal. Abnormal sensory action potentials (SAP) were found in 13 patients. On clinical appraisal 11 of these 14 patients had sluggish or absent deep reflexes, although they had no remarkable wasting or paralysis. Seven had, in addition, proprioceptive sensory loss. Three patients had exaggerated deep

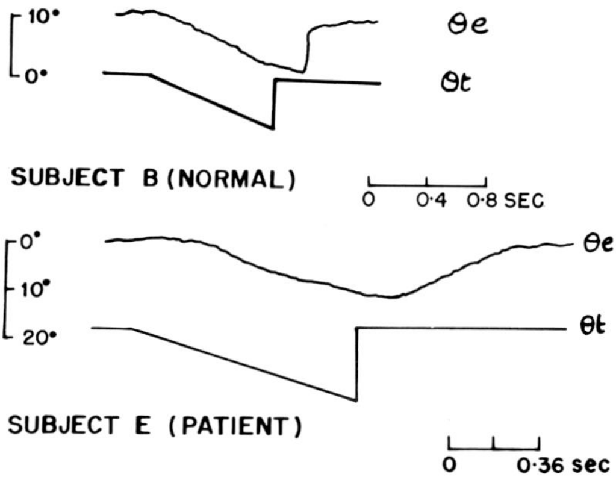

FIG. 4. Eye movement response to ramp step input. Note the similarity in the smooth pursuit (ramp) and the marked difference in the saccadic (step) response in patient and control.

reflexes, especially in the lower limbs, and two of them also had proprioceptive loss. Electromyography revealed denervation in one and abnormal SAP in both. That left one with exaggerated reflexes but no abnormality on EMG.

It is evident that electrophysiological studies indicated lower motor and sensory neuron lesions in 13 of the 14 patients examined. Sural nerve biopsies in 4 patients showed axonal degeneration, predominantly of the large myelinated fibers at an early stage and of practically all fibers at an advanced stage of the disease (Figs. 5a–5c). The sum of EMG and biopsy evidence suggests degeneration of the anterior horn and posterior root ganglion cells, with "dying-back" motor and sensory neuronopathy. Some of these data have already been recorded (45), and more details are soon to be published elsewhere (46).

Pathological Examination and Clinicopathological Correlation

Four autopsy examinations in 3 families have been made; information from one of these has already been reported (43). Histological examination is available in 3 so far. Short case histories of the autopsied propositus are given below; pertinent information is summarized in Tables 1 and 2, and in Figs. 6 to 10.

1. *P.S.J. (Fig. 3a, III, 13)*: The age of onset for this male was 24 years [detailed history recorded earlier (43)]. At age 31, he showed remarkable cerebellar ataxia, dysarthria, slow but full range eye movements without nystagmus, head jerking, absent deep reflexes, bilateral facial weakness, and plantar flexors. ECG, EEG, and CSF were all normal. Electromyography (of face and limb muscles) showed denervation with giant units in some muscles. Spinal motor nerve conduction velocity was normal. A gastrocnemius biopsy showed denervation atrophy. Five years later, the patient was bedridden with gross ataxia, head titubation, vibration loss, distal wasting of limbs, spasticity at the knees, urinary incontinence, mental deterioration, and inability to swallow. The eyes were almost immobile but could be moved reflexly by the doll's eye maneuvre and caloric stimulation, but with no saccadic response. Optokinetic nystagmus was absent; cataracts had appeared. Death occurred 12 years after onset. Inheritance was autosomal dominant.

2. *S.D.H. (Fig. 3b, II, 2)*: This 33-year-old male presented with progressive imbalance, dysarthria, and clumsiness of the hands of 5 years' duration. On examination there was severe limb and trunk ataxia, slow saccades on random and reflex (cold caloric and rotation) eye movements, absence of optokinetic nystagmus, depressed upper limb reflexes, brisk knee and normal ankle jerks, plantars flexor, and fasciculations in the lower limbs. The patient died 7 years later with gross ataxia, vibration loss, peripheral wasting, areflexia, and very slow eye movements. Inheritance was uncertain, possibly recessive.

3. *A.B. (Fig. 3c, II, 6)*: This 25-year-old male presented with imbalance on walking, slurred speech and difficulty in writing of 5 years' duration. Severe cerebellar ataxia, staccato dysarthria, mild bilateral facial weakness, and absent deep reflexes were noted. The plantar reflexes were flexor. There was no nystagmus,

TABLE 1. *Histological examination*[a]

Site	Patient		
	P.S.J.	S.D.H	A.B.
Cerebral hemispheres			
Cerebrum (especially frontal)	+ +	(+)	N
Hippocampus, thalamus	N	N	N
Hypothalamus, striatum	N	N	N
Pallidum, amygdala	N	N	N
Midbrain			
Substantia nigra	N	+ + +	+ + +
Red nucleus, III–IV nuclei	N	N	N
Pyramidal tract	N	N	N
Pons			
Nuclei pontis	+ + +	+ +	+ + +
Transverse pontine fibers	+ + +	+ +	+ + +
Middle cerebellar peduncle	+ + +	—	+ + +
V, VI, VII, VIII Nuclei	N	N	N
Medial longitudinal bundle	N	—	N
PPRF (adjacent to VI nucleus)	—	—	N
Pyramidal tract	N	N	N
Medulla			
Inferior olive, olivary fibers	+ + +	+ + +	+ + +
Descending trigeminal tract	+ + +	—	(+)
Fasciculus solitarius	—	—	(+)
Medial leminiscus	—	—	(+)
Pyramids	N	N	N
IX, X, XII Nuclei	N	N	N
Cerebellum			
Molecular layer	+	N	N
Purkinje cell layer	+ + +	+ + +	+ + +
Granular layer	+ +	+	+ +
Central white matter	+ + +	+ + +	+ + +
Dentate nucleus	+ +	+	N
Superior cerebellar peduncle	+	—	N
Spinal cord			
Posterior columns	+ +	N	+ + +
Lateral and anterior columns	N	N	N
Clarke's column	N	N	N
Anterior horn cells			
Cervical	+ +	N	(+)
Thoracic	+ +	+	(+)
Lumbar	+ + +	N	(+)
Posterior roots	—	+	+ + +
Sural nerve biopsy	—	—	+ + +

[a] +, Slight degeneration/demyelination; + +, moderate degeneration; + + +, severe degeneration; (+), questionable change; N, normal; —, unreported.

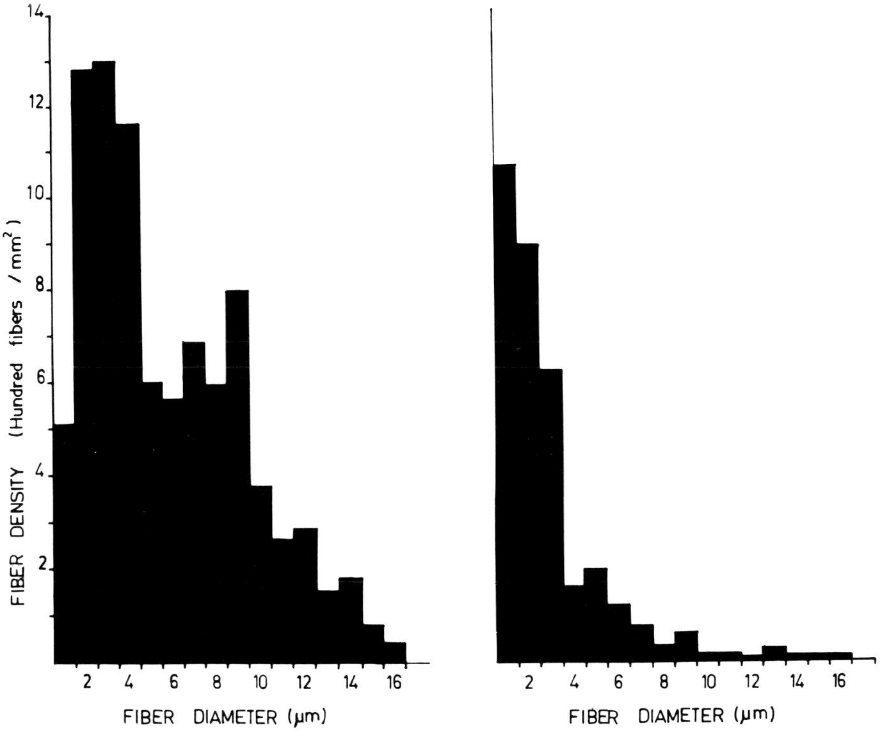

FIG. 5a. Histogram of fiber-diameter distribution of myelinated fibers in sural nerve of: *(left)* control subject (fiber density, 8845/mm^2) and *(right)* patient A.B. (fiber density, 3785/mm^2). Note gross fall out of fibers.

and random and reflex saccadic eye movements were slow. Blinking and head jerking movements were also observed. Optokinetic nystagmus was absent. EMG showed chronic partial denervation of limb muscles with normal nerve conduction velocity; sensory action potentials were absent in the ulnar, median, and both sural nerves. A sural nerve biopsy showed axonal degeneration and severe fallout of all fibers, especially the large myelinated ones (Figs. 5a and 5b). EMG of ocular muscles, EEG, ECG, and CSF were all normal.

Seven years later the patient was bedridden and incontinent of urine. Vibration and position sense were lost in the lower limbs. There was some spasticity at the knees, the plantar reflexes were extensor; and deep tendon reflexes were absent. Bilateral cataracts were present. EMG showed more extensive denervation and evidence of collateral sprouting. The motor conduction velocity remained normal; SAPs were absent. The patient died 16 years after onset. One sister (Fig. 3c, II, 5) died very recently, 16 years after onset of an exactly similar disease; her brain showed the gross changes of olivopontocerebellar atrophy. The pattern of inheritance was autosomal dominant.

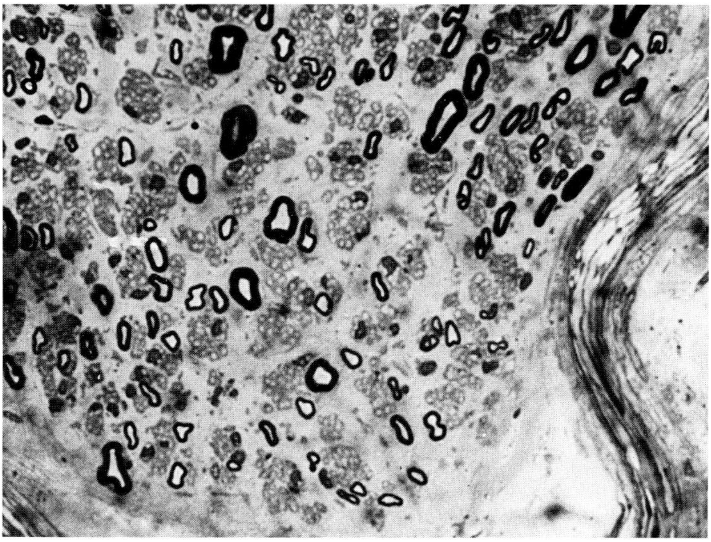

FIG. 5b. Semithin section of sural nerve of patient A.B. showing gross fall out of myelinated fibers (toluidene blue, ×530).

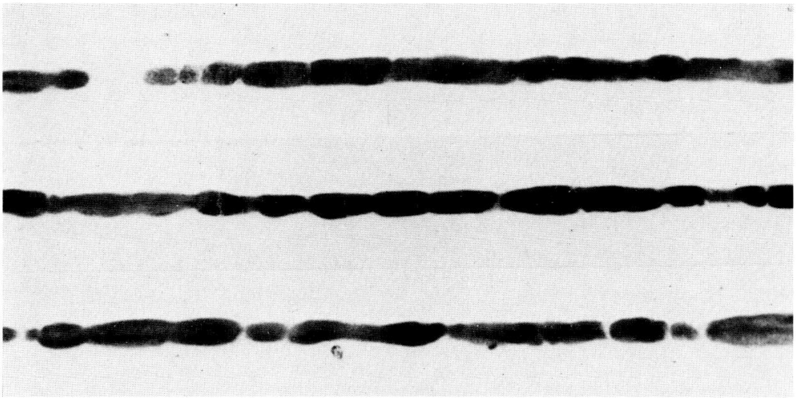

FIG. 5c. Portions of teased fiber from another patient showing axonal degeneration (osmium tetroxide).

Pathological Findings

Gross examination of all 4 brains showed severe olivopontocerebellar (Fig. 6) and mild cerebral atrophy with ventricular dilatation. The brain weight was considerably reduced. Histology revealed severe atrophy of the basis pontis and cerebellar white matter (Figs. 7 and 8) (Table 1). The Purkinje cell loss was more remarkable than that of the granular layer, and in patient A.B. where the observation

TABLE 2. *Clinicopathological findings of autopsied cases*

	Mass and Scherer (24)	Sigwald et al. (36,37)		Sears et al. (33)	Koeppen and Hans (18)[b]	Koeppen et al. (19)[b]		N. H. Wadia (Unpublished data), Case 1	Wadia (43)	
		Case 1	Case 2			Case II,2	Case III,3		Case 2	Case 3
Clinical finding[a]										
Sex	F	F	F	*b*	M	F	F	M	M	M
Age at death (yr)	38	84	82	–	61	59	35	37	40	36
Cerebellar ataxia	+	+	+	+	+	+	+	+	+	+
Slow saccade	+	+	–	+	+	+	–	+	+	+
Involuntary movements	–	–	–	–	+	+	–	–	–	–
Dementia	–	–	–	+	–	+	+	+	–	–
Posterior column loss	–	+	+	–	–	+	+	+	+	+
Absent deep reflexes	+	+	+	–	–	+	+	+	+	+
Lower motor neuron lesions	–	+	+	–	+	–	–	+	+	+
Extensor plantar response	+	±	–	–	–	+	+	–	–	+
Site of cell or fiber loss[a]										
Olives, pontine-nuclei, cerebellar cortex	+	+		+	+	+	+	+	+	+
Dentate	–	–	+	–	+	–	–	+	+	–
Substantia nigra	–	+	±	+	–	+	+	–	+	+
Posterior columns	+	+	+	–	+	+	+	+	–	+
Anterior horn cells	–	+	+	–	–	+	+	+	–	±
Lateral columns	–	–	–	–	–	–	–	–	–	–

[a]Present (+); absent or unreported (–); doubtful (±).
[b]Review of records and autopsy.

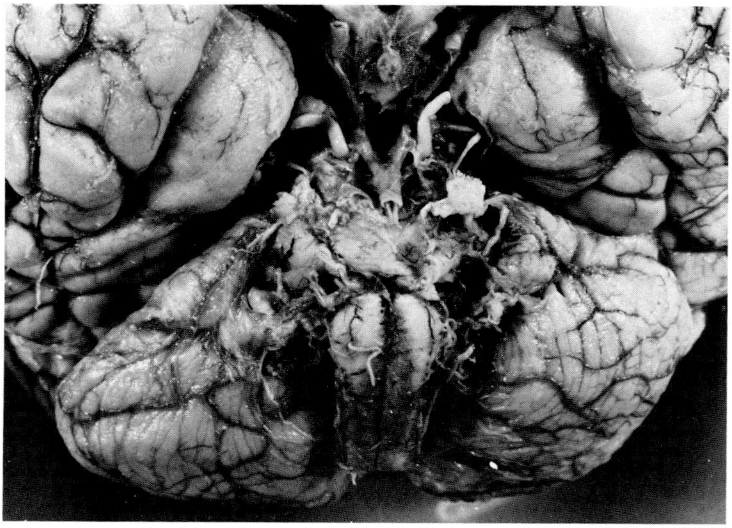

FIG. 6. Brain of patient A.B. showing remarkable atrophy of cerebellum and pons. The olives are not clearly seen.

was specifically made, the vermis was more affected than the hemispheres while the flocculus was relatively spared (Fig. 8b). The additional degeneration of the substantia nigra (Fig. 9), the dentate nucleus, the frontal cortex, and the anterior horn cells was variable and occurred in different combinations. Unfortunately, insufficient examination of the posterior root ganglia was made; however, the remarkable degeneration of the posterior columns and atrophy of posterior roots gave indirect evidence of degeneration of these neurons. In A.B., a gross degeneration of the posterior columns throughout the cord (Fig. 10), a devastating loss of posterior root fibers, and a severe fallout of myelinated fibers of the sural nerve suggest a primary degeneration of the posterior ganglion neurons, with dying-back degeneration of their central and peripheral axons. The spinocerebellar and pyramidal tracts, the oculomotor nuclei, and the medial longitudinal fasciculus were intact.

Clinicopathological Correlation

The areflexia seems to have resulted from degeneration of the posterior root ganglia rather than from loss of anterior horn neurons. The more extensive information gathered by EMG and sural nerve biopsies of other patients brings this out more clearly. The autopsies, however, failed to explain the terminal spasticity at the knees and bulbar palsy in case 1; the wasting of limbs, areflexia, and absent proprioceptive sensibility in case 2, and the terminal lower limb spasticity in case 3. Nor did they show the lesion or lesions responsible for the slow eye movements.

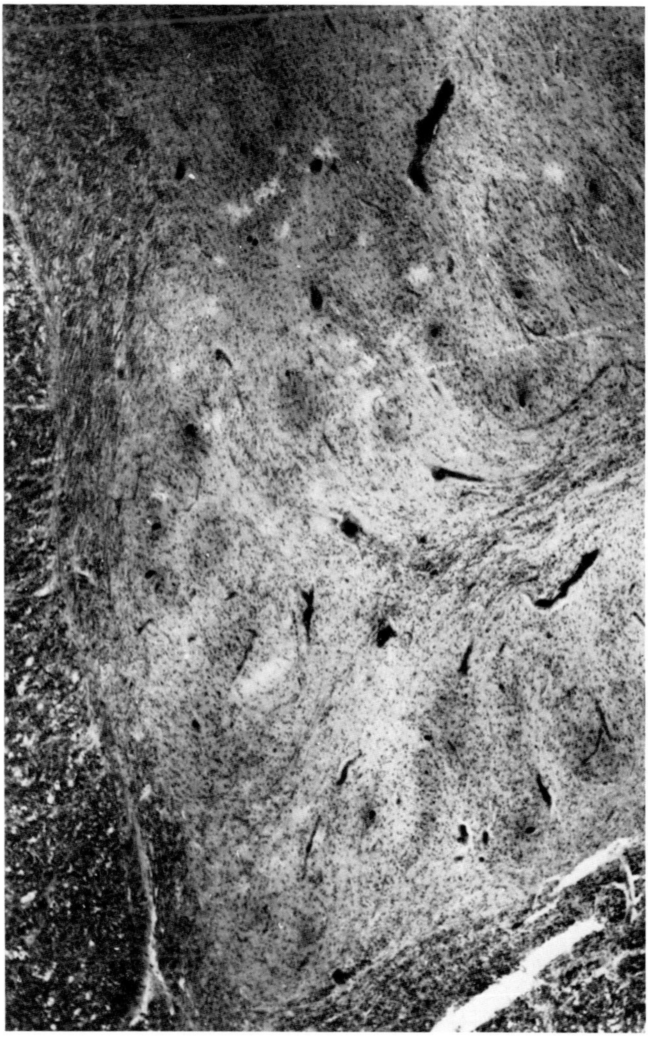

FIG. 7. Section through the olive showing loss of nerve cells and central myelin (Klüver-Barrera, ×60).

The degenerative changes described are not different from those generally seen in other varieties of OPCA with normal eye movements. Until an additional degenerative lesion in a specific set of neurons concerned with oculomotor function is shown in this group of patients, the clinicopathological correlation regarding this feature will remain speculative. Finally, it is notable that severe degeneration of the substantia nigra in 2 patients was not reflected by parkinsonian symptoms during life.

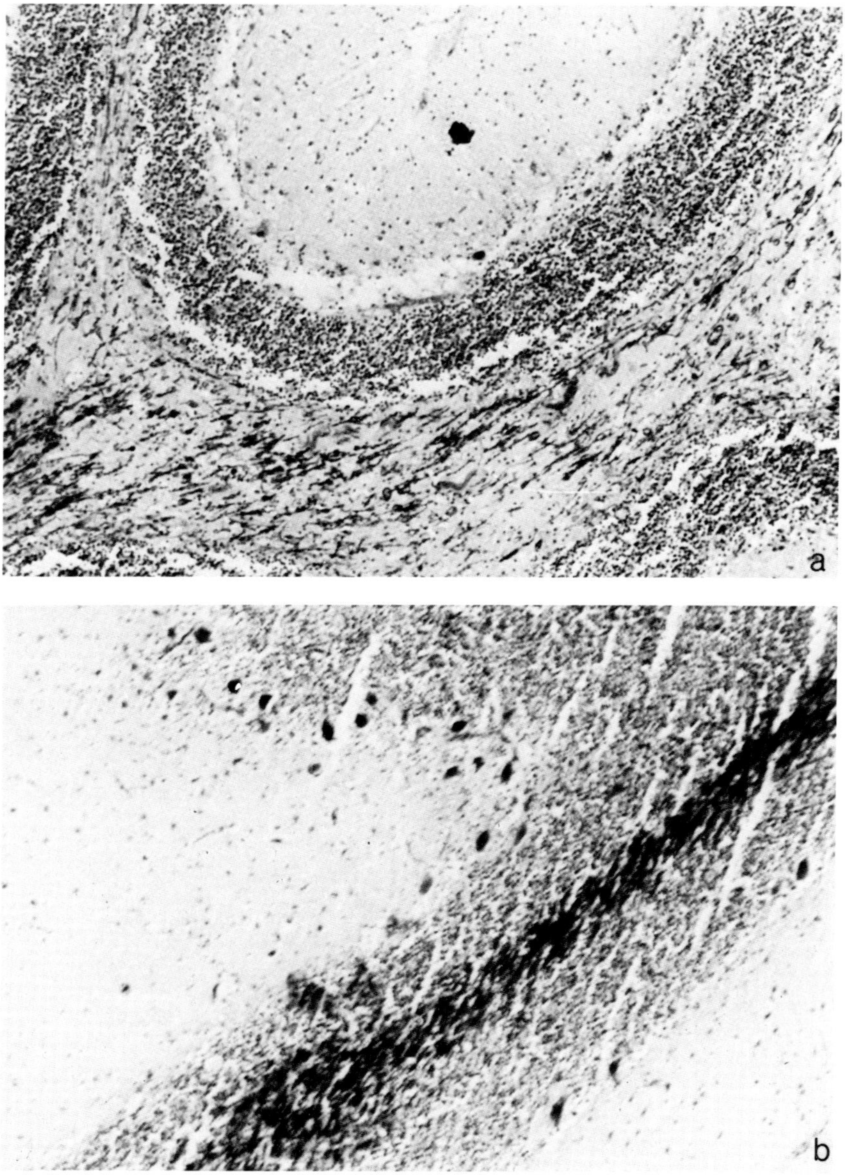

FIG. 8a: Section through cerebellum showing severe loss of Purkinje cells and of central myelin (Klüver-Barrera, × 126). **b:** Section of nearby flocculus showing relative preservation of Purkinje cells and of central myelin (Klüver-Barrera, × 126).

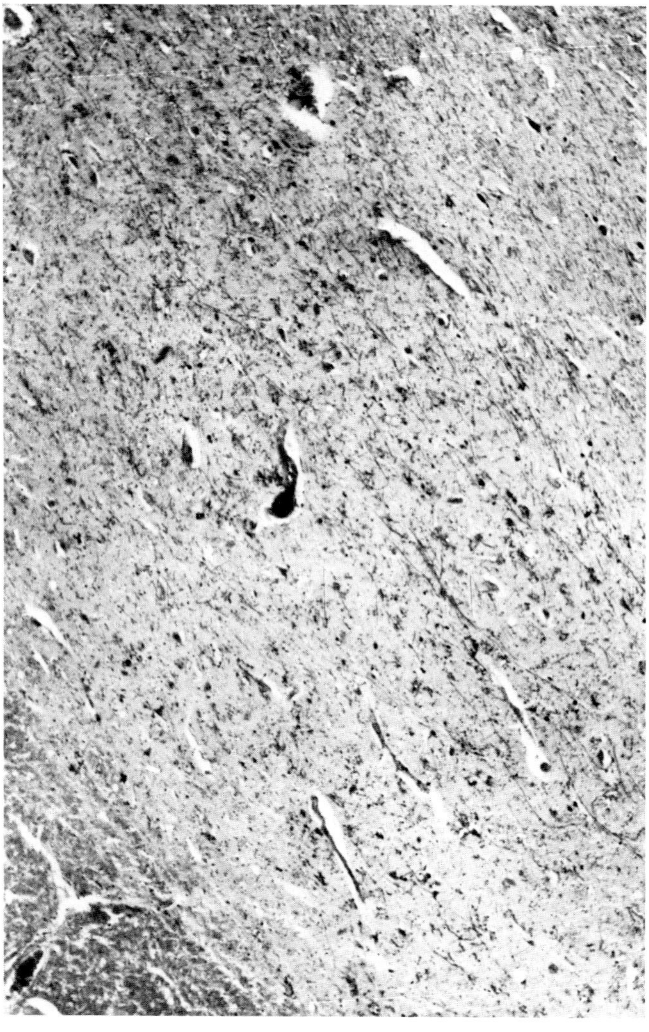

FIG. 9. Substantia nigra depleted of large pigmented cells (Klüver-Barrera, ×60).

SURVEY OF AVAILABLE LITERATURE

Case Reports

Patients Studied at Autopsy (Table 3)

Germany. Family of Mass and Scherer (24)

A German female aged 33 years, developed progressive imbalance, dysarthria and poor memory. She was diagnosed 2 years later as having multiple sclerosis. Five years later, severe symmetrical cerebellar ataxia, absent tendon reflexes and

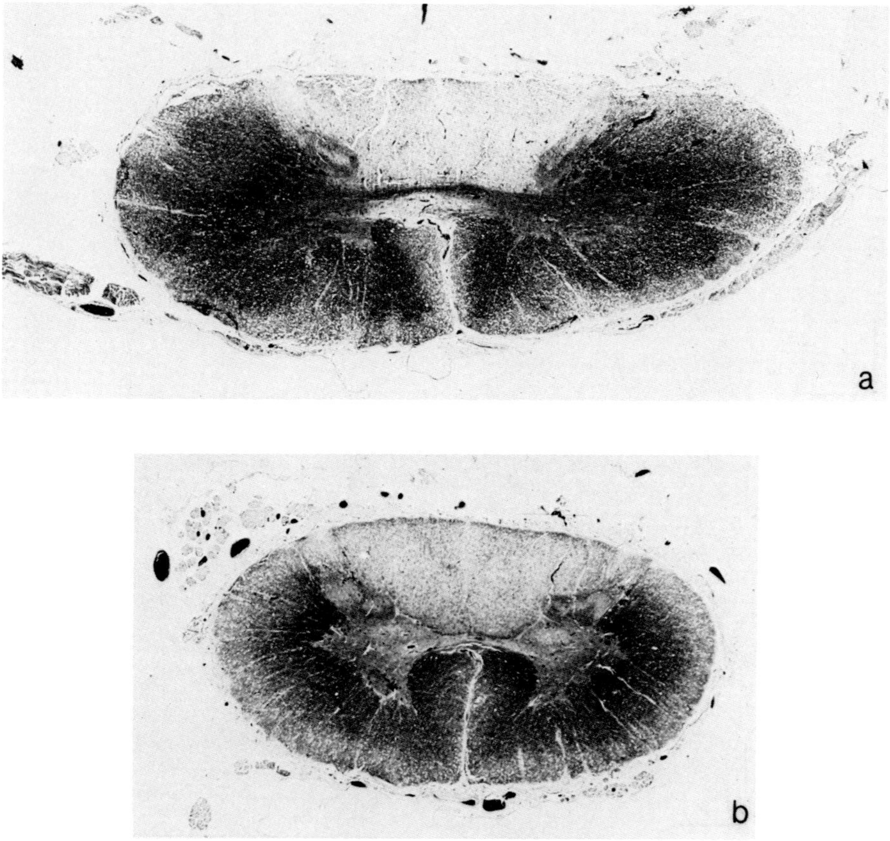

FIG. 10. Myelin stained sections of lower cervical **(a)** and lumbar **(b)** spinal cord showing gross degeneration of the posterior columns.

plantar extensors were noted. "Eye movements in all directions full but slow, when the patient spontaneously or on command looked to one side, or when following a moving object or on converging". There was no nystagmus. Caloric stimulation and rotation caused deviation of the eyes to one side without nystagmus. Borderline temporal pallor of the optic discs and definite narrowing of the visual fields was observed. The patient worsened and died five years later. Autopsy revealed degeneration of the olivary, pontine, Purkinje, granular, globosus, and emboliformis neurons. The dentate nucleus and substantia nigra were preserved. Severe demyelination of the posterior columns and roots, but no degeneration of anterior horn cells was noted. No other member of the family were affected.

France. Family of Sigwald et al. (36,37)

A French woman developed progressive ataxia at the age of 73 years. Her last examination 2 years before death at 84 years showed remarkable cerebellar ataxia

TABLE 3. *Survey of literature*

Country	Reference	Families	Members examined and affected	History of similar illness of other members[b]
Canada	Sharpe (34)	2	3	—
England	Oppenheimer (27, 28)	1	2 (1[a])	—
France	Cambier et al. (7)	1	1	—
	Sigwald et al. (36, 37)	1	2[a]	1
Germany	Mass and Scherer (24)	1	1[a]	—
India	Kini and Venugopal (16)	1	2	3
	N. H. Wadia (Unpublished up-to-date data)	24	32 (4[a])	23
	R. S. Wadia et al. (47)	5	9	7
Italy	Avanzini et al. (2)	1	1	—
Japan	Ozawa et al. (29)	3	4	—
Scotland	Koeppen et al. (19)	1	4 (2[a])	—
Taiwan	Lai and Hung (22)	1	1	—
U.S.A.	Koeppen and Hans (18)	1	9 (1[a])	—
	Murphy and Goldblatt (26)	1	Several	—
	Sears et al. (33)	1	3[a]	—
	Singh et al. (35)	1	1	3
	Starkman et al. (39)	1	17	—
	Zee et al. (49, 50)	2	2	1

[a]Autopsy proven.
[b](—) Not recorded.

with wasting, absent deep tendon reflexes, and loss of vibration and postural sense in the lower limbs. Babinski's sign was doubtful. Voluntary and reflex eye movements were slow. Autopsy showed OPCA, with degeneration of the substantia nigra and locus ceruleus (with Lewy bodies). There was also degeneration of the posterior columns of the spinal cord, anterior horn cells, and Clarke's columns. Her sister, who died at the age of 82, had developed a very similar disorder at the age of 71 years except that her ocular movements were not slow. Autopsy examination of the brain showed degeneration of the dentate nuclei with sparing of the cerebellar cortex, nuclei pontis, and olives. A third sister reportedly had progressive cerebellar ataxia, but details were not available. Genetic inheritance was not discussed.

United States. Family of Sears et al. (33)

Three members of an American family of unrecorded ancestry with slow eye movements and olivopontocerebellar atrophy were examined. "Saccadic eye movements completely absent with voluntary, optokinetic or caloric stimulation; observations confirmed by electronystagmography" (33). Dementia starting with impairment of recent memory progressed to a vegetative state. Postmortem study showed typical changes of OPCA and also degeneration of the substantia nigra and subthalamic nucleus. An unusual feature was extensive cerebral cortical atrophy. The nuclei of the cranial nerves III, IV, and VI and the median longitudinal fasciculus were intact. Spinal cord examination was not mentioned. Inheritance was autosomal dominant.

Clinical Details of Patients, with Autopsy of a Sibling or Parent

United States. Family of Koeppen and Hans (18)

Geneological data on 8 generations of a Scottish family were made available. The fourth generation migrated to the United States. Six members of generations IV and V were considered "affected" because their records showed diagnoses of cerebellar degeneration, Marie's ataxia, locomotor ataxia, adult onset cerebellar ataxia, or disseminated sclerosis. A male (generation V, case 3) aged 61 years had ataxia, athetosis, and atrophic leg muscles. "[His] eyes were slow to follow and extra ocular movements were restricted" (18). He was not examined by the authors. Autopsy revealed severe degeneration of the Purkinje, granular, pontine, and inferior olivary neurons and lesser involvement of the dentate nuclei. The cerebellar white matter, transverse pontine fibers, olivary hilum, and dorsal columns of spinal cord were demyelinated. The spinal cord grey matter was intact.

Two cousins (VI, 2; VI, 7) aged 52 and 59 years with reportedly affected mothers were examined. They complained of progressive ataxia for 20 years. Findings included slow eye movements, head jerking, absence of the fast component of caloric and optokinetic nystagmus, athetoid movements, areflexia, and normal sensation.

The daughter (VII, 3) of one, aged 27 years, had mild ataxia and slow eye movements like her father and uncle, without being aware of it.

Scotland. Family of Koeppen et al. (19)

The propositus (case III, 1) was a male, 49 years of age, with progressive imbalance, dysarthria, and clumsiness of the hands for 10 years. Examination showed moderately severe ataxia. It also showed selective defect of saccadic movements with pursuit full but slow, a staring look, normal doll's eye maneuvre, absence of optokinetic nystagmus, localized fasciculation in the upper limbs, absence of tendon reflexes, right extensor plantar response, slight impairment of vibration in the feet, and athetoid hand postures.

His mother (case II, 2) was fifty-nine years old at death. Her records revealed a 10-year history of progressively severe ataxia and dysarthria, choreiform movements of the upper limbs, terminal dementia, areflexia, a right extensor plantar response, and absence of vibration sense at the ankles. Oculomotor examination was not mentioned beyond the statement that there was "no nystagmus." Postmortem study revealed degeneration of the Purkinje granular layer cells of the cerebellum, substantia nigra, pontine, and posterior and inferior olivary nuclei. There was demyelination of the cerebellar white matter, transverse pontine fibers, and hilus and periphery of the inferior olivary nuclei. The dentate nuclei were normal, but the hilus appeared pale in myelin preparations. In the spinal cord, there was demyelination of the posterior columns and degeneration of the anterior horn cells.

His sister (case III, 3) died at age 35 after 14 years of progressive cerebellar ataxia with terminal mental changes and double incontinence. The tendon reflexes were absent, but the reflexes were extensor with hypertonia of all limbs. Vibration sense was absent at the ankles. Oculomotor examination was not mentioned. The postmortem findings were "very similar to mother's."

His son (case IV, 2) was examined at age 24, 4 years after onset. He had mild dysarthria, gross finger-nose ataxia, and "some abnormality of saccadic eye movements as his father." All deep reflexes were absent. The plantars reflexes were flexor.

Clinical Details without Autopsy

India

(1) Family of Kini and Venugopal (16): The propositus was a Hindu male, 40 years of age with progressive cerebellar ataxia of 11 years' duration, which began with gait imbalance. He had a "staring look and the ocular movements were sluggish." There was paresis of upward gaze. His daughter, age 16, had a similar but milder ataxia for 1 year, with a "curious fixed gaze with slow movements of eyes." No ocular examination was done. No other abnormal signs were noted. There was a history of ataxia in his mother, a maternal uncle, and his son. OPCA was suspected. *(2) Five families of R. S. Wadia et al. (47):* Nine members of 5 families were examined and a history of 7 more affected members was elicited. The clinical features were similar to those described by Wadia and Swami (41). Age at onset was 6 to 53 years. Cerebellar ataxia was seen in all. Slow eye movements with abnormal ocular reflex responses were found in 8. "Amyotrophy," hyporeflexia, vibration loss, brisk reflexes with plantar extensor, optic atrophy, and chorea were also seen. Motor nerve conduction velocity done in one patient was normal. The authors drew attention to a familial case in whom eye movements were normal with early cerebellar ataxia and to another in whom slow eye movements would have been missed if the family history had not been known. The disease appeared to be autosomal dominant in 4 families and sporadic in 1.

France. Family of Cambier et al. (7)

This report concerned a French male, aged 26 years, with progressive cerebellar ataxia of 11 years' duration, distal limb wasting, action myoclonus, and slow viscous horizontal ocular movements. EOG showed "aboliton of horizontal jerks, induced by either voluntary, automatic (optokinetic nystagmus), or reflex (vestibular) stimuli." Voluntary upward vertical movements were slow. Pursuit movements were normal. EMG gave evidence of denervation with large motor units. The distal latency in the external popliteal nerve was delayed. CT scan showed a large fourth ventricle and prepontine cistern. The mother and sister also had progressive ataxia, but no mention was made of ocular dysfunction. The suggested diagnosis was OPCA with a less likely possibility of the Ramsay-Hunt syndrome.

Japan. Three families of Ozawa et al. (29)

(a) A Japanese male, 30 years of age, had "head jerking," progressive imbalance, and dysarthria for 7 years. Clinical and electrooculographic recording showed normal pursuit and slow saccades in all directions of gaze with a maximum horizontal velocity of 30°/sec. Optokinetic nystagmus and the fast phase of the caloric response were absent. There were signs of bilateral symmetrical cerebellar disorder, "weak" tendon reflexes, and a positive Babinski's sign. The nonconsanguineous parents and 4 brothers were normal. On pneumoencephalography the fourth ventricle and cisterna magna were enlarged. EMG showed a "giant" polyphasic pattern in the extremities. OPCA was diagnosed. (b) A Japanese male, 44 years of age, presented with incontinence and progressive cerebellar disorder of 2 years' duration. Clinical findings included mild dementia, ataxia confined to the lower limbs, dysarthria, and slow spontaneous and reflex eye saccades (with normal pursuit). No pathological reflexes were reported. Extensive investigations (EEG, EMG, angiography, pneumoencephalography) showed no abnormality. There was asymptomatic postural hypotension. The diagnosis was OPCA or Shy-Drager syndrome. (c) A Japanese female aged 30 years, had narcoleptic attacks since age 7 and when reading "raised and lowered" her head. Symptoms of cerebellar disorder had been present since high school. Slow comprehension and abnormal cerebellar signs were found. The saccade was mildly slow through a full range, but the electrooculogram revealed that the horizontal maximum angular velocity was reduced by one-half. Vertical eye movements were even slower and accompanied by constant blinking. Reflex eye movements were normal. Her brother, aged 25 years, had no cerebellar ataxia, but his eye movements were "similar to his sisters." She was the eldest of 3 children and her nonconsanguineous parents were normal. The diagnosis was familial spinocerebellar degeneration.

Taiwan. Family of Lai and Hung (22)

A Chinese female, aged 38 years, had a progressive disorder of gait for 8 years and of speech for 3 years. Examination revealed bilateral cerebellar ataxia, a staring facial expression, slow voluntary eye movements and head jerking. Optokinetic nystagmus was absent, but normal eye movements were easily elicited by the doll's eye maneuvre. Vibration sense was impaired in the left foot. The deep reflexes were normal; plantar reflexes, flexor. "A prominent familial occurrence of dominant inheritance" was mentioned. The diagnosis was OPCA.

United States

1. Family of Starkman et al. (39): Thirty-two of the 70 living members of this American family of Italian descent were examined. Autosomal dominant inheritance was evident. "Ten had abnormal eye movements as well as signs of spinocerebellar degeneration"; 1 had only abnormal eye movements and 6 had only signs of spinocerebellar degeneration. Fifteen relatively young members were unaffected. Classical slow voluntary and reflexly induced saccades with normal pursuit was described along with ataxia, hyperreflexia in the lower limbs, and posterior column deficit. The family was compared with those of Wadia and Swami.

2. Family of Singh et al. (35): The propositus of an American Black family, a female aged 23 years, had progressive severe symmetrical cerebellar ataxia from

age 12. Classical slow saccades, head jerking, and delayed arrival of the eyes to the target were all present. Eye movements were easily elicited by the Doll's eye maneuvre. Optokinetic and caloric nystagmus were absent. There was some cogwheel rigidity of the limbs, but no other abnormal signs were noted. EEG was normal, but a pneumoencephalogram showed cerebellar and cerebral atrophy. Her father's case notes recorded a progressive ataxia of 11 years' duration before his death at age 49. There was no reference to abnormal ocular movements. His brother's notes showed that he had been severely handicapped in 8 years by cerebellar ataxia beginning at age 29. "Conjugate lateral gaze was slow and incomplete." A pneumoencephalogram revealed generalized ventricular dilatation. Their mother was reported to have had tremor and slurred speech. Their 2 brothers were unaffected. The family was compared with those of Wadia and Swami.

3. Two families of Zee et al. (49): (a) An American girl, age 14 (racial ancestry not mentioned) had progressive wasting of the distal musculature and difficulty in running for 4 years. Head jerking was noticed, but no ocular complaints were noted. The family history was negative. Findings included mild scoliosis, pes cavus, cerebellar signs, distal limb atrophy and weakness, areflexia, extensor plantar responses, postural loss in the lower limbs, and loss of vibration sense in all limbs. The random and command eye movements were full but slow, the horizontal movements being more severely affected. Blinking, head jerking, and a lagging of the eyes behind the head on target fixation were described. Reflex eye movements were full, but with a slow saccadic response. Pursuit movements were normal; CSF and EEG were normal. Motor nerve conduction was impaired. A muscle biopsy showed denervation; the sural nerve, "decreased myelinated fibers." (b) An American male (racial ancestry unrecorded) age 19 years, had progressive cerebellar ataxia for 10 years. His mother had progressive incoordination and unsteady gait of unspecified duration before she died of breast cancer at the age of 42. Positive findings on examination included moderate cerebellar ataxia, areflexia, and flexor plantar responses. EMG–NCV and EEG were normal. Voluntary eye movements were slow in all directions, the least affected was downward gaze. Convergence was intact and pursuit movements were normal. Blinking, head jerking, and head-eye lag were noticed. Defective saccades were seen on optokinetic, caloric, and rotatory stimuli.

The authors concluded after extensive oculometric examination and computer simulation of eye movements that both these patients had OPCA, though clinically the first appears to resemble Friedreich's ataxia.

4. Family of Murphy and Goldblatt (26): An American woman, 61 years old (ancestry not mentioned), had progressive instability of gait since her late 30s and incoordination of the upper limbs and dysarthria in her early 50s. Examination showed severe cerebellar ataxia, slow but full-range voluntary eye movements, depressed tendon reflexes in the lower limbs, impaired vibration sense, and flexor plantars responses. Over the years she became bedridden; the voluntary eye movements became slower; the oculocephalic reflex became hyperactive; the tendon

reflexes were lost; and distal wasting of limbs with some blunting of all sensory modelities, grimacing, and moderate dementia appeared. Electrooculographic records confirmed the reduced velocity of saccades and an increased latency before onset of movement on command, and absence of saccades on optokinetic and caloric stimulation. EMG showed chronic and active denervation with normal motor conduction velocities. There were family members of both sexes affected by similar ataxia in 3 consecutive generations, but no comment was available on their eye movements.

Other Relevant Information

Sharpe (34) briefly reported a quantitative analysis of oculomotor function which showed paresis of all fast eye movements "in a syndrome of spinocerebellar ataxia similar to that described by Wadia and Swami . . . [where] macular degeneration, dementia, were variable manifestations of this disorder in a black man and his son, and in a white girl of Greek descent" living in Canada. Avanzini et al. (2) studying ocular motility in patients with cerebellar diseases, mentioned slow saccades in a patient they describe as clinically very similar to that reported by Wadia and Swami, and 4 others with a clinical diagnosis of OPCA.

Garcin and Man (10) described "viscous" voluntary eye movements in spinocerebellar degeneration of various types including Friedreich's ataxia, but did not mention OPCA. However, clinically diagnosed Friedreich's ataxia could well turn out to be OPCA at autopsy, as was found in the Schut family (31). Garcin and Man (10) refer to cases of ocular disorder in cerebellar degeneration in the earlier literature (1929–1956). From among them, the family of Gentili and Zambonelli alone resembled ours. They published a family of 93 subjects with hereditary degenerative cerebellar disease; in 4, lateral eye movements took place with a remarkable slowness which the authors described as tonic.

Several reports from Japan related to slow eye movements have appeared in the last decade (9,14,15,48). Although oculometric records were available, other clinical details were insufficient for documentation. The authors have, nevertheless, compared their cases with those of Wadia and Swami (41). Sobue (38) wrote that a few additional, similar cases have been reported in the Annual Japanese Neurological Congress.

Oppenheimer (28) found OPCA with chronic demyelinating neuropathy and severe posterior column degeneration in a 61-year-old Englishman with a 30-year history of progressive ataxia. Recently, his 37-year-old daughter, who had cerebellar ataxia, was recalled for examination and was "found to have full eye movements and difficulty in following fast moving objects with her eyes." These features had been missed earlier: "Unfortunately, not much is recorded about the father's eye movements." More details about him are mentioned in another report of Oppenheimer (27), referred to as case 10.

Finally, attention has also been drawn by colleagues from all over India in the last 10 years to similar cases under their care.

Mention of families resembling those described here is pertinent. Brown (6) was the first to note ocular signs in spinocerebellar degeneration in an American family with autosomal dominant inheritance. In one of his cases autopsied by Barker (3), Brown mentioned that "all movements of ocular muscles and all pupillary reflexes are sluggish" but the patient also had "marked static ptosis, greater in the left eye, with incoordinate overaction of the levator". No mention was made of the reflex eye movements. The overall description of the rest of the family, including 2 other autopsied members (3,25) indicated that diplopia, bilateral ptosis, partial or total ophthalmoplegia, squint, pupillary abnormalities, early optic atrophy, and pyramidal tract signs formed the clinical picture. The 3 postmortem examinations showed degeneration in the dorsal columns of the cord, the direct spinocerebellar tracts, and Clarke's columns. There was anterior horn cell atrophy in 1. There was little, if any, degeneration of the brainstem and cerebellum. As we have always maintained (41), Sanger-Brown ataxia is different from what is described here.

Schut (31) made a passing reference to 1 female member of his large family of Dutch ancestry, whose ocular movements were performed slowly. She had slight ptosis and enophthalmos, but no nystagmus. She presented with spastic paraplegia and mild late ataxia, and was classified as "hereditary spastic paraplegia." No autopsy was done. Clinically, she too is different. Yet it is interesting that in the same pedigree, Schut classified other members as Friedreich's disease and hereditary cerebellar ataxia (subgroups A and B) pointing to a wide intrafamilial variability. No slow eye movements were detected. Autopsy of some members of these 2 groups showed OPCA with posterior column degeneration (31,32). Does this family of OPCA belong to the group described above with slow eye movements observed in 1 and perhaps not present or detected in the others? This is relevant because Landis et al. (23) reviewing this family some years later simply mentions "apractic" eye movements in as many as 8 of 9 new members, pointing out that this eye movement abnormality was not mentioned in the earlier generations by Schut. In 1 of the 2 recorded histories they state that "she had left medial and inferior rectus palsies. Her eye movements were slow and coarsely saccadic, suggestive of oculomotor apraxia." Comment on this important family is difficult. It seems that though OPCA has been pathologically shown, the ocular and other clinical signs are different from those discussed in this chapter; however, semantic differences and clinical misinterpretation of "ocular apraxia" and "slow eye movements" may contribute to clinical misclassification.

Similarly, attention must be drawn to a family of autosomal dominant inheritance first seen in 1955, by Alajouanine et al. (1) and later by Bonduelle et al. (5). The mother, her eldest son, and 2 of her daughters had progressive cerebellar ataxia, myoclonic jerks, absent deep reflexes, posterior column disorder, mild distal wasting (denervation on electromyography), and a positive Babinski's sign to a variable degree in each. The mother's eye movements were not recorded. The son had restricted voluntary upward gaze and full but slow lateral gaze and convergence. The older affected daughter had no significant abnormality, but the younger had slow (viscous) eye movements. Clinically, the differential diagnosis suggested fell between the Ramsey-Hunt syndrome and Friedreich's ataxia, but autopsy of the older sister showed OPCA with degeneration of the substantia nigra, the posterior columns, the anterior horn cells, and Clarke's column of the spinal cord. This family, like that of Schut mentioned above, might belong to the group under discussion here but for the intrafamilial differences in the disorder of ocular movements and insufficient observations or recording of details.

Finally, Gerstenbrand and Weingarten (11) described a family with 15 ataxic members in 4 generations. Conjugate gaze paralysis, with diplopia and ptosis and restricted eye movements in some members, was the predominant disorder. There was no mention of slow eye movements. Besides this, Parkinsonism, obvious dementia, and myoclonus formed important features. A clinical diagnosis of OPCA was mentioned, and though no autopsy was available in this pedigree, OPCA was found in another closely related family with a similar ataxic disorder. Though earlier (43) we had mentioned this family as belonging to the group described here, a closer reading has raised some points of doubt.

CONCLUSIONS

The families reviewed here form a group. The majority showed autosomal dominant heredity affecting both sexes though sporadic cases have been recorded; our series has also suggested the possible occurrence of a recessive trait. The average age at onset and the duration of the disease was the same in our patients and in the others where information was available. Progressive cerebellar ataxia and slow eye movements were the identifying signs in all. Spinal cord or peripheral nerve (lower motor and sensory neuron) affection, as evidenced by areflexia, proprioceptive sensory loss, and occasional distal atrophy, terminal mental deterioration [except in the family of Sears et al. (33), where it was severe], bilateral facial weakness, pyramidal signs, involuntary movements, and subclinical optic atrophy occurred variably. Early cataracts and kyphoscoliosis were very occasionally seen. Pes cavus and cardiac or electrocardiographic abnormalities were not recorded. Cambier et al. (7) mentioned myoclonic jerks in their patient. Macular degeneration was seen by Sharpe (34) alone, and there was coincidental narcolepsy in 1, and asymptomatic postural hypotension in another case of Ozawa et al. (29). Autopsy showed OPCA in every family. Degeneration was also seen in the posterior columns, substantia nigra, anterior horn cells, and dentate nuclei in that order of frequency (Tables 1 and 2). Sigwald's family showed degeneration additionally of the Clarke's column. The lateral columns were consistently spared.

The clinicopathological evidence shows that the slow eye movements result from a supranuclear disorder of ocular function. A wide variety of ocular signs have been described with different types of cerebellar degenerations (41,49,50), and it is not always easy to distinguish them. Slow eye movements may miss detection early in the disease. This was evident in some families already mentioned (19,26,28,35), where earlier examination of older generations mentioned no ocular disorder, but then detected perhaps as a result of greater awareness in the recent generations. It is also likely that the oculomotor disorder can be misinterpreted as oculomotor apraxia or other supranuclear, inter- or infranuclear ophthalmoplegias, especially at a late stage of the disease. The absence of ocular symptoms, squint, ptosis, and pupillary abnormality and the full range of slow voluntary and reflex movements in all directions with head jerking are useful pointers. The oculometric record, the full clinical picture, and family history become helpful in the more difficult cases. It is important to note that in 3 families (36,37,39,47), slow eye movements were not seen in some ataxic members, while both ocular and cerebellar signs were found in others. However, as pointed out (47) this was usually early in the disease, and no mention has been made of oculometric recording of these atypical members. Starkman et al. (39) even mentioned the rare case of the patient with slow eye movements without cerebellar ataxia in his family.

Though no satisfactory pathological demonstration of neuronal degeneration causing the slow eye movement has been shown, conjectures as to its location have been made by almost all reporters since Mass and Scherer (24). Current opinion points to the region of the paramedian pontine reticular formation rostral to the abducens and third nerve nuclei. In this regard, it is worth mentioning that among the autopsied cases (Table 2), the only one (Sigwald, case 2) who had no degeneration of the olives, nuclei pontis, or cerebellar cortex did not have slow eye movements though ataxia was remarkable. All others including her sister (case 1 of Sigwald) had slow eye movements and ataxia. Yet the role, if any, of the frontotegmental descending tracts, or of the cerebellum, has not been clarified. That similar slow eye movements occur in Huntington's chorea (40) and Wilson's disease (17), where no significant brainstem lesions have been demonstrated, needs also to be explained. It is possible that in a multisystem disorder like OPCA, degeneration of more than 1 set of neurons is operative in slowing the saccade.

It appears that spinal cord and peripheral nervous system involvement is the rule rather than the exception in both the dominant and sporadic cases, though clinically the only evidence may be areflexia. Generally, accounts of patients with spinocerebellar degenerations do not reflect careful assessment of the peripheral nervous system either by repeated clinical and electromyographic examination through the course of the disease or by sural nerve biopsy. Whereas this is not always possible or necessary, our experience is that the relevant physical signs may appear at any stage, and electromyography and/or sural nerve biopsy may reveal subclinical disease. Thus, 22 out of our 37 patients had depressed deep reflexes even on initial clinical examination, and 13 out of 14 examined electromyographically showed lower motor/sensory neuron lesions. Similar observations have been made in more than one-half the reviewed families, which were often less extensively studied. Similarly, 2 of our 3 histologically examined autopsies, and all those reviewed showed changes in the spinal cord except that one described by Sears et al. (33) (where probably the spinal cord was not examined). Fallout of large, and in the advanced stage practically all, myelinated fibers in the sural nerve biopsy was seen in our patients and was also noted by Zee et al. (49). These observations suggest that there is a dying-back of the central and peripheral axons because of a selective degeneration both of the large neurons in the dorsal root ganglia and, less frequently, of the anterior horn cells—a sensory and motor neuronopathy.

In accepting that clinical, pathological, and genetic heterogeneity exists and that classification of "familial ataxias" is difficult (4,8,12,30), the families here described nevertheless form an identifiable subentity. The autopsies place them firmly among "the olivopontocerebellar atrophies", with the ataxia, the specific ocular disorder, and the clinical or subclinical affection of the spinal lower motor/sensory neurons essentially forming the consistent clinical picture. The genetic pattern is autosomal dominant. Our fully studied case A.B. is representative of this group. Although some autopsies show additional degeneration of the substantia nigra or of the dentate nuclei, this does not prevent its pathological identification. Similarly, a certain degree of clinical or genetic variation does not really lead to misclassification of this disorder during life. It is agreed that there will be individual cases where a major clinical variability, e.g., absence of slow eye movements, absence of ataxia, or presence of excessive spinal cord signs such as spasticity or atrophy, will make accurate diagnosis difficult. A later examination of the patient or family members may be more revealing. Starkman's family (39) is a good example. Oculometric recording of eye movements and electromyography or sural nerve biopsy may add useful subclinical information. Apart from these rare exceptions, few inter- and intrafamilial variations as well as formes frustes have been described.

It has been stated (13) that Sanger-Brown commented on the presence of slow eye movements in his family, but the sources cited therein (3,6) did not reveal OPCA. We have yet to come across a carefully recorded case of cerebellar ataxia with slow saccade where OPCA has not been found at autopsy in the patient or in an affected member of the family even if the clinical diagnosis during life was otherwise.

It is known (8,12,20,30) that OPCA is a pathologically recognized group with variable clinical and occasionally even genetic expression. The group described here would form a separate subentity under the Konigsmark and Weiner classification (20). If we use the older classification of Greenfield (12) the balance of evidence based on age at onset, family history, and spinal cord affection would place most of our families into the "Menzel type of hereditary ataxia," rather than that described by Dejerine and Thomas (12). Yet the fallibility of such divisions is too well known to reiterate. For example, where would we put our sporadic cases or, for example, autopsied case reported above of S.D.H. with doubtful recessive inheritance, with clinical signs of lower motor/sensory disorder but with little changes in the spinal cord at autopsy? Perhaps such classifications are best abandoned, and we should merely identify recognizable recurrent clinicopathological patterns, of which this is one.

In summary, this variety of usually autosomal dominant cerebellar ataxia with slow voluntary eye movements and frequent lower motor/sensory neurone signs occurs in both sexes and in many races, religions and regions, though apparently it is more frequent, or is more frequently recognized, among Indians.

ACKNOWLEDGMENTS

I thank the Dean, Dr. S. Y. Deodhare, of J. J. Group of Hospitals and Grant Medical College, Bombay, for permission to use the records and Dr. Meher Desai for helping to gather and complete the information over the years. The pathological examinations were made by Drs. D. K. Dastur and David Oppenheimer, neuropathologists of Bombay and Oxford; the electromyography by Dr. P. N. Wadia; and the sural nerve study by Drs. S. M. Katrak and Lata Mehta. I acknowledge their reports gratefully. Figures and photographs were made by the Medical Education Department of Glaxo Laboratories (India) limited, Bombay. Final thanks are due to V. B. Lacca for her secretarial assistance.

REFERENCES

1. Alajouanine, M. Th., Scherrer, J., Contamin, F., Marteau, R., and Calvet, J. (1955): A propos de l'association "Dyssnergia cerebellaris myoclonica" de R. Hunt et hérédo-dégéneration spino-cérébelleuse type Friedreich. Etude clinique et électromyographique d'un cas. *Rev. Neurol. (Paris)*, 93:577–581.
2. Avanzini, G., Girotti, F., Crenna, P., and Negri, S. (1979): Alterations of ocular motility in cerebellar pathology. An electro-oculographic study. *Arch. Neurol.*, 36:274–280.
3. Barker, L. F. (1903): A description of the brains and spinal cord of two brothers dead of hereditary ataxia. Cases 18 and 20 of the series in the family described by Dr. Sanger Brown. *Trans. Assoc. Am. Physicians*, 18:637–709.
4. Bobowick, A. R., and Brody, J. A. (1975): Epidemiology of neurodegenerative system disorders. In: *Handbook of Clinical Neurology*, Vol. 21, Part 1, edited by P. J. Vinken, G. W. Bruyn, and J. M. B. V. Dejong, p. 14. North-Holland, Amsterdam.
5. Bonduelle, M., Escourolle, R., Bouygues. P., Lormeau, G., and Gray, F. (1976): Atrophie Olivo-ponto-cérébelleuse Familiale Avec Myoclonies. Les Limites de la dyssynergie cérébelleuse Myoclonique (Syndrome de Ramsay-Hunt). *Rev. Neurol. (Paris)*, 132(2):113–124.
6. Brown, S. (1892): On hereditary ataxy, with a series of twenty-one cases. *Brain*, 15:250–268.
7. Cambier, J., Masson, M., and Prier, S. (1978): Étude électrooculographique d'un cas d'abolition des saccades horizontales avec viscosité du regard au cours d'une hérédo-dégénérescence cérébelleuse. *Rev. Neurol. (Paris)*, 134(8-9):461–470.
8. Eadie, M. J. (1975): Olivo-ponto-cerebellar atrophy. In: *Handbook of Clinical Neurology*, Vol. 21, Part 1, edited by P. J. Vinken, G. W. Bruyn, and J. M. B. V. Dejong, pp. 415–449. North-Holland, Amsterdam.
9. Fujita, T., and Tsubaki, T. (1975): Slow eye movements (Viscosite). *Adv. Neurol. Sci.*, 19:1010–1011 (Abstr.).
10. Garcin, R., and Man, H. X. (1958): Sur la lenteur particulière des mouvements conjugués des yeux observée fréquemment dans les dégénérations cérébelleuses et spino-cérébelleuses: La "viscosité" des mouvements volontaires. *Rev. Neurol. (Paris)*, 98:672–673.
11. Gerstenbrand, F., and Weingarten, K. (1962): Beitrag zum Problem der Systematrophien des Kleinhirns. *Wien. Klin. Wochenschr.*, 74:702–705.
12. Greenfield, J. G. (1954): *The Spino-cerebellar Degenerations*. Blackwell Scientific, Oxford.
13. Harding, A. E. (1982): The clinical features and classification of the late onset autosomal dominant cerebellar ataxias. A study of 11 families, including descendents of "The Drew family of Walworth." *Brain*, 105:1–28.
14. Hirayama, K., Hattori, T., Kumada, H., and Komatsuzaki, A. (1978): *Familial Spino-cerebellar Degeneration with Slow Eye Movements*. Annual report of Research Committee on SCD by the Ministry of Health and Welfare, Japan.
15. Kanehisa, Y., Suda, M., Yagi, K., Beppu, H., and Uono, M. (1979): A heredo-familial spino-cerebellar degeneration with slow eye movements—A study of 5 cases. *Clin. Neurol. (Tokyo)*, 19:209–216 (Abstr.).
16. Kini, P. M., and Venugopal, N. S. (1967): Hereditary cerebellar ataxia. Report of a family. *J. Assoc. Physicians India*, 15:369–371.

17. Kirkham, T. H., and Kamin, D. F. (1974): Slow saccadic eye movements in Wilson's disease. *J. Neurol. Neurosurg. Psychiatry*, 37:191–194.
18. Koeppen, A. H., and Hans, M. B. (1976): Supranuclear ophthalmoplegia in olivo-ponto-cerebellar degeneration. *Neurology*, 26:764–768.
19. Koeppen, A. H., Hans, M. B., Shepherd, D. I., and Best, P. V. (1977): Adult-onset hereditary ataxia in Scotland. *Arch. Neurol.*, 34:611–618.
20. Konigsmark, B. W., and Weiner, L. P. (1970): The olivopontocerebellar atrophies: A review. *Medicine*, 49:227–241.
21. Kulkarni, S. A., and Wadia, N. H. (1975): Model of an oculomotor subsystem. *Int. J. Biomed. Comput.*, 6:1–31.
22. Lai, M. L., and Hung, T. P. (1979): A clinical study of spinocerebellar degeneration amongst Chinese in Taiwan. *Bull. Neurol. Soc. (Taiwan)*, 4:65–67.
23. Landis, D. M. D., Rosenberg, R. N., Landis, S. C., Schut, L., and Nyhan, W. L. (1974): Olivo-pontocerebellar degeneration: Clinical and ultrastructural abnormalities. *Arch. Neurol.*, 31:295–307.
24. Mass, O., and Scherer, H. J. (1933): Zur Klinik und Anatomie Einiger Seltener Klinhirnerkrankungen. *Z. Gesamte Neurol. Psychiatr.*, 145:420–444.
25. Meyer, A. (1897): The morbid anatomy of a case of hereditary ataxy. *Brain*, 20:276–289.
26. Murphy, M. J., and Goldblatt, D. (1977): Slow eye movements, with absent saccades, in a patient with hereditary ataxia. *Arch. Neurol.*, 34:191–195.
27. Oppenheimer, D. R. (1980): Lateral horn cells in progressive autonomic failure. *J. Neurol. Sci.*, 46:393–404.
28. Oppenheimer, D. R. (1981): *Personal communication.*
29. Ozawa, T., Naito, M., Takasu, T., Warabi, T., and Yamagami, Y. (1974): Disorders of saccadic eye movement in cerebellar degeneration. *Jpn. J. Ophthalmol.*, 18:363–380.
30. Pratt, R. T. C. (1967): *The Genetics of Neurological Disorders.* Oxford University Press, London.
31. Schut, J. W. (1950): Hereditary ataxia. Clinical study through six generations. *Arch. Neurol. Psychiatry*, 63:535–567.
32. Schut, J. W., and Haymaker, W. (1951): Hereditary ataxia: A pathological study of five cases of common ancestry. *J. Neuropathol. Clin. Neurol.*, 1:183–213.
33. Sears, E. S., Hammerberg, E. K., Norenberg, M. D., Wilson, B., and Nellhaus, G. (1975): Supranuclear ophthalmoplegia and dementia in olivopontocerebellar atrophy: A clinico-pathologic study. *Neurology*, 25:395 (Abstr.).
34. Sharpe, J. A. (1976): Global paresis of saccadic eye movements in spinocerebellar degeneration. *Can. J. Neurol. Sci.*, 3:155–156 (Abstr.).
35. Singh, B., Ivamoto, H., and Strobos, R. J. (1973): Slow eye movements in spinocerebellar degeneration. *Am. J. Ophthalmol.*, 76:237–240.
36. Sigwald, J., Lapresle, J., Raverdy, Ph., and Recondo, J. (1963): Atrophie cérébelleuse familiale avec association de lésions nigériennes et spinales. *Rev. Neurol. (Paris)*, 109:571–573.
37. Sigwald, J., Lapresle, J., Raverdy, P., and Recondon, J. (1964): Atrophie cérébelleuse familiale avec association de lésions nigériennes et spinales. *La Presse Med.*, 72(10):557–562.
38. Sobue, I. (1982): *Personal communication.*
39. Starkman, S., Kaul, S., Fried, J., and Behrens, M. (1972): Unusual abnormal eye movements in a family with hereditary spinocerebellar degeneration. *Neurology*, 22:402 (Abstr.).
40. Starr, A. (1967): A disorder of rapid eye movements in Huntington's chorea. *Brain*, 90:545–564.
41. Wadia, N. H., and Swami, R. K. (1971): A new form of heredofamilial spinocerebellar degeneration with slow eye movements (nine families) *Brain*, 94:359–374.
42. Wadia, N. H. (1973): An indigenous form of heredo-familial spinocerebellar degeneration with slow eye movements. *Neurology (India) [Suppl. 4]*, 20:561–580.
43. Wadia, N. H. (1977): Heredo-familial spinocerebellar degeneration with slow eye movements—Another variety of olivo-ponto-cerebellar degeneration. *Neurology (India)*, 25:147–160.
44. Wadia, N. H., and Desai, M. M. (1980): A variety of heredo-familial olivopontocerebellar degeneration with slow eye movements commonly seen in India. In: *Proceedings of the International Symposium on Spinocerebellar Degenerations*, edited by I. Sobue, pp. 193–208. University of Tokyo Press, Tokyo.
45. Wadia, N. H., Irani, P. F., Mehta, L. N., and Purohit, A. V. (1980): Evidence of peripheral neuropathy in a variety of heredo-familial olivopontocerebellar degeneration frequently seen in

India. In: *Proceedings of the International Symposium on Spinocerebellar Degenerations*, edited by I. Sobue, pp. 239–250. University of Tokyo Press, Tokyo.
46. Wadia, P. N., Katrak, S. M., Mehta, L. N., and Wadia, N. H. (1983): Peripheral neuronopathy in olivopontocerebellar degeneration with slowed saccades *(in press.)*
47. Wadia, R. S., Amin, R. B., Divate, U. P., Divate, P. G., Sainani, G. S., and Sardesai, H. V. (1976): Autosomal dominant spinocerebellar ataxia with slow eye movements—A common hereditary ataxia in Western India. *J. Assoc. Physicians India*, 24:367–371.
48. Warabi, T., Toyokura, Y., Takasu, T., and Yanagisawa, N. (1974): A familial spinocerebellar degeneration with abnormal slow eye movements in vertical directions. *Neurol. Med. (Tokyo)*, 1:429 *(Abstr.)*.
49. Zee, D. S., Optican, L. M., Cook, J. D., Robinson, D. A., and Engel, W. K. (1976): Slow saccades in spinocerebellar degeneration. *Arch. Neurol.*, 33:243–251.
50. Zee, D. S., Yee, R. D., Cogan, D. G., Robinson, D. A., and Engel, W. K. (1976): Ocular motor abnormalities in hereditary cerebellar ataxia. *Brain*, 99:207–234.

The Olivopontocerebellar Atrophies, edited by R.C. Duvoisin and A. Plaitakis. Raven Press, New York © 1984.

Joseph Disease: An Autosomal Dominant Motor System Degeneration

Roger N. Rosenberg

Department of Neurology, University of Texas Health Science Center at Dallas, Southwestern Medical School, Dallas, Texas 75235

In 1972, two papers described dominantly inherited neurologic disease in two Azorean-Portuguese families residing in Massachusetts. The first report (8) referred to "Machado disease" to acknowledge the proband family in which there was a progressive cerebellar disease with distal extremity atrophy and sensory loss beginning in the fifth decade. A sural nerve biopsy from one patient documented segmental demyelination. The second report (16) described "nigro-spinal-dentatal degeneration with nuclear ophthalmoplegia" in the Thomas family, presenting in the third to fifth decades with gait ataxia, external ophthalmoplegia, facial-lingual fasciculations, elements of spasticity, and extremity rigidity. The neuropathologic features included neuronal loss in the substantia nigra, dentate nuclei, and Clark's column in the spinal cord. Demyelination was present in the posterior columns, lateral corticospinal, and spinothalamic tracts of the spinal cord, most evident in the thoracic portion.

In 1976, Rosenberg et al. (13) described a progressive motor system disease beginning in the second and third decades in another Portuguese family, the Joseph family of California, consisting of 329 persons in nine generations at that time. The clinical picture differed from that of the two previous reports in that Joseph family affected persons had progressive spasticity, lurching unsteadiness of gait due to spasticity (without cerebellar signs), spastic dysarthria, loss of fast saccadic eye movements, ophthalmoparesis for upward gaze, and facial-lingual fasciculations, with prominent dystonia of head, face, extremities, and trunk in some individuals (Figs. 1–3). The neuropathology consisted of neuronal loss in the striatum, substantia nigra, basis pontis, dentate nucleus, cerebellar cortex, and anterior horns of the spinal cord. Cerebrospinal fluid (CSF) homovanillic acid levels were reduced, correlating with neuronal loss in the zona compacta of the substantia nigra. The Joseph family disorder differed from the Massachusetts cases because: (a) there was striatonigral degeneration; (b) dystonia was severe in some patients; and (c) cerebellar signs were not evident in any family member examined in 1975. The disease was also different from olivopontocerebellar degeneration because the medullary inferior olives were unaffected. It was unlike Huntington's disease (HD)

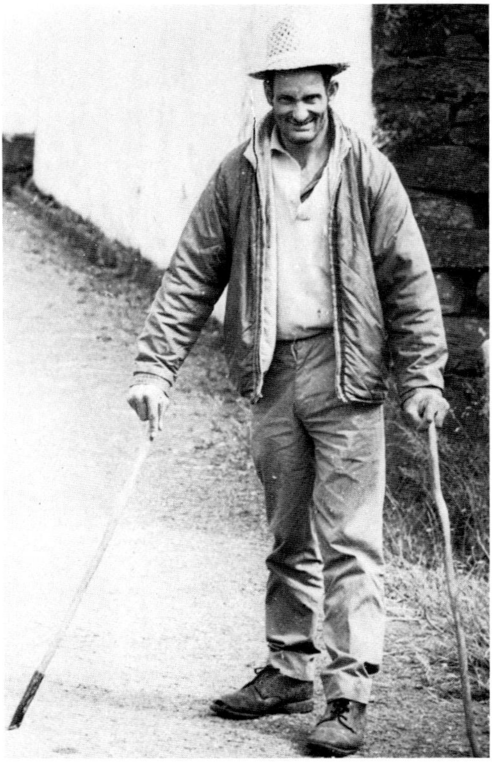

FIG. 1. Patient with Joseph disease, type II, with progressive gait ataxia and spasticity of the legs. This 36-year-old man is patient NS (V,32) in our Sousa family pedigree of the Island of Flores, Azores. He was examined on Flores in June, 1977. (From ref. 11a.)

because intelligence remained normal in all Joseph patients, and the cerebral cortex was histologically normal.

Epidemiologic studies were necessary to establish the spectrum of clinical and neuropathologic findings. The logical place to proceed was in the Azores Islands, particularly on the island of Flores, from which both the Joseph and Thomas families originated. Other suggestions of variable clinical and neuropathologic features were made as personal communications to Dr. Rosenberg from Dr. Coutinho and Dr. Andrade of the Neurology Service, Hospital Santo Antonio, Porto, Portugal. They traveled to Flores in December, 1976, where they found patients with prominent spasticity and extrapyramidal signs and some with cerebellar disorders or peripheral neuropathy. Coutinho and Andrade (1) emphasized types I, II, and III as variants of the autosomal dominant disorder in affected individuals on Flores. Type I corresponded to the typical Joseph phenotype, with only extrapyramidal and pyramidal signs, including dystonia, athetosis, and rigidity with associated spasticity. Type II included patients with cerebellar deficits and spasticity. Type III was

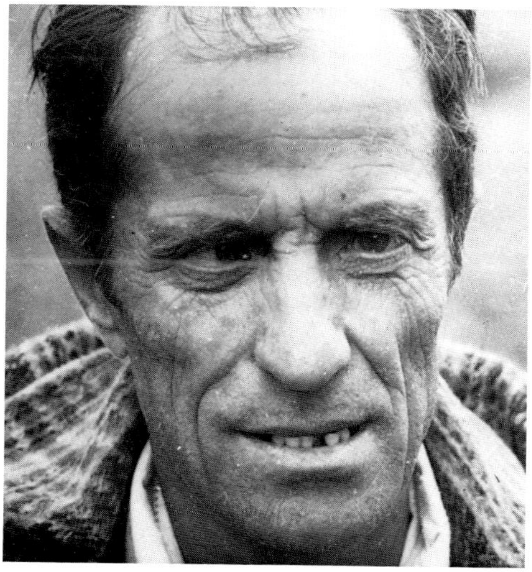

FIG. 2. Patient with Joseph disease, illustrating ophthalmoparesis. The patient is attempting to gaze to the left and has a paresis of the left lateral rectus muscle. He is a type II patient with gait ataxia and a moderate spastic paresis. He was examined in Flores, Azores, in 1977. (From ref. 11a.)

reserved for patients with the Machado phenotype—patients with a dominantly inherited form of motor polyneuropathy and true cerebellar deficits (1,10).

Romanul et al. (9) described another Massachusetts family of Portuguese ancestry with a similar clinical spectrum of gait ataxia, parkinsonian rigidity, ophthalmoparesis, muscle fasciculation, areflexia and associated nystagmus, cerebellar tremor, and extensor plantar responses. Postmortem study of one patient showed striatonigral degeneration with severe neuronal loss and gliosis in the putamen; in another patient, the basal ganglia were normal. Their observations supported the concept of a clinical and neuropathologic variation. It seemed likely that all the reported families of similar ancestry represented a single genetic entity with variable expression, and that a better understanding of this disease might accrue from a visit to Flores and San Miguel, from which the family reported by Romanul et al. (9) migrated.

AZOREAN NEUROEPIDEMIOLOGY

In 1977, Rosenberg and Nyhan joined Coutinho in the Azores to investigate the presence of this genetic disease, especially on the island of Flores. Rosenberg, Nyhan, and Coutinho encountered typical genetic disease as described in the Joseph and Thomas families on Flores in the Sousa family (10) (Fig. 4).

Two main variants of the disease were encountered. Type 1 corresponded to the Joseph phenotype, with spasticity, clonus, hyperreflexia, extensor plantar responses, facial and lingual fasciculations, and nystagmus with ophthalmoparesis beginning

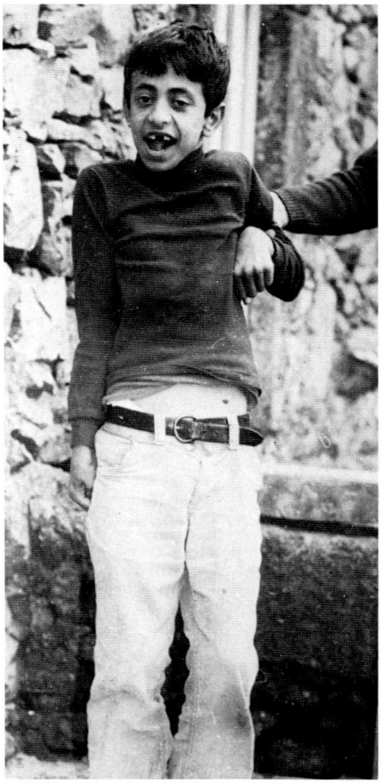

FIG. 3. Patient with Joseph disease, type I, with dystonic posturing of his jaw and left arm. He had evidence of spasticity in his legs and arms. Disease began at age 8 years; he is shown at age 12. He died at age 15. Of note is the fact that his parents were both affected with type II disease, having late onset cerebellar deficits with some leg upper motoneuron signs. (From ref. 11a.)

about age 25. Type II included cerebellar signs, with truncal ataxia and cerebellar deficits of extremities, that began in the early 30s and were less rapid in progression than type I. Typical examples of type I were brothers AS (V,31) age 38, and NS (V,32), age 36 (10). Both noted onset of symptoms in their late 20s, starting with impairment of gait caused by a lurching spasticity. Dysarthria and dysphagia also occurred early. Patient AS developed striking prominence of his eyes, whereas NS did not. Ophthalmoparesis for upward gaze and nystagmus on horizontal gaze were noted. There was stiffness of the arms, spasticity of the legs, and bilateral ankle clonus with extensor plantar responses in one brother and bilateral flexor plantar responses in the other. Both brothers demonstrated dystonia of the face, head, and extremities, exaggerated by talking, standing, and especially walking. Dysphagia and spastic dysarthria were present in both patients.

In the same family was EN (V,38), a 38-year-old woman who was a first cousin of these two brothers; her symptoms began at age 30. She manifested ophthalmoparesis, nystagmus, facial fasciculations and atrophy, spasticity, and increased tone of the legs and hyperreflexia, but with flexor plantar responses. She had truncal ataxia and heel-to-shin and finger-to-nose dysmetria (10).

The husband of EN (V,38) also developed an impaired gait at about age 55. He was examined at age 59; tandem walking was impaired, and there was ataxia of the heel-to-shin maneuver. Their 8-year-old son, Mauricio (VI,63), had impaired

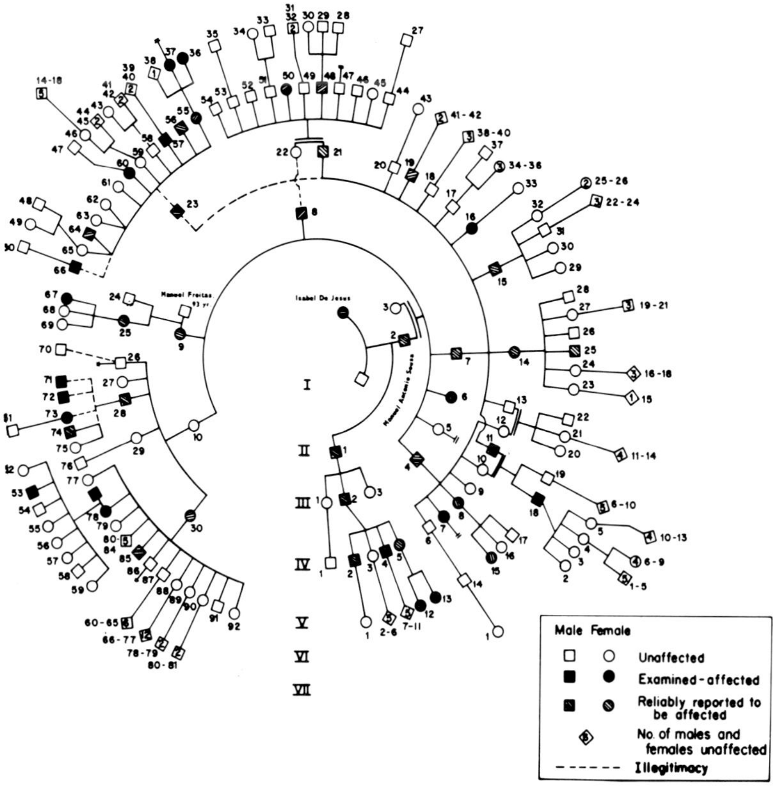

FIG. 4. Sousa family pedigree from the Island of Flores, Azores. Descendants of Manuel Antonio Sousa (II,2) on Flores are shown who indicate dominantly inherited disease of the Joseph disease type. (From ref. 11a.)

coordination of hands, speech, and walking. When we examined him at age 12, there was striking dystonia of facial movements, extremity functions, and walking. He had marked spasticity of the arms and legs, with sustained clonus at the knee and ankle, and equivocal plantar responses. Walking and standing increased the dystonic posturing and elicited superimposed athetotic twisting movements of his hands and face. Drinking water could provoke choking, and his speech was spastic and dysarthric. He was seriously incapacitated, unable to eat or walk unassisted. No cerebellar signs were present (10) (Fig. 3).

Both parents expressed type II disease, with definite cerebellar signs and spasticity, whereas the son expressed a prominent type I form at an early age. It is presumed that he had a double dose of, or was a homozygote for, the mutant autosomal dominant gene and therefore represented the full expression of the disorder. It might be argued that type I disease, with pure extrapyramidal signs of dystonia and athetosis along with clonus, spasticity, and hyperreflexia, but without cerebellar signs, is also a fairly complete expression of the dominant gene. Type

II, having cerebellar signs, a milder clinical course, and later onset (as expressed by the two parents), might represent less complete expression of the gene.

Although we encountered many examples of types I and II disease in the large kindred on Flores, we did not encounter a single example of type III, the Machado form, with peripheral neuropathy, distal atrophy, and cerebellar disorder.

Patient JTS, 67-year-old man, was examined in Santa Cruz. He had a steppage gait and foot drop with absent tendon reflexes in the legs and severe atrophy below the knees. This corresponds to the Machado form, or type III. He indicated that he had a family history of similar illness but could not trace his ancestry sufficiently to relate him to the Machado family in the United States or to the Sousa family manifesting types I and II disease. Type III disease is present on Flores, and patient JTS resembles patients MB (II,7) in the Thomas family; both have polyneuropathy and cerebellar disorder.

Several patients in the Sousa family developed progressive ocular prominence (10). Patient AM (V,36) was a 19-year-old woman who noted ataxic gait at age 15 years and, when examined, had leg spasticity, ankle clonus, flexor plantar responses, and limb ataxia. Her gait was spastic, with lurching from side to side. Her eyes were prominent, and there was ophthalmoparesis and horizontal nystagmus. Ocular prominence also occurred in her mother.

SINGLE GENETIC DISEASE HYPOTHESIS

Synthesizing the data from the Joseph, Thomas, and Sousa families (10), the data of Coutinho and Andrade (1), and the data of Romanul et al. (9), we believe we are witnessing the expression of a single gene that causes (a) early onset disease with pyramidal and extrapyramidal signs (type I), (b) intermediate age of onset and progression, with cerebellar deficits as well as pyramidal and extrapyramidal findings (type II), and (c) later onset, with peripheral neuropathy and cerebellar disorder (type III) (Fig. 5). Dominantly inherited parkinsonism with distal atrophy in one family (11) could constitute a type IV disease. It took a systematic evaluation of the California, Massachusetts, and Flores families, however, to document the variations of clinical expression. The additional neuropathologic findings of Romanul et al. (9), indicating the wider pathologic involvement with striatonigral degeneration in only some patients, also implied varied expression of this mutant gene.

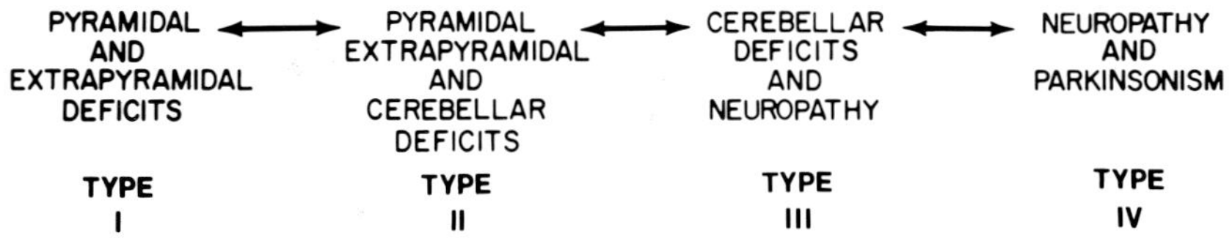

FIG. 5. Spectrum of clinical findings in Joseph disease. It is proposed that a single gene mutation can have clinical and neuropathologic variation, with at least four types now being recognized. (From ref. 11a.)

Alternatively, types I and II may represent one distinct genetic disease with variable cerebellar involvement that is present only on Flores and in descendants from the island. The Machado variant, type III, present in San Miguel, may be a separate dominant entity. The family reported by Romanul et al. (9) was originally from the same region of San Miguel and had typical Machado, or type III, disease. In favor of a single basic genetic mutation, however, were the findings in one autopsied member of the Romanul-Fowler family (9) of a striatonigral degeneration (patient III,7), the presence of parkinsonian features in two others (III,3 and III,7), the fact that two Thomas family members, a family originally from Flores, had type III disease, and, finally, the fact that one Joseph family member, EJ (III,19), may have a variant expression (type III) of the family disorder (Fig. 6A and B). The hypothesis of a single genetic disease seems plausible but lacks the critical support of a biochemical marker that is a constant abnormality regardless of clinical expression.

More recently, two reports have cited this genetic disorder in two families, one in northeastern Portugal (7) and one in New York (3)—a black family traced to North Carolina. They had clinical features similar to those of the Joseph and Thomas families, but neither family had any identifiable linkage to the Azores. Neuropathologic studies are required to prove that these families have the same disease.

It is generally agreed that despite the three major phenotypes, there is only one genetic disorder. Type I disease refers to onset in the second or third decades, with an expression of pyramidal or extrapyramidal features, including spasticity, rigidity, and dystonia. Type II disease includes pyramidal and extrapyramidal findings, with cerebellar ataxia of gait and extremities. Type III disease refers to late onset disease, beginning in the fifth to seventh decades, and expressing progressive cerebellar-type gait ataxia, hyporeflexia, hypotonia, and distal sensory loss and distal atrophy. These three phenotypes are probably clinical variations of the same gene mutation because: (a) all three types have been recorded in each of three separate families; (b) type I disease occurred in a parent, with types I and III in two children (Fig. 7); and (c) type II disease presented in both parents with onset of type I disease in their 8-year-old child, who presumably was homozygous for the dominant gene.

Of historic interest is the fact that when Dawson reexamined a member of his original Machado family (Fig. 8) in May, 1983, 11 years after his report in 1972 (8), the patient had bilateral extensor plantar responses, i.e., Babinski signs in addition to the typical cerebellar deficits. Again, this finding is a unifying feature to link types II and III disease. Thus this Machado family member was a transition patient, supporting the one gene hypothesis.

BIOCHEMICAL FINDINGS

In 1979, Rosenberg et al. (14) published two-dimensional acrylamide gels from one patient and control brain samples. There were several significant changes, with increases of 50,000 and 40,000 molecular weight proteins in patient cerebellum

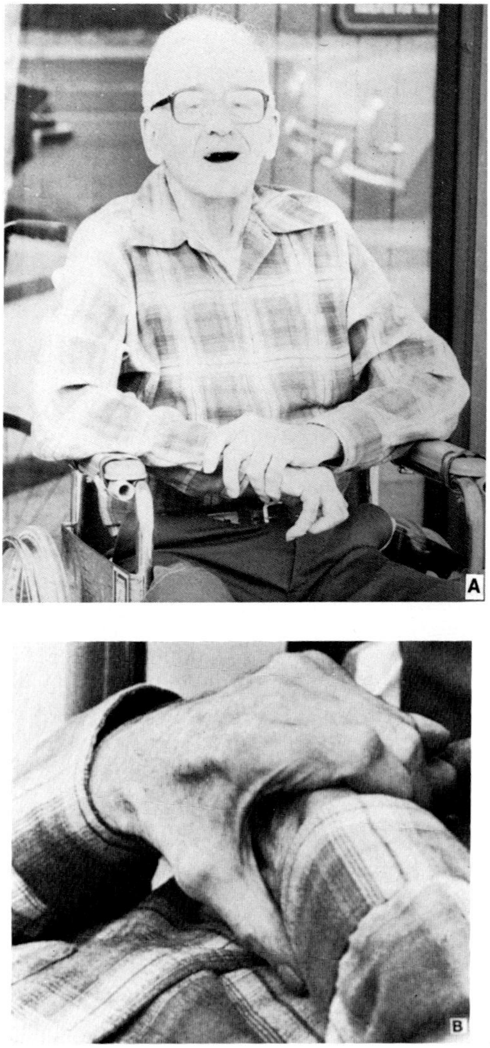

FIG. 6. A: Patient EJ (III,19) (10,13) is shown at age 75 with Joseph disease, type III. Onset of progressive cerebellar deficits began at age 65. (From ref. 11a.) **B:** Atrophy distally at age 75 years. Of note is the fact that he is the grandson of Antone Joseph and is the exception in the Joseph family, having type III disease whereas others in the family express type I disease. (From ref. 11a.)

and putamen corresponding to gliosis seen histologically (Fig. 9). These findings were later confirmed in samples of cerebellum and putamen from five patients (12).

Joseph disease results from neuronal loss with attendant glial reaction and replacement, i.e., gliosis. The disease may occur because the gene mutation results in the loss of a glial trophic factor required for neuronal function. Two changes

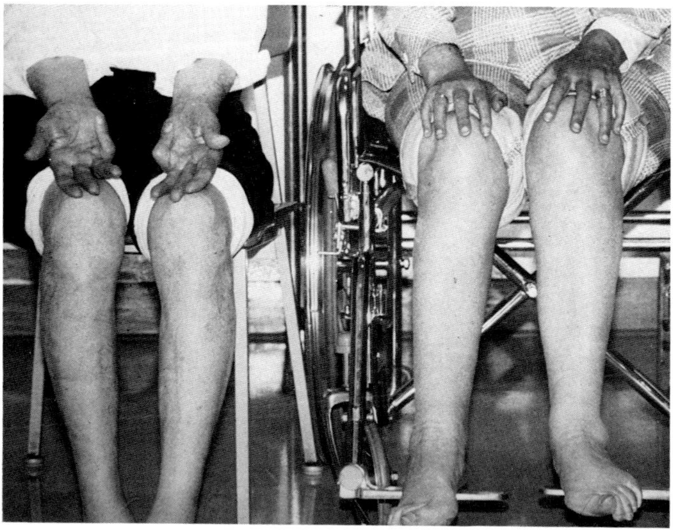

FIG. 7. A brother *(right)* and sister *(left)* having types III and I Joseph disease, respectively. She presented in her late 30s with leg spasticity; he presented in his 60s with progressive cerebellar gait ataxia. He is developing distal extremity atrophy as well, characteristic of type III disease. By history, their mother had type I disease, evidence supporting the hypothesis of a single gene producing either type I or III phenotype. (From ref. 11a.)

would follow. First, glial cells would increase in dynamic compensation to provide an increased total amount of glial factor, but this is ultimately insufficient, resulting in secondary neuronal dysfunction and loss. This view is supported by the evidence of increased Jc, Jd, L_1, L_2, and h proteins, which are synthesized by glia (Fig. 9). Multiple sclerosis plaques are also foci of gliosis, and only these J- and L-specific classes of proteins are increased. The h class of proteins was determined by comigration studies to be glial filamentous acidic proteins (14).

Increased glial proteins might be merely a biochemical reflection of nonspecific gliosis, but these changes may be due to an increased glial protein response per cell and by a total increase in glial numbers, attempting specifically to correct another primary gene mutation. The neuropathology and these biochemical changes are still compatible with the provocative interpretation that Joseph disease and the other dominant ataxias are the result of a genetic mutation that causes the loss of glial trophic factor, leading to neuronal loss and glial reaction. A genetic reciprocal interaction between glial cells and neuroblasts had been documented in cell culture (15). A glial gene product induces a repressed neuronal gene and results in the expression of a specific neuronal protein (15). Joseph disease and other dominant ataxias may be the clinical counterpart of defective glial-neuronal interaction.

JOSEPH DISEASE DESIGNATION

A preference for the term "Joseph disease" is generally expressed because it is the largest known pedigree, including more than 600 persons in 10 generations.

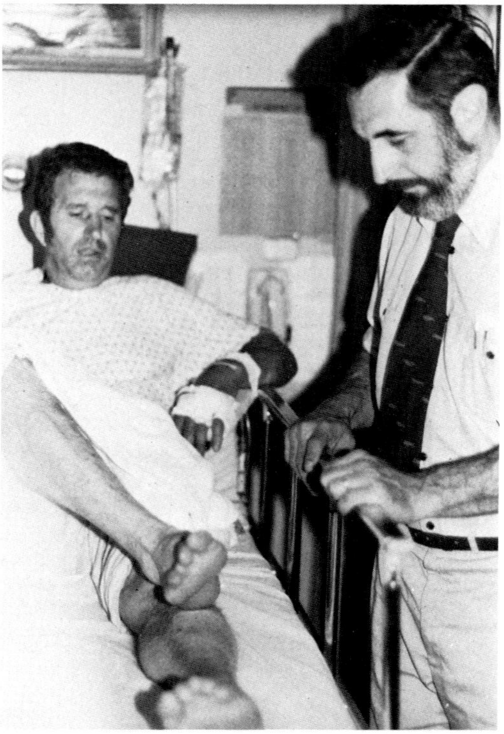

FIG. 8. Dr. David Dawson is examining a member of the original Machado kindred in our May, 1983, Massachusetts Clinic. The patient had extensor plantar responses in addition to cerebellar findings of a type III patient and thus is an important transitional form between types II and III.

The Joseph family includes all three types of disease, and brain samples of all three types show similar protein patterns on two-dimensional gels. It has been possible to reconstruct the spectrum of clinical disease, propose the unitary hypothesis of a single gene mutation resulting in several clinical phenocopies from analysis of this family, and provide direct biochemical evidence in support of this single genotype from brain samples obtained principally from this family. It may be possible to identify expression of disease by patterns of skin fibroblast proteins labeled with ^{35}S-methionine obtained from Joseph family members (12). For these compelling reasons, Joseph disease seems to be the proper designation. The term "Azorean disease" was objected to by physicians and scientists from Portugal, the Azore Islands, the United States, and Canada for the reasons cited above and also because some affected families have no known connection with any Azorean family (7,10). Azoreans and the Portuguese medical community find the term objectionable because of the stigma it gives to the Azorean people.

OLIVOPONTOCEREBELLAR ATROPHY AND JOSEPH DISEASE

There is considerable historic evidence from the explorations and subsequent reciprocal migrations of the Dutch, Portuguese, Portuguese-Azoreans, and Portu-

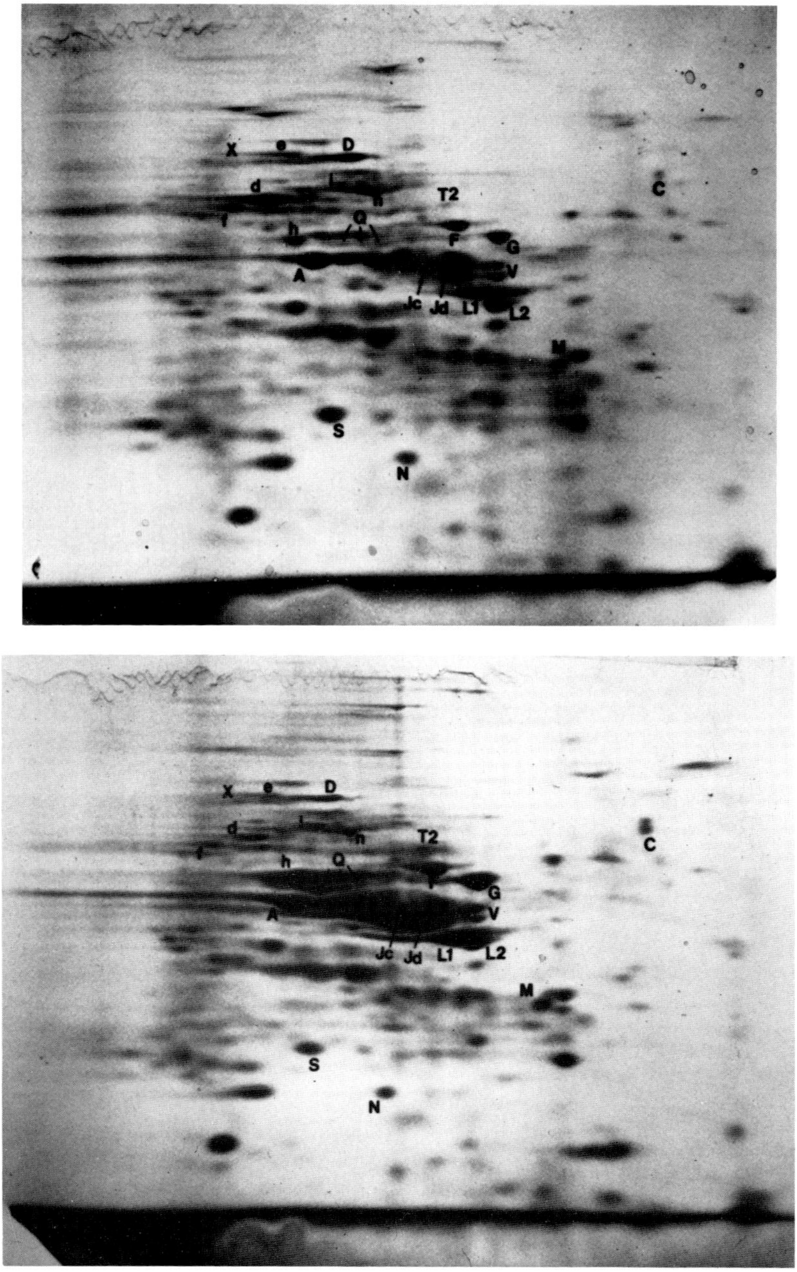

FIG. 9. Two-dimensional gel protein separations of control **(top)** and Joseph disease **(bottom)** cerebellar proteins. This 73-year-old type III patient (EC) was reported previously in detail (14). The patient gel shows a significant increase in the h, J, and L classes of proteins; 1 mg protein from a brain homogenate was added to each gel. (From ref. 11a.)

guese-Brazilians between the 12th and 17th centuries to speculate that autosomal dominant olivopontocerebellar atrophy (OPCA) of the Schut-Swier type (5) (of Dutch origin) and Joseph disease (of the Portuguese) could be the result of the same mutant gene. Clinical and neuropathologic variations of OPCA and Joseph disease, and among families with Joseph disease, could be the result of both heterogenous nonallelic and allelic genetic modification of the mutant gene expression. Population genetic analyses, gene mapping, and precise identification of the altered gene product in patients with both types of disease will be required to resolve this point.

JOSEPH DISEASE AS A UNIQUE SPINOCEREBELLAR DEGENERATION

Joseph disease is a unique, dominantly inherited spinocerebellar degeneration, rarely encountered in ethnic groups other than the Portuguese. Its clinical phenotype includes a specific constellation of features: prominent eyes due to lid retraction, ophthalmoparesis, loss of fast saccadic eye movements, facial and lingual fasciculations without atrophy, dystonia, spasticity and parkinson-like features of tremor-at-rest, bradykinesia, and rigidity. It is a spinocerebellar degeneration with invariant symmetrical degeneration of the cerebellum and thoracic cord in all patients and variable degeneration of the striatum, substantia nigra, basis pontis, oculomotor nuclei, and peripheral nerves. The inferior olives are always spared, thus separating Joseph disease from dominant OPCA. The variation in penetrance and expressivity follows the pattern encountered in other dominantly inherited disorders but was verified only by virtue of neuroepidemiologic, clinical, and biochemical analyses (10–12). Patients with elements of spasticity or parkinsonism, despite associated cerebellar deficits, may benefit from treatment with L-DOPA.

MECHANISMS OF DOMINANT ATAXIAS

It is expected that several molecular bases for the pathogenesis of disease will be uncovered for any given single clinical syndrome. Conversely, any one genotype will include variation of clinical features within a family and between families. The biochemical challenge is formidable, but, with an appreciation of the molecular basis of any of the dominantly inherited neurologic diseases, rapid progress should be made in all the ataxias. Several biochemical clues are emerging. Two other dominant conditions, HD and myotonic muscular dystrophy (MMD), are probably diffuse and universal disorders of cell surface membranes. Biophysical studies of HD and MMD fibroblast, red cell, and lymphocyte membranes indicate alterations in membrane fluidity and dynamics (1). Dominantly inherited neurofibromatosis results in part from defective and elevated serum levels of nerve growth factor and reduced numbers of cell surface receptor sites for lymphocyte epidermal growth factor. These defects may result in improper cell-cell recognition and biochemical cell-cell interaction. Neuronal loss and gliosis, as discussed above, result in HD and Joseph disease; tumor formation occurs in neurofibromatosis, along with such

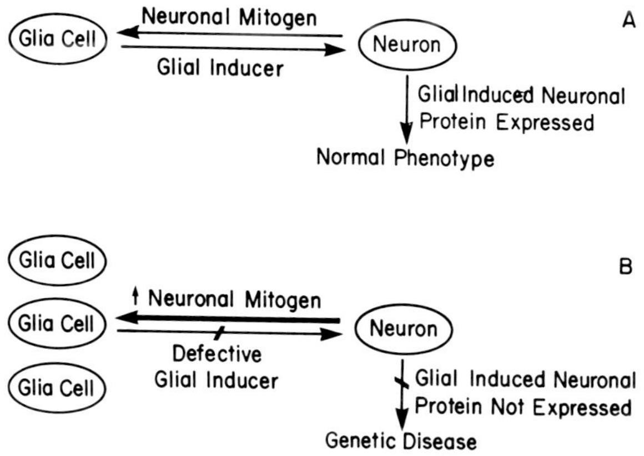

FIG. 10. A model for the biochemical basis of gliosis. It is postulated that glia and neurons form a biochemical unit with reciprocal intercellular biochemical regulation. It is also postulated that glial genes exist that induce neuronal genes for the expression of neuronal proteins; in turn, neurons regulate the glial population by the release of a mitogen at low levels in the normal brain **(A)**. The mutation **(B)** results in the loss of glial inducer for a neuronal protein and, thus, in neuronal degeneration. The neuronal compartment, in turn, secretes increased amounts of mitogen to cause an increase in glial number to provide more glial inducer and more gliatropic support. Gliosis and associated neuronal degeneration, therefore, are the end stage results of a compensatory biochemical interaction between these two cell types. (From ref. 11a.)

other architectonic abnormalities as neuronal heterotopias and cortical disorganization. Glial-neuronal biochemical interactions, so indispensible for neuronal life, fail, perhaps because of cell surface alterations resulting in compensatory glial proliferation. This idea of impaired glial-neuronal interaction is based on these biochemical clues and should be pursued (12).

Viral factors must be mentioned in view of the findings of paracrystalline and myovirus-like structures in neurons of OPCA patients by Landis et al. (6). Furthermore, a dominantly inherited pattern of Creutzfeldt-Jakob disease (CJD) has been reported by Gajdusek and Gibbs, with several patients having ataxia (2). No evidence of vertical transmission has been maintained, and it is assumed that there is increased susceptibility on a genetic basis for the CJD agent. A brain specimen from a Joseph patient was inoculated into primates and other small mammals; as of 1980, no disease resulted in the host animals. The necessity for careful pathologic examination is emphasized, since CJD has now been diagnosed in a family with HD and is suspected in a family with Alzheimer disease. Inoculation of biopsy material from some Alzheimer patients caused spongiform encephalopathy in animals.

Other possible mechanisms productive of the dominant ataxias due to a single gene mutation include: (a) alteration of a subunit of a cell surface receptor site for a neurotransmitter or neuromodulator, (b) alteration of an antigenic site on the cell surface resulting in an autoimmune state, (c) an altered soluble repressor substance within the cell nucleus irreversibly inhibiting the transcription of a gene, (d) altered regulatory enzymatic activity in a crucial biochemical cyclic pathway, (e) enzyme alteration producing a neurotoxin or an inhibitor, and (f) alteration in the intron region of deoxyribonucleic acid (DNA), a region that normally splits the exon portion of a gene and that may be essential for efficiency or rate of ribonucleic acid (RNA) transcription for protein synthesis or for final protein modification by phosphorylation, glycosylation, or methylation.

CONCLUSION

The dominant ataxias are a group of disorders characterized by a regular, progressive, and symmetrical degeneration of the cerebellum and its pathways. Disease results in half the sons and daughters of an affected parent; and, therefore, disease occurs in the heterozygote. Variation in age of onset, clinical findings, neuropathologic features, and penetrance of disease are usual (10–12). New mutations must be rare. Linkage of HLA to the ataxia gene on chromosome 6 in one large family but not others suggests at least two separate genotypes for the OPCAs (4). It is not clear if all the dominantly inherited ataxias are due to a single gene mutation that has entered various ethnic populations and produces different syndromes. Such a supposition is possible but must be supported by a common molecular defect, independent of clinical or neuropathologic variation. Joseph disease is a dominantly inherited ataxia in which it has been demonstrated that a single gene mutation can cause wide variation in phenotype of affected persons within a single family and between families. Increased 50,000 and 40,000 MW classes of proteins have been found in six Joseph disease brains compared to appropriate control brain, as shown on two-dimensional acrylamide gels (12,14). These increased proteins, in part, are glial proteins expressed most abundantly in cerebellum and basal ganglia and represent a glial response to compensate, it is hypothesized, for defective glial-neuronal interaction (11,12,14). The dominant ataxias may be due to allelic mutations within a single gene, resulting in the clinical variation noted. The altered gene product is responsible for an impairment in cell-cell recognition (glial-neuronal biochemical interaction), leading to the characteristic neuropathology of neuronal loss and gliosis (Fig. 10). The finding of the altered gene product in nonneural tissue would provide a marker for effective genetic counseling and elimination of disease in a family in one generation. The goals are now clearly defined, and current research approaches appear promising for new insights into these disorders in the immediate future.

REFERENCES

1. Coutinho, P., and Andrade, C. (1978): Autosomal dominant system degeneration in Portuguese families of the Azores Islands. *Neurology*, 28:703–709.
2. Gajdusek, D. C., and Gibbs, C. J., Jr. (1975): Slow virus infections of the nervous system and the laboratories of slow temperate virus infections. In: *The Nervous System. The Clinical Neurosciences*, Vol. 2, pp. 120–124, edited by D. B. Tower. Raven Press, New York.
3. Healton, E., Brust, J., and Kerr, D. (1979): Familial cerebellar ataxia, dystonia, and abnormal eye movements in a non-Portuguese family. *Neurology*, 29:559–560.

4. Jackson, J., Currier, R., Teraski, P., and Morton, N. (1977): Spinocerebellar ataxia and HLA linkage risk prediction in HLA typing. *N. Engl. J. Med.*, 296:1138–1141.
5. Konigsmark, B., and Weiner, L. (1970): The olivopontocerebellar atrophies: A review. *Medicine*, 49:227–241.
6. Landis, D., Rosenberg, R. N., Landis, S., Schut, L., and Nyhan, W. (1974): Olivopontocerebellar degeneration. *Arch. Neurol.*, 31:295–307.
7. Lima, L., and Coutinho, P. (1980): Clinical criteria for diagnosis of Machado-Joseph disease: Report of a non-Azorean Portuguese family. *Neurology*, 30:319–322.
8. Nakano, K. K., Dawson, D. M., and Spence, A. (1972): Machado disease: A hereditary ataxia in Portuguese immigrants to Massachusetts. *Neurology*, 22:49–55.
9. Romanul, F. C. A., Fowler, H. L., and Radvany, J. (1977): Azorean disease of the nervous system. *N. Engl. J. Med.*, 296:1505–1508.
10. Rosenberg, R. N. (1978): Joseph's disease. In: *Advances in Neurology, Vol. 21, The Inherited Ataxias*, edited by P. Kark, R. N. Rosenberg, and L. Schut. pp. 1–424. Raven Press, New York.
11. Rosenberg, R. N. (1980): Genetic variation and neurological disease. *Trends Neurosci.*, 3:144–148.
11a. Rosenberg, R. N. (1983): Dominant ataxis. In: *Genetics of Neurological and Psychiatric Disorders*, edited by S. S. Kety, L. P. Rowland, R. L. Sidman, and S. W. Matthysse, pp. 195–213. Raven Press, New York.
12. Rosenberg, R. N., Ivy, N., Kirkpatrick, J., Bay, C., Nyhan, W. L., and Baskin, F. (1981): Joseph disease and Huntington disease. Protein patterns in fibroblasts and brain. II. *Neurology*, 31:1003–1014.
13. Rosenberg, R. N., Nyhan, W. L., and Bay, C. (1976): Autosomal dominant striatonigral degeneration: A clinical, pathologic, and biochemical study of a new genetic disorder. *Neurology*, 26:703–714.
14. Rosenberg, R. N., Thomas, L., Baskin, F., Kirkpatrick, J., Bay, C., and Nyhan, W. L. (1979): Joseph disease: Protein patterns in fibroblasts and brain. *Neurology*, 29:917–926.
15. Rosenberg, R. N., Vance, C. K., and Prashad, N. (1978): Differentiation of neuroblastoma, glioma, and hybrid cells in culture as measured by the synthesis of specific protein species: Evidence for neuroblast-reciprocal genetic regulation. *J. Neurochem.*, 30:1343–1355.
16. Woods, B. I., and Schaumburg, H. H. (1972): Nigro-spino-dentatal degeneration with nuclear ophthalmoplegia: A unique and partially treatable clinicopathological entity. *J. Neurol. Sci.*, 17:149–166.

The Olivopontocerebellar Atrophies, edited by R.C. Duvoisin and A. Plaitakis. Raven Press, New York © 1984.

Dominantly Inherited Ataxia with Abnormal Urinary Glycolipid Content

[1]Richard A. Berenberg, *Onur Melen, [2]George F. Howard III, and Donald H. Harter

*Departments of Neurology and *Ophthalmology, Northwestern University Medical School, Chicago, Illinois 60611*

The study of dominantly inherited ataxias is a difficult and complex task. It has been traditional to classify patients on the basis of clinical symptoms and pathologic distribution of neuronal loss. An objective of the various classification schemes has been to group together families that presumably have identical genetic defects. Clearly, this is an inexact exercise (5). Until specific biochemical markers can be found for a defective gene, there can be no definitive scheme of classification. Just as a single genetic mutation may have a wide spectrum of clinical manifestations (13,14), so may different genetic mutations produce the same clinical syndrome. This is illustrated in recessively inherited diseases, such as juvenile spinal muscular atrophy (Kugelberg-Welander diseases), which may result from hexosaminidase deficiency but usually has other causes, presumably also enzyme deficiencies (7). Even in diseases in which specific biochemical abnormalities are known, the relationship between clinical and pathologic features and the biochemical defect is not fully understood. This is true for both genetic diseases, such as abetalipoproteinemia (Bassen-Kornzweig disease) (15), and acquired diseases, such as vitamin B_{12} deficiency. Some biochemical defects can be directly related to the disease process, such as glutamate dehydrogenase (GDH) deficiency (10). In autosomal dominant conditions, however, the abnormalities are less specific. Rosenberg et al. (13), for example, have reported some variation in the protein pattern of cultured skin fibroblasts found on two-dimensional acrylamide gel separations in patients with Joseph disease. Nevertheless, such biochemical abnormalities may provide clues to the pathogenesis of the disease process or at least serve as markers for the underlying genetic defect.

The family that is the basis of this report attracted our attention because of its highly unusual phenotype. The combination of prominent bulbar palsy, axial and limb atrophy, extraocular muscle involvement, unusual facial expression, and predominantly midline cerebellar involvement distinguished these individuals from

[1]Deceased.
[2]Present address: Department of Neurology, Boston University Medical School, 80 East Concord Street, Boston, Massachusetts 02118.

most other reported cases. Having identified an abnormal pattern of glycolipids in the urinary sediment of these patients, we are encouraged to continue our investigations, looking for an intrinsic membrane defect that might relate to the pathogenesis if not the root cause of this disease. These results have been published in abstract form (1).

CLINICAL FEATURES

Fourteen family members in four generations are known to be affected by either personal examination (five) or history (see Fig. 1). The mode of transmission is clearly autosomal dominant. The family originated in Alabama but is now distributed across the United States. The affected father of patient 1 was caucasian, and all reported members are mixed caucasian and black. There is no indication of Portuguese ancestry.

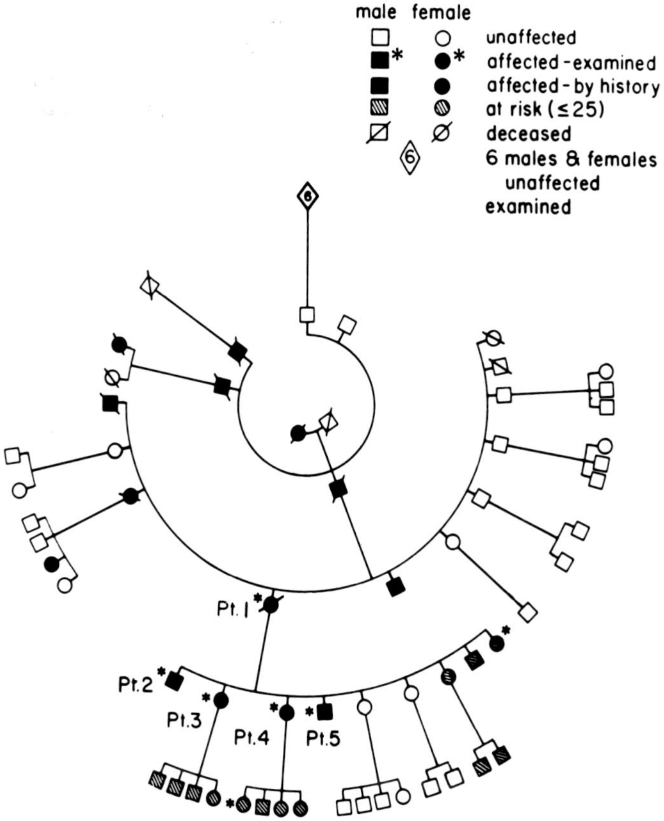

FIG. 1. This pedigree shows autosomal dominant transmission of the disease gene to 14 family members in four generations. The fifth generation is still at risk.

Patient 1

Patient 1 was 60 years old at her death. Onset of neurologic symptoms was in her late teens, with difficulty running. Gradual progression of ataxia and weakness led to marked staggering by age 30 and confinement to a wheelchair at age 40. Arm strength, speech, and vision deteriorated, and recurrent pneumonia developed. On examination age 58, she was wasted, head resting on her chest, and unable to maintain an erect posture while sitting. She communicated by head nodding. Her IQ was Dull Normal, without evidence of dementia on psychometric testing. Visual acuity was 20/200 in the right eye and light perception in the left. Both optic discs were pale, and there was no retinopathy. The eyes were prominent, with a staring expression, and there was bilateral, asymmetrical, and variable ptosis (Fig. 2, left). There was a fixed left exotropia and complete ophthalmoplegia, with no response to oculocephalic maneuver. Jaw and facial muscles were markedly weak. The pharynx was ectatic, with the soft palate hanging low, resting on the tongue. The gag reflex was active. The tongue was weak and atrophic, with occasional fasciculations. Muscle bulk and tone were diminished in all limbs, but atrophy was most severe in the hands. Weakness was moderate in the proximal limbs and severe in the hands, feet, and trunk. Mild dysmetria was present. Reflexes were generally hyperactive but were absent at the ankle. Plantar responses were occasionally extensor. Mild impairment of vibration and position sense in the toes were the only sensory abnormalities. The patient died following hospitalization at a local community hospital for aspiration pneumonia and respiratory arrest. No autopsy was obtained.

Patient 2

This 37-year-old son of patient 1 had onset of symptoms in his early 20s. His clinical course was similar to that of his mother. Mental status was normal. Visual

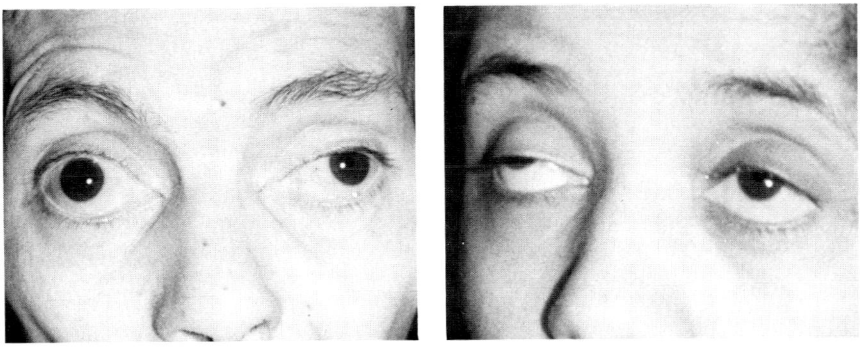

FIG. 2. Left: Left eyelid ptosis and right lid retraction with bilateral contraction of the frontalis muscle are shown in patient 1. At other times, ptosis and lid retraction were on the opposite side or bilateral. Left exotropia is evident on attempted frontal gaze. **Right:** Patient 2 shows bilateral ptosis with frontalis muscle contraction. Within the same few minutes, lid retraction and a prominent staring expression would replace the ptosis on one or both sides.

acuity was 20/20 bilaterally; pupils and fundi were normal. The eyes were prominent, with bilateral lid retraction and mildly weak lid closure. He was unable to open his eyelids for 5 to 10 sec following voluntary closure (apraxia of lid opening). He facilitated the opening by contracting his frontalis muscles. There was conjugate upward and horizontal paresis of saccadic, pursuit, and oculocephalic eye movements. Downward gaze was preserved. Facial and bulbar weakness were severe, with functional anarthria. There was atrophy of distal limb musculature, with moderate proximal weakness, increased tone, and hyperactive reflexes. Truncal ataxia was severe.

Patient 3

This 35-year-old daughter of patient 1 noted difficulty walking at age 19. By her late 20s, she had intermittent diplopia, indistinct speech, dysphagia for liquids, limb weakness, and incoordination. She was unable to walk without support. Visual acuity and pupillary function were normal, although optic pallor was present bilaterally. Lid retraction, with a prominent staring expression, alternated with incomplete ptosis (see Fig. 2B). There was a right hypertropia on right gaze, left hypertropia on left gaze, and some diminution of upward gaze. Saccades were slowed, and there was gaze-evoked nystagmus on horizontal and upward gaze as well as ocular dysmetria. Facial and jaw muscle weakness were severe. The soft palate hung low but elevated briskly on testing the gag reflex. The tongue was small and weak but showed no fasciculations. No speech sounds were produced. Neck and trunk were tilted toward the left. She was unable to maintain an erect posture without support. Muscle tone was increased, more so in the legs, with only mild weakness. All movements were markedly slowed but only slightly ataxic. She was unable to stand because of truncal weakness and instability. Deep tendon reflexes were hyperactive, and plantar responses were extensor. Sensation was normal.

Patients 4 and 5

The 32-year-old daughter and 31-year-old son of patient 1 developed an unsteady gait and slurred speech in their early 20s. Both remained ambulatory and active, despite increasingly ataxic gait. They, too, had prominent eyes and lid retraction but no ptosis. Visual acuity, fundi, and pupils were normal. Patient 4 had a variable esotropia on primary and lateral gaze and exotropia on upgaze. Other eye movements were full, except for diminished convergence. Gaze-evoked jerk nystagmus was present on horizontal and upward gaze. Patient 5 had slowed saccadic velocity, limited upgaze, and horizontal gaze-evoked nystagmus. Dysphagia, facial weakness, mild distal limb weakness with increased tone, hyperactive reflexes, and normal sensation were present. Cerebellar dysfunction in the limbs was minimal compared to the gait disorder.

Among the neuroophthalmologic findings in these patients, the prominence of the eyes, with lid retraction and staring appearance, was most conspicuous. They were noted in all patients and were accompanied by ptosis in two and apraxia of lid opening in a third. Abnormalities of ocular motility ranged from gaze-evoked nystagmus to total immobility of the eyes and included slowed saccades, impaired pursuit and convergence, and alternating vertical divergence (probably alternating skew deviation). Two patients had optic atrophy, and none had pigmentary retinopathy.

The HLA typing of four patients and one unaffected sibling of patient 1 showed no linkage with the disease gene. Computerized tomography scans of patients 1 and 3 showed widening of the superior cerebellar cisterns, normal serum lipoproteins, serum and urinary copper, and urinary amino acids. All patients had normal routine chemistries, red blood cell morphology, urinalysis, thyroid functions, and electrocardiograms.

The electromyograms of patients 1 and 3 showed active denervation in a multisegmental distribution, with increased insertional activity, fibrillations, positive waves, and fasciculations. Some motor unit potentials were large and polyphasic. Slight abnormalities of conduction were seen in the posterior tibial and peroneal nerves of patient 1. A muscle biopsy from the quadriceps of patient 3 showed small groups of atrophic fibers involving types I and II equally, indicative of denervation.

URINARY GLYCOLIPID ANALYSIS

Methods

Urinary glycolipids in 24-hr collections from patients 1, 3, 4, and 5 and controls (two female, one male) were studied in the laboratory of Dr. Sen-Itiroh Hakamori (Seattle, Washington). The membrane fraction was sedimented at $12{,}000 \times g$ and kept frozen prior to analysis. The specimens were homogenized and extracted in chloroform/methanol (2:1). The soluble fractions containing the glycolipid were acetylated and purified on a fluorisil resin column. Following deacetylation, the glycolipids were spotted on TLC (silica gel 60) plates and developed in chloroform/methanol/water (60:35:8). Glycolipid concentration was corrected for original urine volume. The chloroform/methanol-insoluble protein fraction was taken up in 1% SDS (2 ml/liter original urine volume). Aliquots were run on a 5 to 14% polyacrylamide gradient gel.

Results

There was a general increase in the amounts of both lipid and protein fractions (greater than twofold) in patients 1, 3, and 4 versus controls. The increased glycolipid was present primarily in bands which comigrated with ceramide trihexoside and asialo GM2. There was also an increase in the total amount of the more polar lipids. Neither the quantity of lipid nor its specific pattern was of the type seen in lipid storage disease, such as Fabry's disease (3). The youngest patient, a male, had more glycolipid and protein than the male but not the female controls. Cultured fibroblasts from patient 3 contained normal amounts of alpha-galactosidase A and B.

DISCUSSION

The clinical manifestations of multisystem neurologic involvement in this family were highly unusual. The illness began at the end of the second or early in the third decade, with ataxia of gait of midline cerebellar type. Toward the end of the third decade, brainstem signs appeared, involving ocular, facial, and bulbar functions. In the fourth decade, the patients became wheelchair bound because of truncal instability; facial, bulbar, and limb weakness progressed, with increasing lower motoneuron involvement. The most advanced case had such severe truncal and neck muscle weakness that she was unable to hold her head erect. There was no evidence of intellectual deterioration, significant sensory loss, generalized peripheral nerve dysfunction, or basal ganglia involvement.

The predominant oculomotor abnormalities derived from involvement of supranuclear pathways in the brainstem and cerebellum. There were also signs of nuclear and/or infranuclear origin, such as ptosis. In two patients, ptosis alternated with lid retraction in the fellow eye, complying with Hering's law of equal innervation. Two others had lid retraction and impaired upgaze without ptosis, characteristic of mesodiencephalic dysfunction. The most unusual finding was the apraxia of lid opening in patient 2, a clearly supranuclear phemonenon, which was described previously by Goldstein and Cogan (4) in patients with generalized cerebral and basal ganglia disorders. Gaze-evoked horizontal and upbeating nystagmus and decreased saccadic velocity in the same directions imply involvement of the paramedian pontine reticular formation and/or its projections and both medial longitudinal fasciculi. The horizontal and upgaze paresis in patient 2 was likely of supranuclear origin because of preserved downgaze. However, the lack of reflex eye movements in the most affected case (patient 1) suggests nuclear or infranuclear disease in addition to advanced supranuclear gaze abnormalities. Pregeniculate involvement of the optic pathways was indicated by optic disc pallor in two patients, one of whom had visual loss.

All these features of multisystem disease have been described in varying combinations in other individuals with autosomal dominant ataxias. Schut (14) described some members of an extensive family with significant limb and bulbar atrophy as well as prominent eyes. Stephens et. al. (16) also described a family with early onset of ataxia and subsequent limb atrophy and ophthalmoplegia. This family had severe sensory loss. A similar case was described by Pitrangeli et al. (9) with optic atrophy, amyotrophy, ophthalmoparesis, dysphonia, and dysphagia, but with significant peripheral nerve involvement.

Autosomal dominant motor system degeneration in Portuguese families of Azorean origin has been extensively described by a number of authors (2,12,13; see Rosenberg, *this volume*). The present family had similar staring eyes, dysphagia and dysphonia, amyotrophy, and cerebellar ataxia but lacked the dystonic posturing of the type 1 variant, had a much earlier age of onset and more severe amyotrophy than the type II variants, and lacked the peripheral nerve involvement of the type III variants (13). There was no indication of Azorean inheritance in this family from Alabama back as far as four generations. One family, with a condition similar to the type II Azorean disease and without known Portuguese ancestry was reported by Healton et al. (6). The clinical pattern of the family overlaps but is not identical to previously described familial ataxic syndromes.

Urinary glycolipids are derived from the membrane fraction of desquamated renal tubular epithelial cells in the absence of urinary tract infection (3). The twofold increase in total lipid content, but not the proportion of constituent glycolipids, may have been influenced by the number of cells per volume of urine. The prominent glycolipid bands separated by thin layer chromatography were in regions that comigrated with ceramide trihexoside and asialo GM2. These were found only in the three female patients and not in female controls. The glycolipid content of normal urine is so low that prominent bands are never seen (3). The male patient did not show the same result but was also younger and less affected at the time of study. These findings were not of such a degree or specificity to indicate a single enzymatic defect causing lipid storage, such as is seen in Fabry's disease (3). They do suggest an imbalance in membrane glycolipid content, which might have important metabolic and physiologic consequences within the nervous system.

The predominant lipid constituents of cell membranes are phospholipids and cholesterol, which are organized in a bilayer with a nonpolar core and hydrophilic surface (11,17). As reviewed by Maggio et al. (8), the conformation of lipid molecules profoundly affects the biophysical properties of the membrane through their effect on protein elements embedded in the membrane and at the surface. Although glycolipids make up a small proportion of the total membrane lipid, the large polar carbohydrate moieties may significantly affect the packing of the major structural lipids (phospholipids and cholesterol). Thus, the glycolipid content of the membrane influences its permeability to Ca^{2+}, K^{+}, and Na^{+}, thereby affecting neurotransmitter release and electrical activity in neurons. Lipid-protein interactions also control the conformation of glycoprotein moieties at the cell surface, which determines the activity and specificity of cell receptors (for neurotransmitters, neuromodulators, and perhaps trophic substances) and affects antigenicity.

We are now attempting to correlate the biochemical abnormality in renal epithelial cell membranes with the biophysical properties of red cell membranes. Preliminary studies of erythrocyte ghosts from patient 3 using Raman spectroscopy have been performed in the laboratory of Professor John Kauffman at Northwestern University. These have demonstrated consistent differences in the spectra of the patient membranes indicating decreased fluidity of membrane lipids. There was a parallel increase in order for the secondary structure of the membrane protein molecules as indicated by exceptionally prominent Raman bands corresponding to the alpha helical conformation. Decreased membrane fluidity means that the phospholipid molecules are more tightly packed and cannot change their orientation as easily (17). It is known that the glycolipid content can profoundly affect membrane fluidity in artificial membranes (8) and is probably important in natural membranes as well. We are planning to attempt to reproduce the observed changes in the Raman spectra by the addition of glycolipids to normal red cell ghosts.

At the present stage of investigation, it is possible only to suggest that the alteration in glycolipid distribution demonstrated in renal epithelial cells may reflect a similar abnormality in red cells and neural membranes. A significant imbalance in membrane glycolipid content could have profound effects on cell function and viability even if it is only an indirect product of the dominantly inherited gene. The finding of an abnormal content of urinary glycolipids in this family with an unusual and devastating neurologic disease should alert others to look for similar biochemical defects in other patients with inherited ataxia.

ACKNOWLEDGMENTS

Dr. Berenberg is the recipient of a NIH (NINCDS) Teacher Investigator Development Award. We thank Dr. Sen-Itiroh Hakamori (University of Washington, Seattle) for performing the glycolipid analysis and Professor John Kauffman and Michael Rooney (Technological Institute, Northwestern University) for providing a preliminary report on the Raman spectroscopic analysis of the red cell ghosts from patient 3. We particularly express our appreciation to the family that is the subject of this report for their enthusiastic cooperation with all aspects of this investigation.

REFERENCES

1. Berenberg, R. A., Howard, G. F., and Harter, D. H. (1980): Dominantly inherited ataxia with motor neuron disease. *Trans. Am. Neurol. Assoc.*, 105:391–393.
2. Coutinho, P., and Andrade, C. (1978): Autosomal dominant system degeneration in Portuguese families of the Azores Islands. *Neurology*, 28:703–709.
3. Desnick, R. J., Dawson, G., Desnick, S. J., Sweeley, C. C., and Krivitt, W. (1971): Diagnosis if glycophingolipidoses by urinary-sediment analysis. *N. Engl. J. Med.*, 284:739–744.
4. Goldstein, J. E., and Cogan, D. G. (1965): Apraxia of lid opening. *Arch. Ophthalmol.*, 73:155–159.
5. Harding, A. E. (1982): The clinical features and classification of late onset autosomal dominant cerebellar ataxias. *Brain*, 105:1–28.
6. Healton, E. B., Brust, J. C. M., Kerr, D. L., Resor, S., and Penn, A. (1980): Presumably Azorean disease in a presumably non-Portuguese family. *Neurology*, 30:1084–1089.
7. Johnson, W. G. (1982): Hexosaminidase deficiency: A cause of recessively inherited motor neuron diseases. In: *Advances in Neurology, Vol. 36, Human Motor Neuron Diseases*, edited by L. P. Rowland, pp. 159–164. Raven Press, New York.
8. Maggio, B., Cumar, F. A., and Caputto, R. (1981): Molecular behaviour of glycosphingolipids in interfaces: Possible participation in some properties of nerve membranes. *Biophys. Biochim. Acta*, 650:69–87.
9. Pitrangeli, A., Gessini, L., Jandolo, B., and Occhipinti, E. (1981): Atypical hereditary spinocerebellar degeneration. Description of a case with familial study. *Ital. J. Neurol. Sci.*, 4:387–390.
10. Plaitakis, A., Nicklas, J., and Desnick, R. J. (1980): Glutamate dehydrogensase deficiency in three patients with spinocerebellar syndrome. *Ann. Neurol.*, 7:297–303.
11. Robertson, J. D. (1981): Membrane structure. *J. Cell Biol.*, 91:189s–204s.
12. Romanul, F. C. A., Fowler, H. L., Radvany, J., Feldman, R. G., and Feingold, M. (1977): Azorean disease of the nervous system. *N. Engl. J. Med.*, 296:1505–1508.
13. Rosenberg, R. N., Nyhan, W. L., Coutinho, P., and Bay, C. (1978): Joseph's disease: An autosomal dominant neurological disease in the Portuguese of the United States and the Azores Islands. In:

Advances in Neurology, Vol. 21, The Inherited Ataxias, edited by R. A. P. Kark, R. N. Rosenberg, and L. J. Schut, pp. 33–57. Raven Press, New York.
14. Schut, J. W. (1950): Hereditary ataxia: Clinical study through six generations. *Arch. Neurol. Psychiatry*, 63:535–568.
15. Schwartz, J. F., Rowland, L. P., Eder, H., Marks, P. A., Osserman, E. F., Hirschberg, E., and Anderson, H. (1963): Bassen-Kornzweig syndrome: Deficiency of serum B-lipoprotein. *Arch. Neurol.*, 8:108–124.
16. Stephens, J., Hoover, J. L., and Denst, J. (1958): On familial ataxia, neural amyotrophy, and their association with progressive external ophthalmoplegia. *Brain*, 81:556–566.
17. Zwaal, R. F. A. (1981): Structure and function of blood cell membranes. *Pediatr. Res.*, 8:1143–1149.

The Olivopontocerebellar Atrophies, edited by R. C. Duvoisin and A. Plaitakis. Raven Press, New York © 1984.

Four Biochemically Different Types of Dominantly Inherited Olivopontocerebellar Atrophy

Thomas L. Perry

Department of Pharmacology, University of British Columbia, Vancouver, British Columbia, Canada V6T 1W5

In 1970, Konigsmark and Weiner (13) subdivided the olivopontocerebellar atrophies (OPCAs) into five different disorders based on clinical and neuropathologic features and on mode of inheritance. Four are inherited as autosomal dominant disorders. Other chapters of this book provide updated material on the classification of the OPCAs and on their clinical characteristics. In my laboratory, we have been able to carry out biochemical studies on autopsied brain from a number of OPCA patients, thanks to the curiosity of two clinical neurologists and the meticulous attention they paid to obtaining and freezing autopsied brain rapidly after death.

When one or several types of neurons undergo premature death in human brain, the neuronal loss may cause a localized decrease in the content of specific neurotransmitters or in the activities of their synthesizing enzymes. This is the case in Parkinson's disease, where loss of dopaminergic nigrostriatal neurons is accompanied by decreased dopamine content and diminished activity of tyrosine hydroxylase in the substantia nigra, caudate nucleus, and putamen (10). In Huntington's chorea, premature loss of several specific neuronal populations results in a lowered content of γ-aminobutyric acid (GABA) in the corpus striatum, globus pallidus, substantia nigra, and other regions (1,25), decreased activity of its synthesizing enzyme, glutamic acid decarboxylase (1,2), and a reduced content of substance P in the globus pallidus and substantia nigra (8).

The dominantly inherited forms of OPCA seem to be particularly well suited to a search for abnormalities in the contents in autopsied brain of several different amino acids. Amino acids are likely to be the neurotransmitters of seven major types of cerebellar neurons (7,15). GABA is almost certainly the inhibitory neurotransmitter of most of the efferent Purkinje cells (20,28,31), and it may be the neurotransmitter of one or more of the three types of inhibitory interneurons in the cerebellar cortex: the basket, stellate, and Golgi cells (28,31). Taurine content of the cerebellar cortex is much higher than in other human brain regions (22), however, and experimental evidence from laboratory animals (14,16,19) suggests that taurine rather than GABA might be the inhibitory neurotransmitter of the stellate cells. Recent studies also suggest that some of the Purkinje cells may utilize taurine as an inhibitory neurotransmitter (4).

Glutamic acid is probably the excitatory neurotransmitter of the afferent mossy fibers and of the granule cells with their parallel fibers (9,16,29). Finally, aspartic acid may be the excitatory neurotransmitter of the climbing fibers, whose cell bodies lie in the inferior olivary nuclei and whose axons ascend to synapse with the dendrites of Purkinje cells in the molecular layer of the cerebellar cortex (18,34). The only known cerebellar neurons that do not utilize an amino acid as neurotransmitter are the noradrenergic neurons, which rise from the brainstem to synapse in the cerebellar cortex with the Purkinje cells (3).

We reported earlier on abnormalities in the amino acid contents of the cerebellum and other brain regions in 10 patients who died with various forms of dominantly inherited OPCA (26). The observed differences led us to conclude that at least three different disorders were represented in this material. This chapter updates our earlier study and is based on the biochemical differences observed in quantitative amino acid analyses of autopsied brain from 16 patients representing five different pedigrees of OPCA inherited in autosomal dominant fashion.

OPCA PATIENTS

Table 1 summarizes some of the genetic and diagnostic features of the OPCA patients studied. Six patients were from the C pedigree, a large pedigree in the southern United States in which at least five successive generations have been affected with OPCA-I (5). The disorder in pedigree C is HLA-linked, with the mutant gene located on chromosome 6 (11,12). The clinical picture and the neuropathologic changes in two of the six autopsied patients in this pedigree were described earlier (23). Biochemical studies were also carried out on a cerebellar biopsy of a seventh member of pedigree C.

The two patients in pedigree O belong to an unrelated family in the northern United States in which at least three successive generations have been affected with a disorder classified as OPCA-I (13), based on its clinical and neurologic

TABLE 1. *Dominantly inherited OPCA patients*

No. of patients	Pedigree	Successive generations affected	Clinical diagnosis[a]	Usual age at death (years)	HLA linkage
6	C	5	OPCA-I	40–60	Yes
2	O	3	OPCA-I	60–70	?
4	A	4	OPCA-I	40–70	No
3	S	6	OPCA-IV	30–40	Yes
1	R	2	OPCA, unclassified	70–80	

[a]OPCA classification of Konigsmark and Weiner (13).

features. Linkage of the mutant gene to the HLA locus has neither been established nor excluded in pedigree O (33).

The four patients in pedigree A belonged to an unrelated family in the southern United States in which at least four successive generations have been affected with a cerebellar disorder compatible with OPCA-I (13) in clinical and neuropathologic characteristics. The mutant gene in pedigree A is not linked to the HLA locus (12).

The three patients in pedigree S belonged to an unrelated family in the northern United States in which at least six successive generations have been affected by a cerebellar disorder that has been classified as OPCA-IV (13). The clinical details of this disorder were described more than 30 years ago by Schut (30). Linkage of the mutant gene in pedigree S to the HLA locus has recently been claimed. The single patient in pedigree R is from an unrelated Canadian family in which at least two successive generations have been affected with an unclassified form of OPCA. Genetic linkage has not been explored in pedigree R.

METHODS

Collection of Brain Specimens

Autopsied brain specimens from the 16 patients presented in Table 1 were frozen at −80° C within 6 hr after death (15 within 4 hr of death), shipped to our laboratory on dry ice, and maintained frozen at −80° C until they were dissected and processed for amino acid analysis. Autopsied brain from control adults was similarly handled.

Biopsy specimens of apparently normal cerebellar cortex were obtained from eight control subjects who underwent neurosurgical removal of posterior fossa tumors and (with informed consent) from one patient in pedigree C. The cerebellar biopsies were immersed in liquid nitrogen within 10 sec of excision and were then held at −80° C or lower until analyzed.

Amino Acid Analyses

Weighed brain specimens were homogenized and deproteinized in 0.4 M perchloric acid, as described elsewhere (22,24,25). Free amino acids and other ninhydrin-positive compounds were identified and quantitated on a Technicon automatic amino acid analyzer using a single cation exchange column and a lithium citrate buffer elution system (27). This method gives a good resolution of the four cerebellar amino acid putative neurotransmitters from adjacent compounds which are unresolved with conventional amino acid analyzer systems. Taurine was clearly separated from both glycerophosphoethanolamine and phosphoethanolamine; aspartic acid was separated from both γ-glutamyl-glutamic acid and from reduced glutathione; glutamic acid was separated from both asparagine and glutamine; and glycine was separated from oxidized glutathione. Without this sort of resolution, quantitation of taurine, aspartate, and glutamate in brain is meaningless.

RESULTS

Abnormalities were found in the contents of the four known or putative amino acid neurotransmitters—GABA, aspartic acid, glutamic acid, and taurine—in the autopsied brains of all 16 OPCA patients. No abnormalities were encountered in the contents of the remaining 32 amino compounds measured, and they are not described here.

A brief discussion is in order as to the probable relationship between brain contents of GABA, aspartic acid, glutamic acid, and taurine during life and the contents of these compounds found in autopsied brain. Incubation experiments in our laboratory have shown that taurine and glutamate contents do not differ in living and postmortem human brain (24). GABA content rises rapidly after brain death, reaching a maximum level by 2 hr and then remaining stable for at least 120 hr thereafter. The aspartate content of human brain remains unchanged for the first 4 hr after death but then rises rapidly in refrigerated but unfrozen brain (24).

Since the death-to-freezing intervals for brains of OPCA patients were all between 1 and 6 hr, we compared taurine, glutamate, and GABA contents with those of a large group of adults who died without neurologic or psychiatric disease and whose brains were frozen between 1 and 30 hr after death. It was necessary to compare the aspartate contents of the OPCA brains with a separate group of control subjects whose brains had been frozen within 6 hr of death. This separate control group included both neurologically normal and abnormal patients, but none of the latter had any disorder known to involve abnormalities of aspartate in brain. Mean ages were similar for both groups of control subjects and for the OPCA patients.

GABA

GABA contents of cerebellar cortex, dentate nucleus, and substantia nigra are shown for the 16 OPCA patients in Fig. 1, together with the mean $\pm$ 2 SD for the control subjects. Five of eight patients from pedigrees C and O and all four patients from pedigrees S and R had GABA contents in the dentate nucleus >2 SD below the control mean. This reflects a marked loss of Purkinje cells in these patients, since Purkinje neurons terminate in synapses in the deep cerebellar nuclei, especially the dentate nucleus. Only one of the four patients from pedigree A exhibited a marked reduction of GABA content in the dentate nucleus, thus suggesting that loss of Purkinje cells was less severe in affected members of pedigree A.

GABA contents of the cerebellar cortex were somewhat reduced in most of the OPCA patients (Fig. 1). The GABA content of cerebellar cortex was 1.65 ± 0.08 μmoles/g wet weight (mean $\pm$ SEM) in 26 control subjects, 1.14 ± 0.13 in the eight patients from pedigrees C and O, and 0.88 ± 0.08 in the four patients from pedigrees S and R. Mean GABA content of cerebellar cortex was significantly decreased compared to controls in both these groups ($p<0.01$). Cerebellar cortex GABA content was not significantly reduced in the four patients from pedigree A.

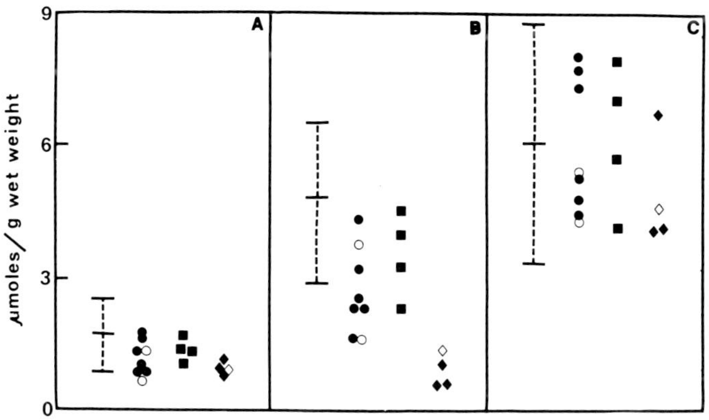

FIG. 1. GABA contents of autopsied brain from 16 OPCA patients: the *vertical dashed line* on the left of each panel indicates the mean ± 2 SD for neurologically normal controls; (●) patients from pedigree C; (○) patients from pedigree O; (■) patients from pedigree A; (◆) patients from pedigree S; (◇) patient from pedigree R. **A:** Cerebellar cortex. **B:** Dentate nucleus. **C:** Substantia nigra.

Reduced GABA levels in cerebellar cortex may reflect loss of either cell bodies of Purkinje neurons or inhibitory interneurons, or both.

GABA content of the substantia nigra is illustrated in Fig. 1 simply to indicate that GABA content was perfectly normal in another brain region where GABA content is characteristically high. GABA values were also normal in all other examined regions of the OPCA patients' brains.

Aspartic Acid

Figure 2 shows the aspartic acid contents of three brain regions for the 16 OPCA patients. For the cerebellar cortex, mean ± 2 SD values are shown for both autopsied control brain (with death-to-freezing intervals less than 6 hr) and biopsied control brain. It can be seen that the aspartate contents of patients from pedigrees C and O and from pedigrees S and R are low not only when compared to values for autopsied control brain but even when compared to biopsied control cerebellar cortex. The aspartate content of autopsied cerebellar cortex was 1.32+0.16 µmoles/g wet weight (mean ± SEM) in 26 control subjects, 0.55 ± 0.06 in the eight patients from pedigrees C and O, and 0.45 ± 0.17 in the four patients from pedigrees S and R. Mean aspartate content of the cerebellar cortex was significantly decreased compared to controls in both these groups ($p<0.05$). Aspartic acid content in the inferior olivary nucleus was also somewhat reduced in single patients from pedigrees C, S, and R, but there was no significant reduction of mean olivary aspartate content in these two patient groups. By contrast, Fig. 2 shows that aspartate contents were normal in both the cerebellar cortex and the inferior olivary nucleus in the four patients from pedigree A.

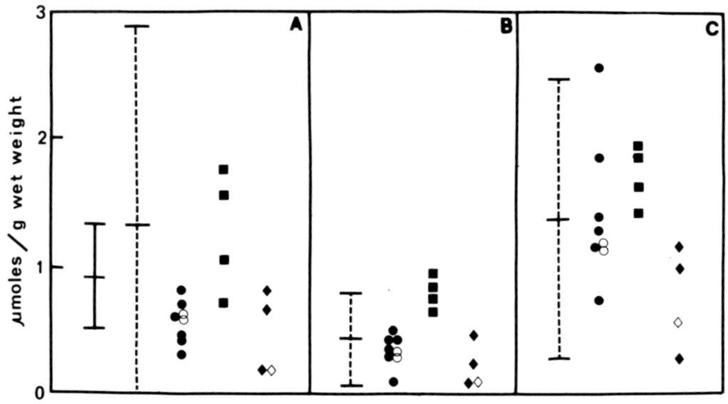

FIG. 2. Aspartic acid contents of autopsied brain from 16 OPCA patients. The *vertical dashed line* on the left of each panel indicates the mean ± 2 SD for control subjects. The death-to-freezing interval for all patients and control brains was <6 hr. The *vertical solid line* in the panel for cerebellar cortex indicates the mean ± 2 SD for *biopsied* control cerebellum. Patient symbols are the same as in Fig. 1. **A:** Cerebellar cortex. **B:** Inferior olive. **C:** Frontal cortex.

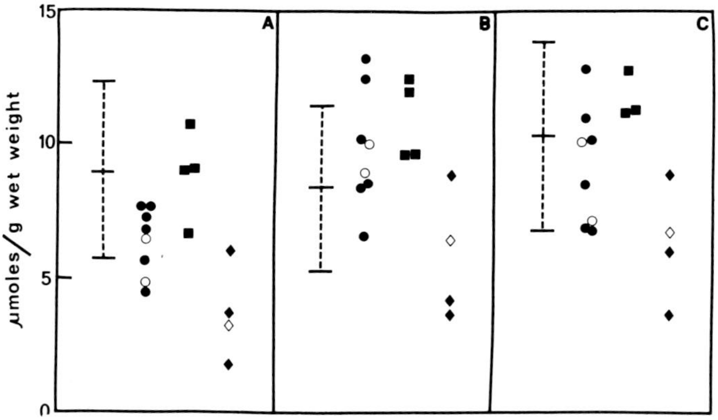

FIG. 3. Glutamic acid contents of autopsied brain from 16 OPCA patients. The *vertical dashed line* on the left of each panel indicates the mean ± 2 SD for neurologically normal controls. Patient symbols are the same as in Fig. 1. **A:** Cerebellar cortex. **B:** Frontal cortex. **C:** Caudate nucleus.

Glutamic Acid

Figure 3 shows the glutamic acid contents of the cerebellar cortex and of two other brain regions where glutamate content is normally high for the 16 OPCA patients. Glutamate content in cerebellar cortex was markedly reduced in three of the eight patients in pedigrees C and O and in all four patients in pedigrees S and R. In addition, some patients in pedigrees S and R had unusually low glutamate contents in the frontal cortex and caudate nucleus. Cerebellar cortical glutamate content was 9.05 ± 0.32 µmoles/g wet weight (mean ± SEM) in 26 control subjects but was reduced to 6.44 ± 0.45 in the eight patients from pedigrees C and O and to 3.75 ± 0.89 in the four patients from pedigrees S and R. These reductions in mean glutamate content of the cerebellar cortex were both highly significant ($p<0.001$). The mean glutamate contents for the four patients in pedigrees C and O were also significantly lower in the frontal cortex (26 control subjects, 8.34 ± 0.31; four patients, 5.77 ± 1.19; $p<0.01$) and in the caudate nucleus (31 control subjects, 10.36 ± 0.32; four patients, 6.34 ± 1.09; $p<0.001$). Glutamate content of the cerebellar cortex and of other brain regions was normal in the four patients from pedigree A.

Taurine

Figure 4 shows the taurine contents of cerebellar cortex and of two other representative brain regions for the 16 OPCA patients. Taurine contents in cerebellar cortex were normal in all the patients from pedigrees O, A, S, and R; however, the individual values for cerebellar cortical taurine are somewhat elevated in patients from pedigree C. Whereas 26 control subjects had a taurine content in this region of 2.65 ± 0.20 μmoles/g wet weight (mean ± SEM), mean cerebellar cortical taurine content was 4.08 ± 0.34 ($p<0.01$) in the six patients from pedigree C. Although the two patients from pedigree O resembled the six patients from pedigree C with respect to cerebellar cortical GABA, aspartate, and glutamate contents, they clearly differed from the pedigree C patients in having low normal taurine levels in the cerebellar cortex.

Biopsy Studies

Amino acids were quantitated in a cerebellar cortical biopsy from a single living patient from pedigree C and were compared with values from control subjects undergoing cerebellar cortical biopsies. The contents of both aspartic and glutamic

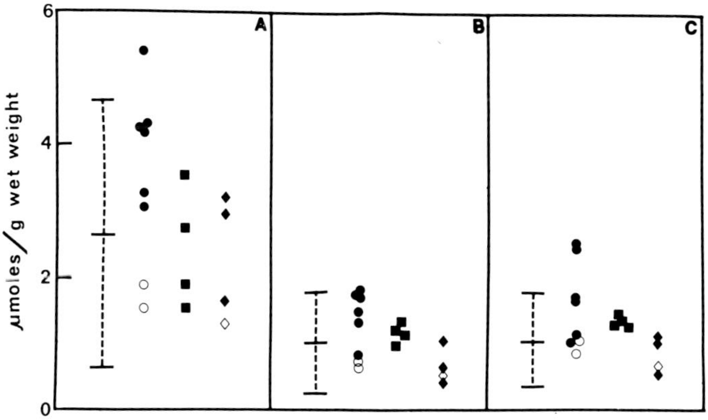

FIG. 4. Taurine contents of autopsied brain from 16 OPCA patients. The vertical dashed line on the left of each panel indicates the mean ± 2 SD for neurologically normal controls. Patient symbols are the same as in Fig. 1. **A:** Cerebellar cortex. **B:** Frontal cortex. **C:** Substantia nigra.

acids were reduced and resembled the values for autopsied cerebellar cortex for patients from pedigree C shown in Figs. 2 and 3 (26).

The activities of two enzymes involved in the synthesis of aspartic acid were determined in biopsied cerebellar cortex from the pedigree C patient and from control subjects. Activities of pyruvate carboxylase, the enzyme that converts pyruvate to oxaloacetate, and of aspartate aminotransferase, the enzyme that converts oxaloacetate to aspartate, were both found to be normal in the cerebellar cortex of this OPCA patient (26).

DISCUSSION

Based on the biochemical findings in the brains of these OPCA patients, it is possible to delineate as many as four different cerebellar disorders, each inherited as an autosomal dominant. Such a biochemical classification may not be any more hazardous than classifications based solely on symptoms or neuropathologic findings (13). The biochemical characteristics of these four postulated disorders are summarized in Table 2. Three of them have been classified clinically by the neurologists and neuropathologists who have observed them as OPCA-I. Yet genetic analyses have shown (Table 1) that one of these disorders is HLA-linked and one is not, while the presence of HLA-linkage is not yet determined for the third.

TABLE 2. *Four biochemically different types of OPCA*

Disorder	Pedigree	Clinical diagnosis[a]	Biochemical abnormalities[b]		Cerebellar neurons affected
1	C	OPCA-I	Cerebellar cortex	ASP ↓	Climbing fibers (?)
				GLU ↓	Mossy fibers (?); granule cells (?)
				TAU ↑	Stellate cells (?)
				GABA ↓	Inhibitory interneurons (?)
			Dentate nucleus	GABA ↓↓	Purkinje cells
2	O	OPCA-I	Cerebellar cortex	ASP ↓	Climbing fibers (?)
				GLU ↓	Mossy fibers (?); granule cells (?)
				GABA ↓	Inhibitory interneurons (?)
			Dentate nucleus	GABA ↓↓	Purkinje cells
3	A	OPCA-I	Cerebellar cortex	None	
			Dentate nucleus	GABA ↓	Purkinje cells
4	S & R	OPCA-IV	Cerebellar cortex	ASP ↓↓	Climbing fibers (?)
				GLU ↓↓	Mossy fibers (?); granule cells (?)
				GABA ↓	Inhibitory interneurons (?)
			Dentate nucleus	GABA ↓↓	Purkinje cells
			Other brain regions	GLU ↓	?

[a]OPCA classification of Konigsmark and Weiner (13).
[b]ASP, aspartic acid; GLU, glutamic acid; TAU, taurine; GABA, γ-aminobutyric acid; single arrow (moderate) and double arrow (marked), increase or decrease acid content.

Disorder 1

Disorder 1, found in pedigree C, is characterized by decreased aspartate, glutamate, and GABA contents in the cerebellar cortex and by decreased GABA content in the dentate nucleus. Taurine content is increased in the cerebellar cortex. These biochemical changes could be accounted for by loss of Purkinje cells (GABA reduced in the dentate nucleus) and of one or more inhibitory interneurons (GABA reduced in the cerebellar cortex). Since aspartic acid may be the excitatory neurotransmitter of the climbing fibers (18,34), the reduced aspartate content in the cerebellar cortex could be accounted for by loss of climbing fibers. The reduced glutamate content in the cerebellar cortex could result from the loss of either the afferent mossy fibers or the granule cell interneurons with their parallel fiber terminals. Glutamic acid is probably the excitatory neurotransmitter in these two types of neurons (9,16,29). The increased taurine content of the cerebellar cortex in disorder 1 might be explained by the persistence of one type of inhibitory interneuron (when other inhibitory interneurons had died off) or by a compensatory overactivity of one of the inhibitory interneurons. It is of interest that there is some evidence from experimental animals that taurine may be the inhibitory neurotransmitter of the stellate cells (14,16,19). Glial hypertrophy in a cerebellar cortex that had suffered multiple neuronal loss would not account for the increased taurine content in disorder 1, since glia do not have an unusually high taurine content.

Disorder 2

Disorder 2, the form of OPCA found in pedigree O, exhibits the same cerebellar biochemical abnormalities as disorder 1. Thus patients from pedigrees C and O have been grouped together in Figs. 1–4. However, taurine content is not elevated in disorder 2. If it could be shown that the mutant gene in pedigree O was not HLA-linked (linkage has neither been established nor excluded to date), this would strengthen the classification of disorder 2 as a separate form of OPCA.

Disorder 3

The disease found in pedigree A is clearly different from disorders 1 and 2, even though it also has been classified as OPCA-I. It is not HLA-linked and, therefore, must be different from disorder 1. Although there is reduced content of GABA in the dentate nucleus in disorder 3, reflecting some loss of Purkinje cells, this abnormality is less severe than in the three other forms of OPCA summarized in Table 2. In addition, there are no abnormalities of aspartate, glutamate, or taurine content in the cerebellar cortex.

Disorder 4

Disorder 4 is the disease found in patients of pedigree S, who have been classified clinically as having OPCA-IV. It is assumed that the single patient from unrelated pedigree R has the same disorder, since the biochemical findings are similar.

Disorder 4 is characterized by a greater reduction of aspartate and glutamate content in the cerebellar cortex than is seen in disorders 1 and 2, by a greater reduction of GABA content in the dentate nucleus (probably representing marked loss of Purkinje cells), and by a reduction of glutamate content in other brain areas, notably the cerebral cortex and the striatum. The physiologic significance of this more widespread glutamate deficiency is not apparent.

Priorities for Future Investigation

The four biochemically distinct disorders we have found in a relatively small collection of autopsied brains from OPCA patients suggest that there are further disorders yet to be found among the various types of OPCA. It will be important to measure amino acid neurotransmitters, especially in the cerebellum, in autopsied brain from pedigrees other than those studied in this laboratory. Do neurochemical abnormalities, or the lack of abnormalities, in them correspond to those described here? Are there additional biochemical disorders consistent within a pedigree? Careful correlation of clinical features and neuropathologic findings with demonstrated biochemical findings remains a high priority and will require good research collaboration among clinical neurologists, neuropathologists, and neurochemists. Do the fine histologic abnormalities corroborate the loss of specific populations of cerebellar neurons postulated in Table 2?

Research must also be directed to the causes of progressive neuronal loss in the dominantly inherited forms of OPCA. Possible mechanisms by which the mutant gene could cause premature neuronal death in heterozygotes include the coding of the gene for an abnormal protein in cell membranes or producing defective DNA repair. It is of interest that in ataxia telangiectasia, a recessively inherited disorder characterized by progressive cerebellar ataxia, there is an inherited defect of DNA repair, which causes impaired survival of cultured fibroblasts exposed to ionizing radiation (21). We have found, in a single ataxia telangiectasia patient, a depletion of glutamate in the cerebellar cortex and a depletion of GABA in the dentate nucleus, as severe as those described here for disorder 4 (27a). However, it is difficult to understand how a defective DNA repair mechanism or an abnormal protein in cell membranes can cause the premature death of certain populations of cerebellar neurons while most neurons in other brain regions remain intact.

Could the neuronal loss in the dominantly inherited forms of OPCA be caused by specific neurotoxins which bind to the receptors on certain types of cerebellar neurons? Might such neurotoxins, of either endogenous or exogenous origin, be incompletely destroyed as a result of subnormal degrading enzyme activity in patients heterozygous for the mutant genes? The ability of 3-acetylpyridine to kill climbing fibers in experimental animals (6), and of phenytoin to damage Purkinje cells in human and animal brain (17,32), make the possible role of neurotoxins worth exploring in the OPCAs. If one were fortunate enough to identify an exogenous neurotoxin as responsible for neuronal death in a form of OPCA, it might be possible to delay or even prevent onset of the disorders among persons genetically at risk.

ACKNOWLEDGMENTS

I thank Dr. Robert D. Currier and Dr. Lawrence J. Schut for providing most of the autopsied brain specimens which made this study possible. Mrs. Shirley Hansen and Dr. Kenneth Berry carried out accurate dissections of frozen brain, and Mrs. Maureen Murphy provided valuable technical assistance. This research was supported by grants from the Medical Research Council of Canada.

REFERENCES

1. Bird, E. D., and Iversen, L. L. (1974): Huntington's chorea: Post-mortem measurement of glutamic acid decarboxylase, choline acetyltransferase and dopamine in basal ganglia. *Brain*, 97:457–472.
2. Bird, E. D., Mackay, A. V. P., Rayner, C. N., and Iversen, L. L. (1973): Reduced glutamic-acid-decarboxylase activity of post-mortem brain in Huntington's chorea. *Lancet*, 1:1090–1092.
3. Bloom, F. E., Hoffer, B. J., and Siggins, G. R. (1971): Studies on norepinephrine-containing afferents to Purkinje cells of the rat cerebellum: I. Localization of the fibers and their synapses. *Brain Res.*, 25:501–521.
4. Chan-Palay, V., Palay, S. L., and Wu, J.-Y. (1982): Sagittal cerebellar microbands of taurine neurons: Immunocytochemical demonstration by using antibodies against the taurine-synthesizing enzyme cysteine sulfinic acid decarboxylase. *Proc. Natl. Acad. Sci. USA*, 79:4221–4225.
5. Currier, R. D., Glover, G., Jackson, J. F., and Tipton, A. C. (1972): Spinocerebellar ataxia: Study of a large kindred. I. General information and genetics. *Neurology*, 22:1040–1043.
6. Desclin, J. C., and Escubi, J. (1974): Effects of 3-acetylpyridine on the central nervous system of the rat, as demonstrated by silver methods. *Brain Res.*, 77:349–364.
7. Eccles, J. C., Ito, M., and Szentagothai, J. (1967): *The Cerebellum as a Neuronal Machine*. Springer-Verlag, New York.
8. Gale, J. S., Bird, E. D., Spokes, E. G., Iversen, L. L., and Jessel, T. (1978): Human brain substance P: Distribution in controls and Huntington's chorea. *J. Neurochem.*, 30:633–634.
9. Guidotti, A., Biggio, G., and Costa, E. (1975): 3-Acetylpyridine: A tool to inhibit the tremor and the increase of cGMP content in cerebellar cortex elicited by harmaline. *Brain Res.*, 96:201–205.
10. Hornykiewicz, O. (1973): Parkinson's disease: From brain homogenate to treatment. *Fed. Proc.*, 32:183–190.
11. Jackson, J. F., Currier, R. D., Terasaki, P. I., and Morton, N. E. (1977): Spinocerebellar ataxia and HLA linkage: Risk prediction by HLA typing. *N. Engl. J. Med.*, 296:1138–1141.
12. Jackson, J. F., Whittington, J. E., Currier, R. D., Terasaki, P. I., Morton, N. E., and Keats, B. J. B. (1978): Genetic linkage and spinocerebellar ataxia. In: *Advances in Neurology, Vol. 21: The Inherited Ataxias: Biochemical, Viral, and Pathological Studies*, edited by R. A. P. Kark, R. N. Rosenberg, and L. J. Schut, pp. 315–318. Raven Press, New York.
13. Konigsmark, B. W., and Weiner, L. P. (1970): Thc olivopontocerebellar atrophies: A review. *Medicine*, 49:227–241.
14. Krnjević, K., and Puil, E. (1976): Electrophysiological studies on actions of taurine. In: *Taurine*, edited by R. Huxtable and A. Barbeau, pp. 179–189. Raven Press, New York.
15. Llinas, R. R. (1975): The cortex of the cerebellum. *Sci. Am.*, 232:56–71.
16. McBride, W. J., Nadi, N. S., Altman, J., and Aprison, M. H. (1973): Effects of selective doses of X-irradiation on the levels of several amino acids in the cerebellum of the rat. *Neurochem. Res.*, 1:141–152.
17. Mimaki, T., Deshmukh, P. P., and Yamamura, H. I. (1980): Decreased benzodiazepine receptor density in rat cerebellum following neurotoxic doses of phenytoin. *J. Neurochem.*, 35:1473–1475.
18. Nadi, N. S., Kanter, D., McBride, W. J., and Aprison, M. H. (1977): Effects of 3-acetylpyridine on several putative neurotransmitter amino acids in the cerebellum and medulla of the rat. *J. Neurochem.*, 28:661–662.

19. Nadi, N. S., McBride, W. J., and Aprison, M. H. (1977): Distribution of several amino acids in regions of the cerebellum of the rat. *J. Neurochem.*, 28:453–455.
20. Obata, K. (1976): Association of GABA with cerebellar Purkinje cells: Single cell analysis. In: *GABA in Nervous System Function*, edited by E. Roberts, T. Chase, and D. B. Tower, pp. 217–222. Raven Press, New York.
21. Patterson, M. C., Anderson, A. K., Smith, B. P., and Smith, P. J. (1979): Enhanced radiosensitivity of cultured fibroblasts from ataxia telangiectasia heterozygotes manifested by defective colony-forming ability and reduced DNA repair replication after hypoxic γ-irradiation. *Cancer Res.*, 39:3725–3734.
22. Perry, T. L., Berry, K., Hansen, S., Diamond, S., and Mok, C. (1971): Regional distribution of amino acids in human brain obtained at autopsy. *J. Neurochem.*, 18:513–519.
23. Perry, T. L., Currier, R. D., Hansen, S., and MacLean, J. (1977): Aspartate taurine imbalance in dominantly inherited olivopontocerebellar atrophy. *Neurology*, 27:257–261.
24. Perry, T. L., Hansen, S., and Gandham, S. S. (1981): Postmortem changes of amino compounds in human and rat brain. *J. Neurochem.*, 36:406–412.
25. Perry, T. L., Hansen, S., and Kloster, M. (1973): Huntington's chorea: Deficiency of γ-aminobutyric acid in brain. *N. Engl. J. Med.*, 288:337–342.
26. Perry, T. L., Kish, S. J., Hansen, S., and Currier, R. D. (1981): Neurotransmitter amino acids in dominantly inherited cerebellar disorders. *Neurology*, 31:237–242.
27. Perry, T. L., Stedman, D., and Hansen, S. (1968): A versatile lithium buffer elution system for single column automatic amino acid chromatography. *J. Chromatogr.*, 38:460–466.
27a. Perry, T. L., Kish, S. J., Hinton, D., Hansen, S., Becker, L. E., and Gelfand, E. W. (1984): Neurochemical abnormalities in a patient with axtaxia-telangiectasia. *Neurology*, 34:187–191.
28. Roberts, E. (1979): New directions in GABA research: I. Immunocytochemical studies of GABA neurons. In: *GABA-Neurotransmitters: Pharmacochemical, Biochemical and Pharmacological Aspects*, edited by P. Krogsgaard-Larsen, J. Scheel-Krüger, and H. Kofod, pp. 28–45. Academic Press, New York.
29. Roffler-Tarlov, S., and Sidman, R. L. (1978): Concentrations of glutamic acid in cerebellar cortex and deep nuclei of normal mice and weaver, staggerer and nervous mutants. *Brain Res.*, 142:269–283.
30. Schut, J. W. (1950): Hereditary ataxia: Clinical study through six generations. *Arch. Neurol. Psychiatry*, 63:535–568.
31. Storm-Mathisen, J. (1976): Distribution of the components of the GABA system in neuronal tissue: Cerebellum and hippocampus—effects of axotomy. In: *GABA in Nervous System Function*, edited by E. Roberts, T. Chase, and D. B. Tower, pp. 149–168. Raven Press, New York.
32. Utterback, R. A., Ojeman, R., and Malek, J. (1958): Parenchymatous cerebellar degeneration with Dilantin intoxication. *J. Neuropathol. Exp. Neurol.*, 17:516–519.
33. Whittington, J. L., Keats, B. J., Jackson, J. F., Currier, R. D., and Terasaki, P. I. (1980): Linkage studies on glyoxalase-I (GLO), pepsinogen (PG), spinocerebellar ataxia (SCA 1), and HLA. *Cytogenet. Cell Genet.*, 28:145–150.
34. Wiklund, L., Toggenburger, G., and Cuénod, M. (1982): Aspartate: Possible neurotransmitter in cerebellar climbing fibers. *Science*, 216:78–80.

The Olivopontocerebellar Atrophies, edited by
R. C. Duvoisin and A. Plaitakis. Raven Press,
New York © 1984.

Clinical Features of Sporadic (Dejerine-Thomas) Olivopontocerebellar Atrophy

Louis R. Caplan

Department of Neurology, Michael Reese Hospital and Medical Center, Chicago, Illinois 60616

Andre Thomas, in his doctoral thesis of 1897, probably reported the first detailed case description of a patient with olivopontocerebellar atrophy (OPCA). In retrospect, this patient was atypical; at necropsy, in addition to the usual cerebellar, pontine, and olivary atrophy, there was loss of anterior horn cells in the eighth cervical segment of the spinal cord, a finding manifested clinically by hand muscle atrophy (6). Three years later, Dejerine and Thomas (7) reported a description of the clinical and pathologic features of a disease they called OPCA. This original description has recently been translated by Hochberg (7), making it more accessible to English-speaking readers. The report began with a detailed clinical and pathologic description of a 53-year-old female newspaper dealer who had a progressive illness lasting 3 years that was characterized by gait ataxia, abnormal speech, altered affect, clumsy hands, and dribbling of urine. Autopsy showed striking atrophy of the cerebellum, basis pontis, brachium pontis, and medullary olives, described by the authors as "systematic degenerative atrophy without sclerosis or inflammation." Also included was a second, clinically similar patient, a 44-year-old farmer examined by Dejerine. Dejerine and Thomas meticulously reviewed prior reports of patients with cerebellar abnormalities and discussed how the new syndrome differed from past cases and probably represented a distinct entity. Critchley and Greenfield (5) and later Eadie (8) reviewed in detail the clinical and pathologic features of the sporadic nonfamilial form of OPCA, which is often referred to as Dejerine-Thomas disease after the original authors. This review of the clinical features of sporadic OPCA is based on the personal observations of a series of patients studied at the Michael Reese Hospital in Chicago.

CLINICAL FEATURES

The earliest sign of nervous system dysfunction in this disorder is usually an alteration in gait. At first, balance is impaired; sudden unexpected falls make the patients feel less secure on their feet. These falls are often attributed by the patient to fatigue or "weakness of the legs." Examination at this early stage does not corroborate any paralysis or weakness; there is unsteadiness or lurching on turns, with unexpected and unpredictable veering from a straight course. Stance is widened. When the toe is aimed at an outstretched object or the heel is guided down the shin, slight incoordination is noted. Rapid movements of the feet, such as toe tapping, are performed clumsily and with an irregular slapping rhythm. Deep tendon reflexes are exaggerated. Gait abnormalities may be the sole evidence of dysfunction for the first 1 or 2 years of the illness. Walking difficulty progresses, so that the patient generally becomes bed- or chair-confined after a few years. When examined at this later, more advanced stage, the gait abnormality is no longer limited to cerebellar system dysfunction. Rigidity of truncal muscles, small steps, and spasticity complicate the cerebellar abnormality. Plantar reflexes are by this time extensor, and toe and foot movements are grossly incoordinated and ataxic. The gait ataxia is not usually accompanied by any cephalic sensation of giddiness, dizziness, or vertigo but is described by the patient as an inability to reliably control the feet.

Incoordination of the upper extremities usually is the next problem noted by the patient. The fingers become clumsy and lose agility for finer movements. Ataxia on finger-to-nose testing and intention tremor are documented on examination. Later, as the disease progresses, handwriting becomes illegible, and the patient has difficulty buttoning shirts, cutting food, and manipulating small objects. Superior extremity dysfunction usually is less prominent than the abnormalities in the lower extremities. Later in the course of progression of OPCA, a parkinsonian-like rigidity of the arms and legs supervenes. Although the arms are stiff and often held flexed, a pill rolling or other parkinsonian-like tremor usually does not occur.

Speech abnormalities are always severe and often so characteristic that the diagnosis can be suggested by listening to the patient on the telephone. Initially, speech is hoarse, somewhat nasal, and breathy, with unreliable volume modification. Slurred syllables, with one word running into the next, give the voice a "drunken ring." Later, volume becomes reduced. Eventually, the patient speaks in a barely audible, breathy whisper. Articulation is effortful and strained. Critchley and Greenfield (5) characterized the speech in one patient as sounding "as if he were talking while being throttled." Interestingly, some patients, although unable to produce louder speech volume when exhorted, have spoken freely in their sleep or when pinched. The variability of voice volume occasionally leads to the false initial impression of hysterical dysphonia in some patients. The articulatory defect in OPCA is quite distinct from the hypophonic tachyphemic speech of Parkinson's disease, and later is usually separable from the scanning, poorly modulated speech associated with multiple sclerosis and alcoholic cerebellar degeneration.

Autonomic dysfunction is also a prominent feature in some but not all patients with OPCA. The most common autonomic system symptoms relate to micturition. Critchley and Greenfield (5) commented on urinary incontinence as an early and frequent symptom in OPCA, in contrast to patients with other cerebellar system degenerations (2). The index patient of Dejerine and Thomas (6) had constant dribbling of urine and constipation. Eadie (8), in his large review, wondered if urinary incontinence could be due to associated dementia, but our own experience (4) of prominent sphincter dysfunction early in the clinical course in intellectually preserved patients led us to attribute the urinary abnormalities to involvement of descending long tracts in the spinal cord or to degeneration of the intermediolateral cell columns of the cord. Geary et al. (9) did not mention urinary symptoms in their patient, but an extreme degree of trabeculation of the bladder was found at postmortem examination. The earliest urinary symptom is frequency often followed by incontinence. Cystometrograms may show uninhibited bladder contractions at this stage. Catheter dependence is common. Urinary stasis may lead to urinary tract infections and stone formation. Death can follow urosepsis. Rectal sphincter dysfunction also occurs, usually in the form of severe constipation, but also in the form of rectal incontinence.

Postural hypotension also occurs in some patients with OPCA and, in fact, may dominate the clinical picture. Giddiness, lightheaded sensations, and faintness are frequently mentioned. Three personally observed patients have had severe postural hypotension that greatly limited their ability to ambulate (4). Bannister et al. (2,10) noted postural hypotension and other signs of autonomic dysfunction in patients with a widespread degenerative disease they called multiple system atrophy. Some of these patients have necropsy evidence of gross atrophy of the pons, brachium pontis, olives, and cerebellum, as well as degenerative changes in the basal ganglia and intermediolateral cell columns of the spinal cord. Analyses of patients with multiple system atrophy have demonstrated abnormal baroregulatory and cardioregulatory reflexes, postural hypotension, abnormal responses to Valsalva maneuvers, lack of sinus arrhythmia, loss of pressor and cardiac rate response to stress, and lack of sweating when ambient pressure rises (1). In addition, resting plasma norepinephrine levels are generally low although dopamine-beta-hydroxylase activity is indistinguishable from control patients (3). Other authors have not commented on postural hypotension or autonomic dysfunction in OPCA. Apparently, autonomic changes occur in some but not all patients with OPCA and are quite variable. It is likely that autonomic signs may occur only in a special subgroup of patients with OPCA with more widespread degenerative changes.

Dysphagia appears at about the same time as abnormalities in speech. Choking, effortful swallowing, and regurgitation make swallowing arduous. Fluids are occasionally regurgitated, and aspiration may occur. The patient at first lengthens the intervals between meals and later begins to eat and drink less. Some patients eventually require gastrostomy for adequate maintenance of nutrition. In my experience, dehydration, inanition, and aspiration pneumonia are frequent complications of the dysphagia.

Extrapyramidal, parkinsonian-like manifestations are quite frequent, and the patients are often given the diagnosis of Parkinson's disease or at least of idiopathic parkinsonism; terminally, they dominate the clinical picture. Fixity of facial expression, diminished tongue, lip, and facial movements, and constant drooling mimic parkinsonism. The limbs also stiffen and may be held in flexion postures. One personally examined patient developed severe neck dystonia with torticollis, making it virtually impossible for her to sit upright in a chair. The trunk becomes immobilized and gait is slow, short-stepped, and shuffling. A typical resting tremor may occasionally appear but is minimal and may be easily overlooked. Despite these parkinsonian features, the signs of pyramidal tract involvement and cerebellar dysfunction distinguish OPCA from paralysis agitans. The prominence of gait disturbance described as unsteady walking is unusual for Parkinson's disease.

Occasional patients complain of burning or dysesthetic feelings, but abnormalities of sensation are rarely detectable on examination. Nystagmus is variable; more often, gaze is saccadic, and rhythmic ocular oscillations are not prominent. Deep tendon reflexes are usually exaggerated early in the course; in later stages, however, they may be diminished and even lost in the lower extremities. Plantar responses are usually flexor early in the course of the illness, but later usually become extensor. Muscle atrophy and paralysis are rare. Intellectual function has been variable. In the index patient of Dejerine and Thomas (6), intellectual faculties deteriorated as the patient grew feeble. In some patients, mental symptoms can precede other dysfunctions, and severe dementia occasionally dominates the clinical picture (11). In our own experience (4), intellectual dysfunction has been slight and late in appearance. Emotionality and euphoria may occur. As in Wilson's disease, the early facial and speech abnormalities may give the patient an outward appearance of simplicity when formal testing reveals preservation of intellect. As the patient becomes more disabled, apathy and depression are frequently noted and clearly contribute to the disability.

AN ILLUSTRATIVE CASE

An analysis of the evolution of the disease in a typical patient may serve to illustrate the clinical picture:

> V.C., a white female, first noted general slowing of gait, smaller and less clear handwriting, and occasional burning feelings in her legs at age 46. Her symptoms initially improved on L-DOPA treatment. No similar disorder had affected members of her family. Two years later, her gait had worsened, and she developed urinary frequency. Later, she was unable to empty her bladder and would find herself wet. She was catheter dependent for the remainder of her life. A year later, balance had deteriorated, and her arms became so unreliable that she could no longer write or feed or dress herself. She became faint on standing. When examined at age 49, her face was nearly expressionless, and saliva drooled from her mouth. She was alert, and detailed testing of intellectual function was normal. Her voice was hoarse and low in volume. Speech was whispered through a nearly closed mouth; pauses and a "breathy" quality, in addition to slurring of lingual syllables, made her speech scarcely intelligible. She could, with effort, accurately pronounce single words if she did so slowly and carefully; in phrases, the words would run together. She sat stiffly in a chair with her head tilted to the right. Her limbs were stiff but strong. Movements were performed slowly and clumsily, but there was no resting or intention tremor. She could stand with support, but her knees would suddenly buckle, and she would lurch forward or to the side if she attempted to walk. Eye movements were saccadic but full. Deep tendon reflexes were hyperactive, and plantar responses were extensor. Sensation was normal. Blood pressure was 130/90 supine but fell to 110/80 on sitting and 80/65 on standing. Cytometrogram revealed a spastic bladder. Neither manipulation of the dose of L-DOPA, addition of carbidopa (in Sinemet), nor use of other antiparkinsonian medications was

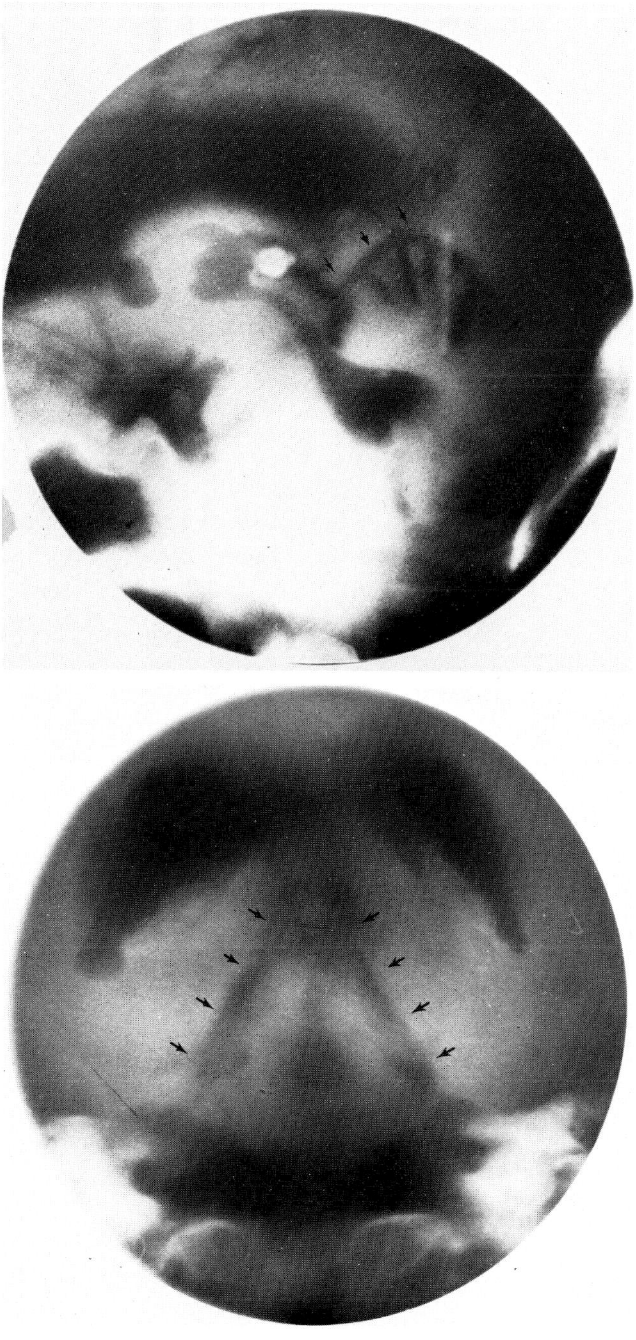

FIG. 1. Top: PEG, lateral view, case 1: large pontine cistern and IV ventricle; small cerebellar folia *(arrows)*. **Bottom:** PEG, A-P view, case 1: Large ambient cistern and small brainstem *(arrows)*.

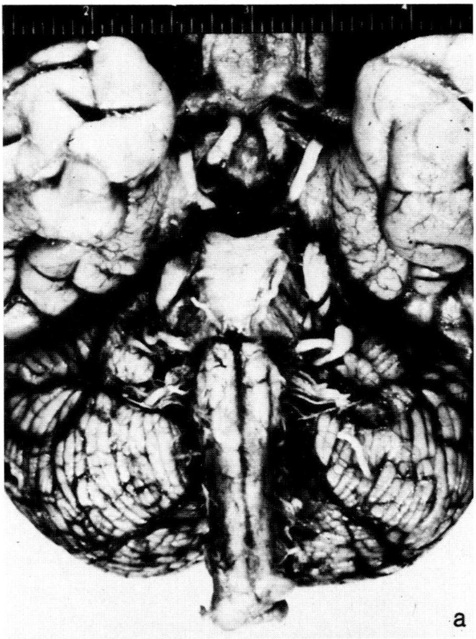
a

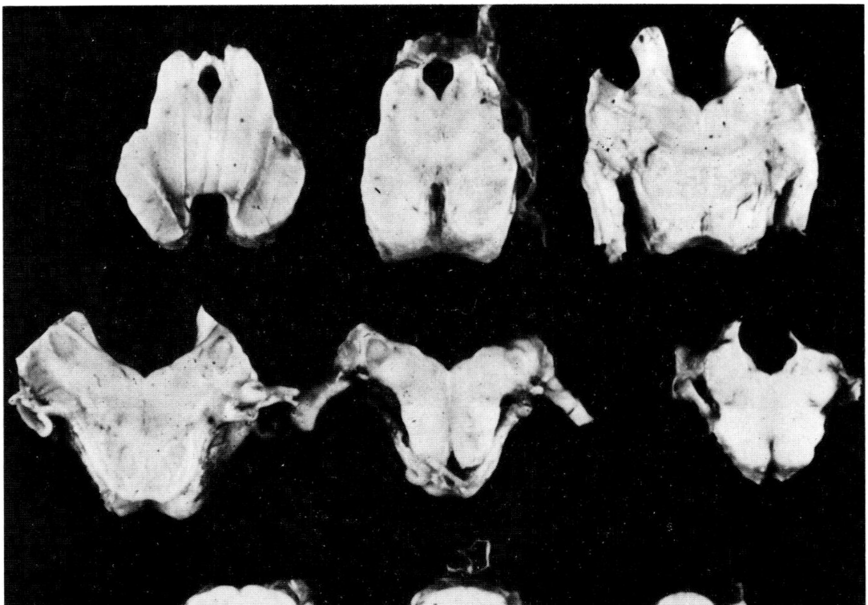
b

helpful. Four years after the onset of her symptoms, her voice was barely audible; there was labile crying and laughing. She developed great difficulty swallowing food or liquids and frequently gagged. Occasional "spells" were described by her husband, and periods of facial grimacing with mouth and lip twitching were seen by physicians. Postural hypotension was consistently demonstrated. Under electrocardiogram (EKG) monitoring, carotid sinus pressure produced no alteration in pulse. An iodine sweat test showed that areas under intense heat did not sweat. Electroencephalograms (EEGs) were normal. Cerebrospinal fluid was under normal pressure; there were no cells, and protein content was 50 mg/dl. A computerized tomography (CT) scan showed slight atrophy of the cerebellum and a large ambient cistern. Pneumoencephalogram (PEG) (Fig. 1) confirmed the large pontine and ambient cisterns and atrophy of the brainstem. During the last 3 years, she was cared for at home by her husband. Although alert to the end, she remained mute and immobile in bed in a helpless state, finally succumbing to pneumonia at age 53.

At necropsy, there was gross atrophy of the basis pontis, brachium pontis, and inferior olives (Fig. 2). The putamen was atrophic and slate gray. The substantia nigra and locus ceruleus were depigmented.

The disorder affects either sex with approximately equal frequency. Onset is usually in middle life. The course generally is slowly progressive. Death is usually due to pulmonary or urinary tract infections and inanition.

DIFFERENTIAL DIAGNOSIS

The differential diagnostic considerations are extensive and depend on the stage of the illness. Early, the major considerations are other disorders of the cerebellum and its connections, such as olivocerebellar degeneration, spinocerebellar degeneration related to carcinoma, multiple sclerosis, cerebellar tumor, and cerebellar infarction. Later, the extrapyramidal and pyramidal dysfunction make these degenerative cerebellar conditions unlikely. Progressive supranuclear palsy usually is associated with more dramatic abnormalities of eye motion with dystonic hyperextension of the neck and does not include cerebellar system abnormalities. In the Shy-Drager syndrome, autonomic symptoms, such as postural hypotension and impotence, precede the signs of parkinsonism and central nervous system (CNS) dysfunction; in OPCA, the autonomic disorder follows or is concurrent with the CNS disturbance. Striatonigral degeneration presents no cerebellar features but rather a primarily bradykinetic parkinsonian syndrome with little or no tremor poorly responsive to levodopa therapy. The CT has proven diagnostically helpful in defining the cerebellar atrophy and widening of the ambient and parapontine cisterns usually found in advanced OPCA. Special attention should be directed to the posterior fossa, scanning with 5 mm sections rather than with the 1 cm sections commonly used in routine CT. Bannister and his colleagues (1–3,10) pointing out the variable involvement of the putamen, locus ceruleus, substantia nigra, and

FIG. 2. a: Case 1, gross view of base of brain. Small cerebellum and nearly absent protuberance of basis pontis. **b:** Case 1, cut sections of brainstem. Marked atrophy of basis pontis and middle cerebellar peduncle.

intermediolateral cell columns of the spinal cord in patients with OPCA at autopsy, have introduced the term multiple system atrophy. They urge including under this catchall designation examples of the Shy-Drager syndrome, OPCA, and forms of striatonigral degeneration with involvement outside the striatum pending the identification of specific etiologies of these entities.

REFERENCES

1. Bannister, R., Davies, B., Holly, E., Rosenthal, T., and Sever, P. (1979): Defective cardiovascular reflexes and supersensitivity to sympathomimetic drugs in autonomic failure. *Brain*, 102:163–176.
2. Bannister, R., and Oppenheimer, D. (1972): Degenerative diseases of the nervous system associated with autonomic failure. *Brain*, 95:457–474.
3. Bannister, R., Sever, P., and Gross, M. (1977): Cardiovascular reflexes and biochemical responses in progressive autonomic failure. *Brain*, 100:327–344.
4. Caplan, L., Thomas, C., Patel, D., Sherman, I., and Kempter, T. (1980): Clinical and CT features of non-familial Olivo-Ponto-Cerebellar Atrophy. *Trans. Am. Neurol. Assoc.*, 105:330–332.
5. Critchley, M., and Greenfield, J. G. (1948): Olivo-ponto-cerebellar atrophy. *Brain*, 71:343–364.
6. Dejerine, J., and Thomas, A. (1900): L'atrophie olivo-ponto-cerebelleuse. *Nou. Iconogr. Saltpet*, 13:330–370.
7. Hochberg, F. (1977): L'Atrophie olivo-ponto-cerebelleuse. (by J. Dejerine and A. Thomas). In: *Neurological Classics in Modern Translation*, edited by D. Rottenberg and F. Hochberg, pp. 219–251. Hafner, New York.
8. Eadie, M. (1975): Olivo-ponto-cerebellar atrophy (Dejerine-Thomas type). In: *Handbook of Clinical Neurology, Vol. 21, System Disorders and Atrophies (Part I)*, edited by P. Vinken and G. Bruyn, pp. 415–431. North-Holland, Amsterdam.
9. Geary, J., Earle, K., and Rose, A. (1956): Olivo-ponto-cerebellar atrophy. *Neurology*, 6:218–224.
10. Spokes, E., Bannister, R., and Oppenheimer, D. (1979): Multiple system atrophy with autonomic failure. *J. Neurol. Sci.*, 43:59–82.
11. Van Bogaert, L., and Bertrand, I. (1929): Une variete d'atrophie olivo-pontine a evolution subaigue avec troubles dementiels. *Rev. Neurol.*, 1:165–178.

The Olivopontocerebellar Atrophies, edited by R. C. Duvoisin and A. Plaitakis. Raven Press, New York © 1984.

Abnormal Metabolism of Neuroexcitatory Amino Acids in Olivopontocerebellar Atrophy

Andreas Plaitakis

Department of Neurology, Mount Sinai School of Medicine, City University of New York, New York, New York 10029

During the past nine decades, a sizable international literature on olivopontocerebellar atrophy (OPCA) has been accumulated. Until recently, this bibliography consisted almost exclusively of reports describing clinical, pathologic, and genetic aspects of the disorder. Although the etiology and pathophysiology of the OPCAs have been addressed by a number of authors (13), concepts introduced in the past, such as "pathoclisis" (16), "abioatrophy" (15), or "catagenic" (27) conditions of the nervous system, have added little to our understanding of the problem. In OPCA, as with other neurologic afflictions with system atrophy, the clue to the problem of pathogenesis is the identification of factors responsible for the selective neuronal degeneration that occurs in these disorders. Their progressive degenerative course is similar to that of genetic diseases in which specific errors of metabolism have been identified (44). Thus specific biochemical defects may underlie the classic structural disorders with system atrophy, but such defects remain unknown for the majority of these conditions. The main difficulty has been the absence of any biochemical leads that could be pursued for elucidating the basic molecular events responsible for the clinical and pathologic expression of these disorders. Most disorders with system atrophy are known to occur sporadically (e.g., Parkinson's disease, Shy-Drager syndrome) or to be genetically transmitted (e.g., Huntington's chorea, Friedreich's ataxia). However, OPCA can be both a sporadic and a familial disorder. When genetically transmitted, OPCA can follow an autosomal dominant or recessive inheritance pattern (30). Although these observations suggest that OPCA encompasses a number of different diseases related to heterogenous etiologic factors, the common neuronal degeneration pattern found in these conditions could result from similar pathogenetic mechanisms.

As with the other inherited disorders, the familial forms of OPCA are expected to depend on genetic factors, such as mutations of enzymes or structural proteins. Detailed below are recent studies in which a lead provided by an animal model was explored; it revealed evidence for deficiency of the enzyme glutamate dehydrogenase (GDH) in a form of OPCA that appears to be recessively inherited. This has been shown to be associated with abnormal systemic metabolism of the major excitatory amino acid glutamate. Alterations in the levels of putative transmitter amino acids have been found in postmortem brain tissues from patients with various types of dominant OPCA (28,29; see Perry, *this volume*). Exploration of the systemic metabolism of these amino acids was undertaken in a family with dominantly inherited OPCA along the above lines of thought; this resulted in the finding of a systemic defect in the metabolism of the other excitatory amino acid, aspartate. Thus systemic defects in the metabolism of neuroexcitatory amino acids may underlie the various forms of OPCA.

GDH DEFICIENCY IN A FORM OF OPCA

Strategy Pursued for Detecting the Enzyme Defect

While searching for animal models of ataxia, we became aware that systemic administration of the nicotinamide antagonist 3-acetylpyridine (3-AP) to rats can result in selective lesioning of the olivocerebellar pathways (12). Treated animals develop long-lasting equilibrium difficulties (ataxia) associated with destruction of inferior olives, olivocerebellar fibers, lower cranial nerve nuclei, and areas of pons and substantia nigra (Table 1). Since the pattern of this selective neuronal degeneration appears to be similar to that found in patients with OPCA (Table 1), 3-AP intoxication in rats was thought to serve as a model for OPCA (31,32). The possibility then was raised that the degenerating neuronal systems in both the animal model and the human disease could respond to a common biochemical factor. Earlier studies (17) had shown that 3-AP intoxication in rats is associated with a substantial incorporation of the toxic agent into the brain NADP system by

TABLE 1. *Pattern of neuronal degeneration in 3-AP intoxication and OPCA*

CNS region	3-AP[a]	OPCA
Inferior olives	+ + + +	+ + + +
Cranial nerve nuclei		
IX, X	+ + +	+ to + + +
XII	+ + +	+ to + + +
VII	+	0 to + +
Pons	+	+ to + + +
Substantia nigra	+	0 to + +
Spinal cord	0	0 to + +

[a]The degree of neuronal degeneration is indicated by the number of plus signs, ranging from 0 (no involvement) to + + + + (complete destruction of neurons of the region). The degeneration pattern of 3-AP toxicity in the rat has been studied by Desclin and Escubi (12) by the use of silver methods; brain morphologic changes as found in the various types of OPCA (13,16,42).

forming 3-APADP in the place of NADP. The produced abnormal nucleotide (3-APADP) was found to be capable of inhibiting a number of NADP(H)-requiring enzymes *in vitro*. These observations suggested that inhibition of these enzymes *in vivo* could be responsible for the neurotoxic effects of 3-AP. In view of these considerations, the possibility was further raised that patients with OPCA may be deficient in one of the above enzymes. This hypothesis was tested by measuring several NADP(H)-requiring enzymes (all known to be inhibited by 3-APADP *in vitro*) in the cultured skin fibroblasts from a patient with a clinical syndrome consistent with OPCA. Results revealed a selective deficiency of the NAD(P)-requiring enzyme GDH, a defect that persisted after several passages of the cultured cells (31,32).

GDH

Mammalian tissues, such as liver, kidney, and brain, are known to possess high amounts of GDH activity (24). The enzyme is thought to have a central role in glutamate metabolism by catalyzing the reversible oxidative deamination of this amino acid to α-ketoglutarate by using NAD or NADP as coenzyme (Fig. 1). This reaction has been thought to be important in maintaining the mitochondrial NAD(P)H/NAD(P) ratio (23), which can be reflected in the cytoplasmic lactate/pyruvate ratio. In the kidney, GDH is known to deaminate glutamate for ammonia production (41). In brain, however, the organ with the highest concentration of glutamate, the

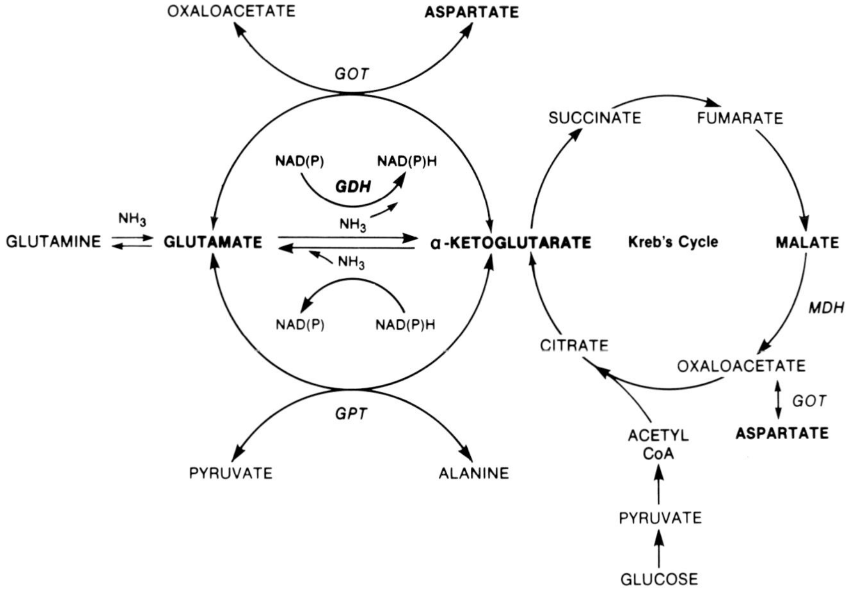

FIG. 1. Metabolic pathways of glutamate and aspartate metabolism in the brain. GDH, glutamate dehydrogenase; GOT, glutamic-oxaloacetic transaminase; GPT, glutamic-pyruvic transaminase; MDH, malate dehydrogenase.

exact function of GDH remains unclear. Earlier studies by Berl (2) suggested that the enzyme favors the synthesis of glutamate by ammonia fixation into α-ketoglutarate in the presence of high concentrations of ammonia. More recent studies by Cooper et al. (8), however, showed little ammonia fixation on α-ketoglutarate in the presence of physiologic concentrations of ammonia. Yu et al. (52) showed that glutamate is oxidized (by GDH) at rather high rates in cultured astrocytes. These observations suggest that in the nervous tissue, GDH may function predominantly in glutamate catabolism (oxidative deamination). These considerations may be of particular importance in understanding the pathophysiology of neuronal degeneration that occurs in GDH-deficient OPCA (see below). Since the metabolism of glutamate appears to be compartmented in the brain (3,4), the function of GDH should be considered within this concept of nervous tissue metabolic compartmentation. Available evidence suggests that the enzyme is associated with at least two pools of glutamate: a "synaptic" pool that is released at the nerve endings during neurotransmission (40), and another that is related to glial cell metabolism (2).

GDH is an allosterically regulated enzyme that has attracted considerable interest because diverse chemical agents have been shown to influence its activity *in vitro* (1,6,39,47–50). Thus steroid hormones, thyroxin, GTP, and high concentrations of NADH can be inhibitory to the enzyme. On the other hand, ADP and the branched chain amino acids L-leucine and L-isoleucine are capable of stimulating GDH *in vitro*. These agents probably influence GDH activity by acting on specific regulatory sites which may be distinct from the catalytic sites of the enzyme (14). In contrast to the rather extensive information available on the *in vitro* modulation of GDH, little is known about the *in vivo* regulation of the enzyme. Such data may be of crucial importance for the development of a rational therapeutic approach for the GDH-deficient OPCA based on the use of enzyme activators.

Phenotypes Associated with GDH Deficiency

Deficiency of GDH was first detected in cultured skin fibroblasts from a patient with progressive cerebellar ataxia, extrapyramidal features, and bulbar nerve dysfunction, a constellation of clinical features thought to be consistent with OPCA (32). Leukocytes from this patient also showed decreased GDH activity. Since white blood cells can be easily prepared from peripheral blood, these preparations were used primarily in subsequent studies. From the initial investigations (33), it became apparent that GDH deficiency is not found in all forms of OPCA. Thus the enzyme defect was absent in the dominant OPCA cases. On the other hand, deficiency of the enzyme was found to correlate with late adult onset OPCA cases, which were either sporadic occurrences or recessively inherited (31–38).

In our latest series (38), GDH activity was determined in leukocytes from 88 patients with various degenerative neurologic disorders affecting primarily the function of the cerebellum and/or the basal ganglia. Twelve patients with slowly progressive multisystem atrophy (MSA) were found to have a partial deficiency of the enzyme (40–55% of control). The clinical characteristics of these patients were similar in many respects to those of late adult onset sporadic OPCA of the Dejerine-Thomas type. These included cerebellar dysfunction, extrapyramidal features (parkinsonism), oculomotor disturbances, dysarthria, corticospinal deficits, anterior horn cell signs, and peripheral neuropathy occurring in various combinations. The disease was familial in seven of these patients and appeared to be sporadic in five. The age of onset of the disease varied from 21 to 73 years (mean, 53.3 years). Difficulty in walking, such as broad-based, ataxic, or small-stepped or shuffling gait, or a combination of both, was the presenting symptom in eight GDH-deficient patients; bradykinesia (slowness of movements) was the presenting symptom in two; aspiration pneumonia (due to bulbar palsy) in one; and diplopia in one. There was considerable variation in the clinical presentation of these patients, particularly in those who were at rather early stages of their illness. In some cases, the extrapyramidal features predominated, suggesting an atypical Parkinson's disease. Others had prominent ataxia, peripheral neuropathy, and/or anterior horn cell signs. In patients with advanced disease state, however, a disorder with multiple system atrophy manifested by a combination of cerebellar, extrapyramical, bulbar, and oculomotor disturbances clearly emerged. In several patients, a dystonic head posturing (head tilt) (Fig. 2) or abnormal body posturing on walking was noted. Other extrapyramidal features were expressionless facies, bradykinesia, cogwheeling rigidity, and "striatal" hand deformities (Figs. 2 and 3). Dysarthria with a monotonous, slurred, dysrhythmic speech was a rather common neurologic feature. In a few patients, speech became markedly hypophonic and barely audible. The oculomotor disturbances seen were gaze-evoked nystagmus, defective pursuit, impaired volitional saccades (usually seen at advanced stages), defective optokinetic responses, and poor suppression of the visual ocular reflex. The peripheral neuropathy was mainly of sensory type, with proprioception (vibration, position sense) of lower extremities being primarily affected. Achilles jerks were depressed or absent in the majority of cases, even in those in which hyperflexia was present elsewhere. Abnormally high arches were observed in several patients (Fig. 4).

Patients with dominant OPCA and a late adult onset sporadic form of MSA associated with orthostatic hypotension and other features of progressive autonomic failure (perhaps representing a Shy-Drager syndrome) (43) were found to have normal GDH activity in leukocytes. In addition, a group of 11 patients with MSA not associated with progressive autonomic failure also had normal GDH activity. One of these patients was found at postmortem examination to have a variant of nigrostriatal degeneration. In contrast to the frequent familial incidence found in patients with GDH deficiency (see below) all cases of MSA with normal enzymatic activity were sporadic occurrences. Patients with typical Parkinson's disease, progressive supranuclear palsy, Huntington's chorea, Friedreich's ataxia, Charcot-Marie-Tooth disease, as well as various types of ataxia not associated with extrapyramidal features had normal GDH activity in leukocytes.

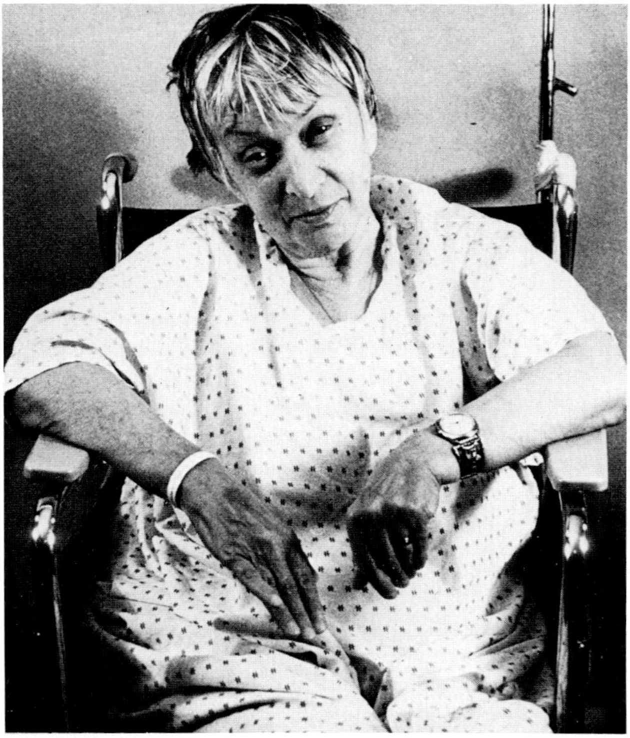

FIG. 2A. A patient with OPCA associated with GDH deficiency. She had the insidious development of gait disturbances (ataxia), incoordination of hand movements, and dysarthria at about age 55. Her condition progressed slowly afterward. Evaluation at age 65 (shown in this illustration) revealed extrapyramidal features, such as expressionless face, "striatal" hand deformity (right hand), with cogwheeling rigidity, head tilt, oculomotor disturbances (slow saccades, impaired pursuit), severe dysarthria, and marked gait and limb ataxia. At this stage, the patient could stand if supported. This patient was one of the subjects of a previous publication (ref. 38, case i).

Deficiency of the Heat-Labile GDH Component in Recessive OPCA

Although mammalian GDH isoenzymes have not been demonstrated, recent studies (38) in our laboratory suggested the presence of two distinct forms of the enzyme in human leukocytes and cultured skin fibroblasts. One form, which is particulate (probably tightly bound to mitochondrial membranes), was found to be largely inactivated by incubation at 47.5° C for 1 hr (heat-labile GDH), whereas the other form, which is soluble, remained stable under the same conditions (heat-stable GDH). These findings are strongly suggestive of the presence of at least two GDH "isoenzymes" in human tissues, which may be determined by heat inactivation.

In our latest study (38), these GDH components were determined in leukocytes from several of the above-described patients. The first step involved the determination of particulate and soluble GDH fractions in patients and controls. Results showed that the decrease in activity was limited to the particulate form of the

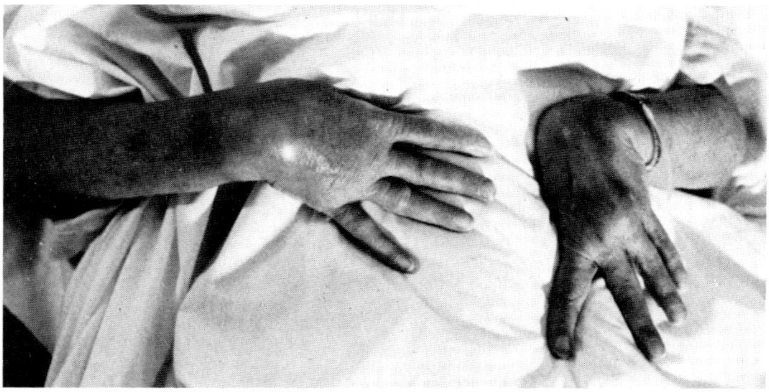

FIG. 2B. Marked postural deformities of upper extremities of the same patient have developed 1½ years later, along with further deterioration in neurologic status due to increasing rigidity-spasticity of all four extremities and bulbar dysfunction. She developed recurrent fevers of unknown origin, generalized body and extremities tremors, and virtual aphoria. She died at age 67; autopsy was not granted. The brain CT of this patient is shown in the chapter by Huang and Plaitakis (case 3, *this volume*).

enzyme, suggesting a defect in the heat-labile GDH. The soluble GDH fraction was not different in patients as compared to controls. In the second step, heat inactivation studies were carried out in whole leukocyte homogenates from nine of the above patients. Results confirmed an almost complete deficiency of the heat-labile enzyme (8% of control activity), whereas the heat-stable GDH was not significantly different in the patients as compared to controls. These data suggest that a mutation in one GDH "isoenzyme" may be the actual gene defect of the disease. Further characterization of the two GDH forms in tissues from patients, obligate heterozygotes, and controls is needed to test this hypothesis.

Studies on Cultured Skin Fibroblasts

Fibroblast lines, obtained by skin biopsy after informed consent, have been established and passed from six patients with late adult onset OPCA. In all, a partial deficiency of total GDH activity was first detected in leukocytes isolated from peripheral blood. As shown in Table 2, determinations of GDH components in leukocytes from these patients revealed an almost complete deficiency of the heat-labile enzyme. Total GDH activity was also significantly decreased (45% of control) in the cultured fibroblasts from these patients (Table 2). In Table 2, leukocyte and fibroblast pellets were prepared as previously described (32) and stored at −80° C until the assays were performed. Special care was taken to remove any excess of physiological saline, used for washing the cells (32), from the tubes with the final pellets prior to their storage. Sodium chloride has been found to influence GDH thermal stability (36a). On the day of analysis, the cells were disrupted by 3 to 4 cycles of freeze–thaw and homogenized in 50 mM tris-HCl (pH 7.40) buffer with a motor-driven glass homogenizer (0.004–0.006-in. clearance; 300 rpm) for 2 to 3 min at 0 to 5° C. Total GDH activity was measured

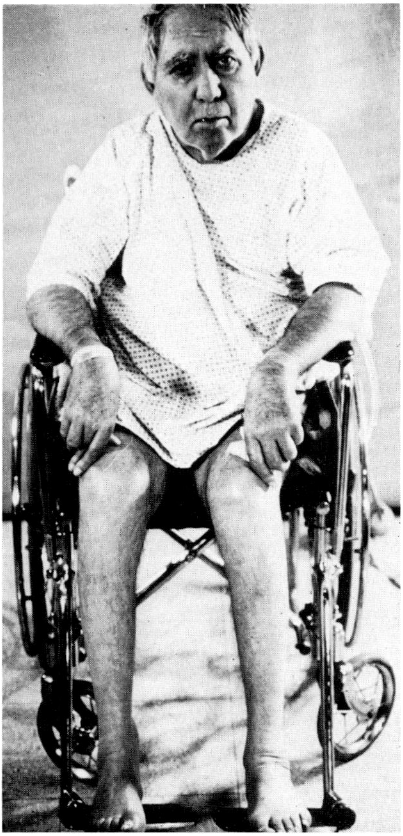

FIG. 3. A 71-year-old patient with OPCA associated with GDH deficiency (older affected brother of family A, Fig. 5). The presenting symptom was diplopia at age 50; this was soon followed by leg weakness and unsteadiness. A neurologic evaluation, done at the early stages of this patient's illness, revealed spasticity predominantly of the lower extremities. The diagnosis of lateral sclerosis was made. Since then, disease progressed slowly, with patient developing increased gait disturbances, incoordination of hand movements, dysarthria, sphincter disturbances, and decreased visual acuity in his mid to late 60s. Neurologic evaluation at age 71 revealed a mild dementia, extrapyramidal features (parkinsonism), oculomotor disturbances, decreased visual acuity, marked dysarthria, ataxia of the upper extremities, marked spastic paraparesis, muscle fasciculations with a degree of amyotrophy, and peripheral neuropathy. This illustration shows parkinsonian features, dystonic posturing of right fingers, and wasting of lower legs. This patient was one of the subjects of a previous publication (case 3 in ref. 32).

fluorometrically at 28° C in whole leukocyte or fibroblast homogenates as previously described (32) with the addition of 1 mM ADP and 0.025% Triton X-100 (final concentrations) to the reaction mixture. For determination of the heat-labile and heat-stable GDH, aliquots of leukocyte homogenates (0.5–0.8 ml, 5–10 mg protein/ml) were transferred to capped Falcon plastic tubes (12 × 75 mm) and incubated at 47.5° C in a Dubnoff incubator with shaking. At exactly 60 min, incubation was discontinued, and portions of homogenates equal to those used for baseline GDH activity (40–60 μl) were removed and assayed in the presence of ADP (1 mM) and Triton X-100 (0.025%). The activity found was considered heat-stable GDH; this was subtracted from the total activity in order to determine the heat-labile GDH. Values represent nanomoles of oxidized NADH per milligrams of protein per hour; mean ± SD; *N*, number of individuals studied. All 16 controls used for the leukocyte studies were healthy adult volunteers. However, of the 17 controls used for the fibroblast studies, 8 were healthy individuals, and 9 were patients with various types of degenerative neurologic disorders not associated with GDH deficiency in leukocytes (diseased controls). For the fibroblast studies, skin was obtained by biopsy after informed consent from patients and controls, and primary

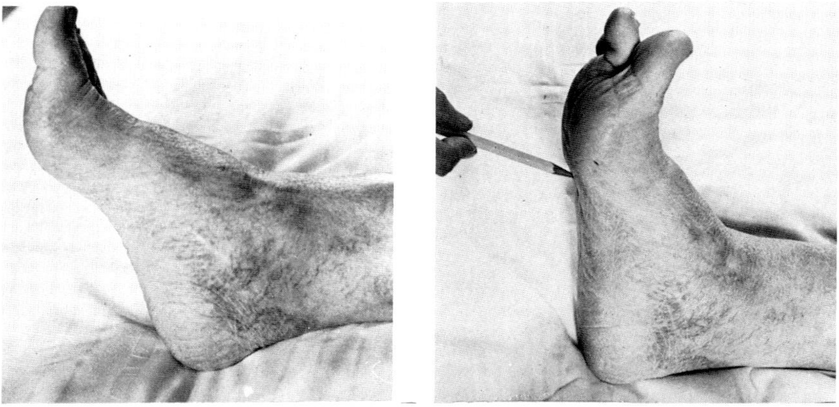

FIG. 4. High arches **(left)** in a 71-year-old patient with parkinsonism associated with cortico-spinal (see Babinski sign, **right**) and cerebellar deficits. One of his brothers (age 70) is similarly affected (pedigree C). Both siblings had deficiency of the heat-labile GDH in leukocytes.

TABLE 2. *Activities of GDH in leuckocytes and cultured skin fibroblasts from patients with recessive OPCA and controls*

	Leukocyte			Fibroblast
Subject	Total	Heat labile	Heat stable	(total)
Control	1,776 ± 205 (*N* = 16)	502 ± 151 (*N* = 16)	1,274 ± 183 (*N* = 16)	7,321 ± 2,408 (*N* = 17)
Patient	1,182 ± 202[a] (*N* = 6)	26 ± 23[a] (*N* = 6)	1,126 ± 201 (*N* = 6)	3,547 ± 543[a] (*N* = 6)

[a]$p < 0.005$.

cultures of these cells were established and passed as previously described (32). Cells from patients and controls were studied after a comparable number ($N = 2$–6) of passages. All assays were done in duplicate, and at least two leukocyte or fibroblast homogenates were studied from each patient.

By showing that the enzymatic defect is also present in cell lines grown *in vitro*, these results suggest GDH deficiency as the primary genetic defect in recessive OPCA. This is supported by metabolic studies (described below) that revealed abnormal glutamate metabolism in patients with GDH-deficient OPCA. Additional studies are now in progress exploring GDH fractions in the cultured cells.

Genetic Aspects

In all patients in whom GDH deficiency was detected in leukocytes, a detailed family history was taken and a pedigree constructed. Every effort was made to study all available surviving family members of these patients. Thus far, we have identified four pedigrees in which the disorder occurred in two or more members. As shown in Fig. 5, affected members with GDH deficiency were siblings of either sex but not parents or offsprings. In one family (Fig. 5, family B), both parents of the patients were available for evaluation. A careful neurologic evaluation failed to detect any abnormal clinical sign in these individuals. These genetic data suggest the autosomal recessive inheritance of the disease. Additional studies are now in progress exploring the two GDH forms in leukocytes and cultured skin fibroblasts from parents or offsprings of affected patients in the above kindreds. Documentation of the carrier state of the enzymatic deficiency in these individuals is required to confirm its recessive inheritance.

ABNORMAL GLUTAMATE METABOLISM IN PATIENTS WITH GDH DEFICIENCY

As already described, decreased GDH activity has been detected in leukocytes and cultured skin fibroblasts from patients with a form of OPCA that appears to be recessively inherited. Thus the genetic defect in these patients is expressed in tissues outside the nervous system, despite the lack of any involvement of these

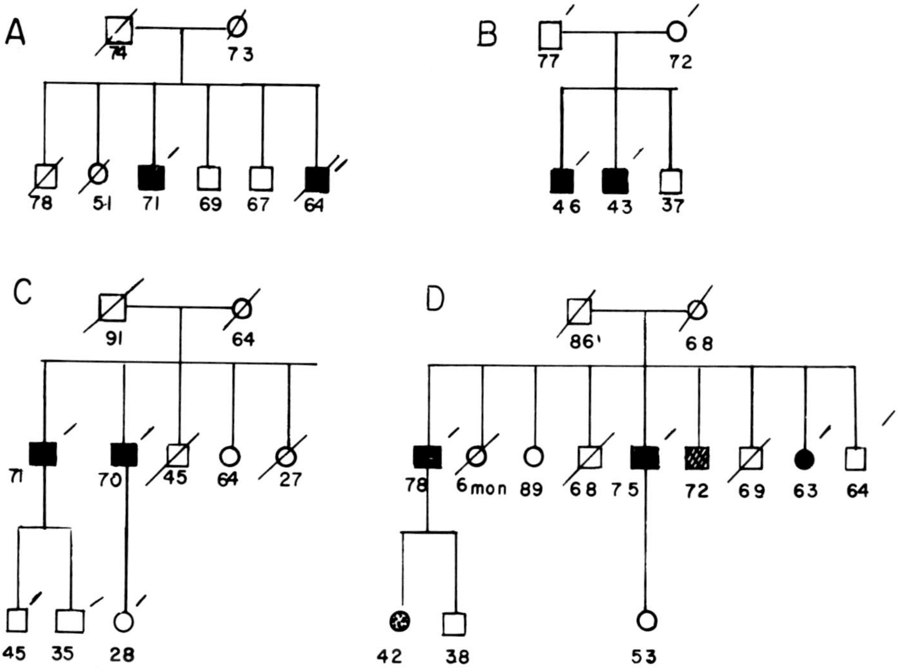

FIG. 5. Fragment pedigrees of families affected by GDH-deficient OPCA: slash (/) indicates individual examined by the author; ages in years are indicated below the symbols. As this figure shows, the disease has been found to affect siblings of either sex without being vertically transmitted. These data are consistent with an autosomal recessive transmission pattern. (Part of the data from refs. 32, 33, and 38.)

tissues that is of clinical significance. We have investigated the possibility of systemic metabolic defects in patients with the enzymatic deficiency. In initial studies (34,35), the levels of the GDH substrates glutamate, α-ketoglutarate, and ammonia were determined in the fasting plasma from GDH-deficient patients as well as from healthy and diseased (non-GDH-deficient neurologic disorders) controls. Results revealed significant increases in plasma glutamate (by 137–149%) and decreases in α-ketoglutarate (by 21–22%) (35,38). These data are consistent with a block at the oxidation of glutamate to α-ketoglutarate (GDH step). These abnormalities were selective, since the levels of other amino acids, as well as those of ammonia, pyruvate, and malate, were not different in the patients as compared to controls (38). In addition, plasma amino acid levels were determined in patients and controls who, after fasting overnight, consumed a standard meal containing 1 g protein/kg body weight. Protein is known to contain about 11% glutamate. At 2 and 4 hr, after ingestion of this meal, plasma glutamate levels rose significantly more in patients than controls (35). Plasma aspartate levels showed similar elevations. A small but significant increase occurred in plasma alanine levels in the GDH-deficient patients 4 hr after the meal, whereas plasma glutamine levels were comparable in the two groups (35).

These results suggested an impaired capacity of the patients to metabolize (oxidize) exogenous (dietary) glutamate, with a resultant increased formation of aspartate and alanine by transamination (Fig. 1). This was confirmed by additional studies involving the oral intake of monosodium glutamate (60 mg/kg body weight) after overnight fasting by patients and controls. Results of these loading tests revealed abnormal elevations in plasma glutamate in the GDH-deficient patients as compared to controls (Fig. 6). Similarly to the protein loading, glutamate intake resulted in elevations in plasma aspartate which were significantly greater in patients than controls, suggesting an intact transamination pathway in these individuals. In contrast, plasma alanine levels did not change after oral intake of monosodium glutamate in patients or controls. These results confirmed previous observations indicating that glutamate absorbed in the form of monosodium glutamate does not enter into the pool of the amino acid that transaminates to alanine, although this has been shown to occur when glutamate is absorbed from protein hydrolysates (22).

Since GDH may function in maintaining the mitochondrial NADH/NAD potentials which can be reflected in the cytoplasmic lactate/pyruvate ratio, this ratio was determined in the plasma of patients and controls after oral glutamate loading. In controls, the lactate/pyruvate ratio increased significantly after monosodium glutamate intake, whereas patients with GDH-deficient OPCA showed a flat curve (35). These results are consistent with the hypothesis that oxidation of the glutamate load in controls (via GDH) produced sufficient amounts of reduced NADH to increase the NADH/NAD ratio. The inability of GDH-deficient patients to respond similarly indicates an impaired capacity of their tissues to oxidize glutamate, which is metabolized primarily by transamination, resulting in increased production of aspartate (Fig. 6).

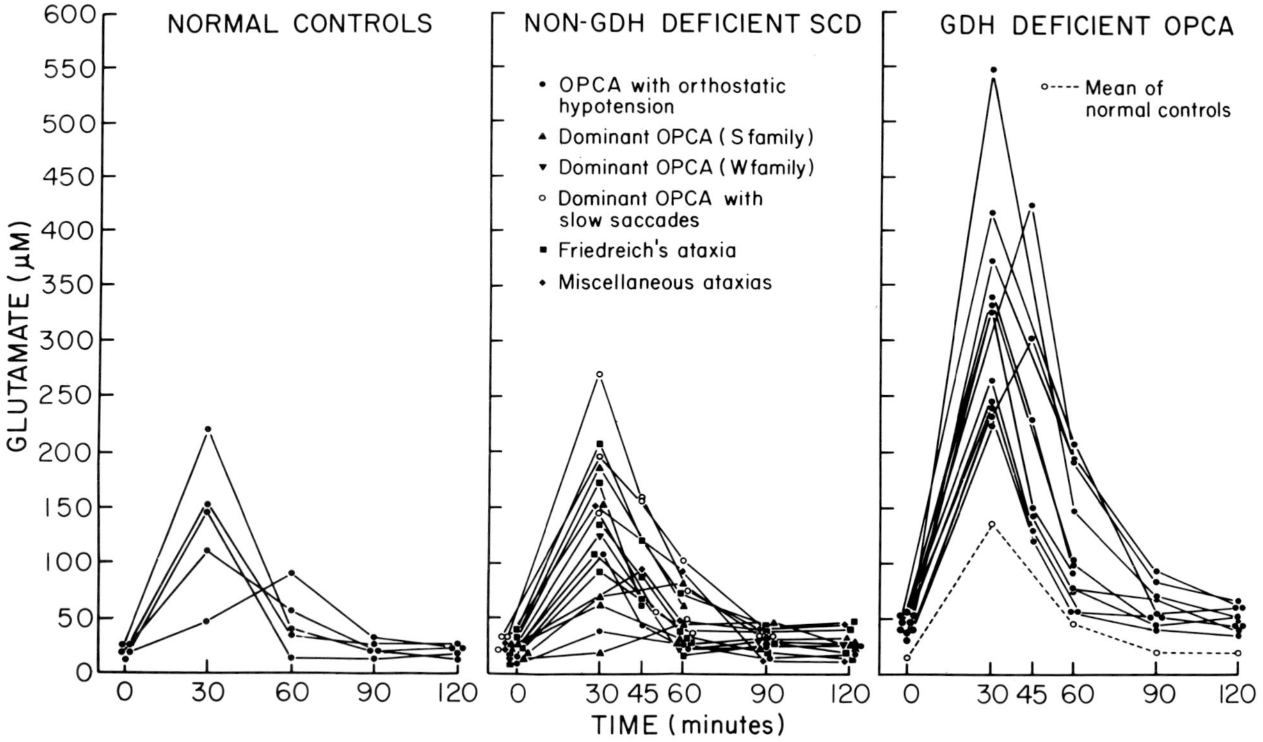

FIG. 6. Glutamate loading tests in patients with GDH-deficient OPCA, healthy controls, and patients with various types of spinocerebellar degeneration (SCD) not associated with GDH deficiency (non-GDH-deficient SCD). The dominant OPCA (S family) includes 5 patients from the Schut kindred (42), whereas the dominant OPCA (W family) is 1 member of the W pedigree (38a). The 3 patients with dominant OPCA associated with slow saccades were from two unrelated families. Patients and controls fasted overnight and the following morning received orally 60 mg/kg body weight of monosodium glutamate dissolved in 100–150 ml of water. At time points indicated, blood samples were drawn, processed, and analyzed, as previously described (35). All individuals were on a regular diet and were not taking any medication at the time of the study.

Besides glutamate and aspartate, no other amino acids changed in the plasma of patients and controls after glutamate loading, except for the significant elevation in plasma taurine levels that occurred in healthy and some of the disease controls (37). Plasma taurine levels did show significant changes in GDH-deficient patients. These results provided additional evidence for an interrelationship between glutamate and taurine metabolism, which appears to be altered in GDH deficiency. The mechanisms of these changes are poorly understood, since no direct metabolic pathway between glutamate and taurine is known. Van Gelder (45,46) has suggested that taurine regulates glutamate metabolism in the brain, and that free glutamic acid increases the release of taurine from synaptosomal preparations. Taurine levels are known to be greater in platelets (which have a high affinity taurine uptake) than in plasma. Thus it is reasonable to postulate that glutamate loading results in plasma taurine elevation by causing its release from platelets (37). Whether or not these observations have a pathophysiologic implication for OPCA is not known at present. It is of interest that Perry et al. (28) have shown an altered balance between aspartate and taurine in cerebellar tissues from patients with a dominant form of OPCA.

Mechanisms of Neuronal Degeneration in GDH-Deficient OPCA

Substantial amounts of GDH activity are present in mammalian brain. Although its exact function in the nervous tissue remains unclear, the enzyme appears to be associated with glia as well as nerve cells. In nerve cells, GDH may be associated with the pool of glutamate that is released as neurotransmitter at the nerve terminals; therefore, it may function in glutamatergic transmission mechanisms. Over the past 25 years, considerable evidence has been accumulated to suggest that glutamate, which appears to be the main excitatory transmitter in the nervous system of vertebrates (11), has neurotoxic potentials when present in this system in excess. Thus Lucas and Newhouse showed in 1957 (18) that systemic administration of monosodium glutamate to experimental animals can result in degeneration of retinal ganglion cells. Olney et al. (25) subsequently showed that systemic administration of acidic amino acids, such as glutamic and aspartic acids, can result in hypothalamic lesions in premature mice. Similar lesions were also found in a premature primate who received monosodium glutamate parenterally (26). In recent years, considerable interest has been aroused by observations indicating that the pattern of neuronal degeneration induced by glutamate, and particularly its potent analogs kainic and ibotenic acids, is similar to that found in some disorders with system atrophy. Thus local injection of these substances into brain regions of experimental animals can selectively destroy local neurons while sparing nerve endings and axons passing from these regions (19). Additional studies (9,10,20,21) further implied that glutamate neurotoxicity may be related to its function as an excitatory neurotransmitter. These observations led to the hypothesis that altered neuroexcitatory mechanisms may be responsible for the neuronal degeneration that occurs in certain disorders with system atrophy.

Since glutamate catabolism is impaired in GDH-deficient OPCA, it is possible that accumulation of this potentially neurotoxic amino acid in the nervous system could be the cause of the selective neuronal degeneration that occurs in this disorder. As described above, GDH is thought to be associated with the pool of glutamate that is released at the nerve terminals as neurotransmitter; therefore, the enzyme could function in glutamatergic transmission mechanisms. Decreased glutamate catabolism at the nerve terminals could result in an increased accumulation of the amino acid released during excitation at the synaptic cleft; this could directly cause degeneration of postsynaptic neurons. Thus, the Purkinje cells that receive glutamatergic innervation by the granule cells (parallel fibers) (Fig. 7) could degenerate in the disease based on this mechanism. Earlier anatomical studies have established that disappearance of cerebellar Purkinje cells is a consistent finding in OPCA (13). This was also true in one case of GDH-deficient OPCA that came to postmortem examination (7). Degeneration of the granule cells and the olivocerebellar fibers (the two systems that maintain direct synaptic contact with the Purkinje cells) could be secondary events attributable to the disappearance of the Purkinje cells (transneuronal degeneration) (9).

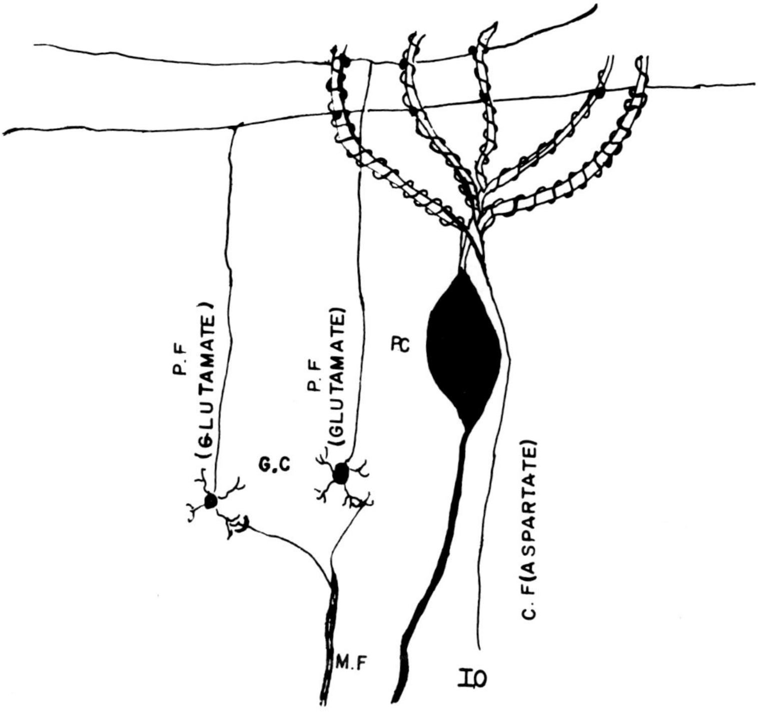

FIG. 7. Projections to the Purkinje cells (PC) thought to utilize neuroexcitatory amino acids as transmitters. The climbing fibers (CF), probably originating from the inferior olives (IO), may be aspartergic (28). On the other hand, the parallel fibers (PF), which originate from the granule cells (GC), may use glutamate as their excitatory transmitter (51). MF, mossy fibers.

We recently studied a significant number of GDH-deficient OPCA cases (Huang and Plaitakis, *this volume*) with the use of the computerized tomography (CT) scan. This provided important insights into the brain structural changes that occur *in vivo* in this disorder. Atrophy of the cerebellum and brainstem, found in this disorder, was consistent with the clinical diagnosis of OPCA. In addition, a marked enlargement of the anterior third ventricle (usually in association with some degree of frontal lobe atrophy) was present in these patients. These latter changes clearly separated GDH-deficient OPCA from the other forms of the disorder that are not associated with the enzymatic deficiency. As discussed in the chapter by Huang and Plaitakis, enlargement of the anterior third ventricle in GDH-deficient OPCA appears to reflect loss of tissue in the hypothalamus and thalamus of these patients. These findings are of particular interest since they appear to represent anatomical correlates of glutamate neurotoxicity in a human disorder in view of the fact that systemic administration of monosodium glutamate to experimental premature animals can selectively damage hypothalamic regions in these animals (5,25,26). Anatomical studies in adult rats treated with monosodium glutamate during their neonatal period revealed enlargement of their third ventricle due to atrophy of the arcuate nucleus and other structures of the hypothalamus (5). These experimental data strongly suggest that atrophy of hypothalamic structures, as demonstrated by CT scan findings, in GDH-deficient OPCA is the result of impaired glutamate catabolism that occurs in this disorder. Therefore, GDH-deficient OPCA appears to be the first adult onset degenerative neurologic disorder with system atrophy for which there is a biochemical basis to account for the selective brain lesion topography. Thus these findings may be of theoretical importance that extends well beyond the problem of the pathogenesis of OPCA.

ABNORMAL ASPARTATE/MALATE METABOLISM IN A DOMINANT OPCA

As already described, OPCA is known to occur sporadically or to be genetically transmitted. The mode of inheritance of the genetic cases can be either autosomal dominant with complete penetrance or recessive. Many of the sporadic cases actually may be recessive (30). These differences in heredity suggest that under the term OPCA are included a number of heterogenous diseases related to different etiologic (genetic) factors. This is supported by the known clinical and even pathologic heterogeneity of OPCA. Nevertheless, all disorders classified as OPCA share some common pathologic features, such as atrophy of the inferior olives, olivocerebellar pathways, cerebellar cortex, and areas of the pons. This degeneration pattern of the various OPCAs may result through common pathogenetic mechanisms. In view of the fact that one form of OPCA (recessive) is associated with abnormal systemic metabolism of the major excitatory amino acid glutamate, it can be hypothesized that other forms of this disorder may be related to alternate but similar metabolic defects.

Along the above lines of thought, we have searched for systemic metabolic defects of amino acid putative transmitters in patients with a dominantly inherited form of OPCA. All these patients were members of a well-studied pedigree known as the Schut family (42). This gave us the opportunity to study eight patients who had the same disease process and genetic background. Three control groups were used. The first was an equal number of sex-matched (of similar age), healthy family members who were not at risk for developing the disease (both parents unaffected; family controls). The second were healthy adult individuals who were not blood related to the affected family (unrelated healthy controls). The third group were patients with nondominant cerebellar degenerations (disease controls). A battery of 18 amino acids and the Kreb's cycle substrates α-ketoglutarate, malate, pyruvate, and lactate were determined in the fasting plasma of these individuals. Results revealed (36) a significant decrease in plasma aspartate levels in the OPCA patients as compared to all three control groups. In about half these patients, plasma aspartate levels were below 2 SD from the mean control values. The decrease in aspartate was selective since the levels of 18 other amino acids and the four Kreb's cycle substrates were not different in the patients as compared to controls. These results suggested a systemic defect in the metabolism of aspartate in this dominant OPCA. Since aspartate can be synthesized from glutamate by transamination (Fig. 1), this pathway was tested by oral glutamate loading tests. Patients and controls received 60 mg/kg body weight monosodium glutamate after overnight fasting. Glutamate absorbed after oral intake of monosodium glutamate appears to be metabolized by oxidative deamination (GDH step) as well as by transamination to aspartate (GOT step) (35). Results revealed comparable elevations in plasma glutamate and aspartate in patients and controls, suggesting that these two pathways were intact in these patients.

Asparate metabolism is also known to be related to that of malate. The so-called "malate shuttle" involves the entrance of malate from the cytoplasm into the mitochondria and the exit of intramitochondrial aspartate to the cytoplasm. This assures that cytoplasmic NADH is converted to NAD to maintain the ratio of NADH/NAD. In view of these considerations, the levels of malate and the aspartate/malate ratio were determined in the plasma of patients and controls who, after overnight fasting, received an oral glucose load (1.75g/kg body weight). Results showed a significant increase in plasma malate and a decrease in the aspartate/malate ratio after glucose intake in patients as compared to controls (36). Since glucose utilization is expected to produce increased amounts of malate via the Kreb's cycle (Fig. 1), as well as an excess of NADH over NAD (which will activate the "malate shuttle"), these results suggested a systemic abnormality in malate/aspartate metabolism in this dominant OPCA. Thus the decreased fasting plasma aspartate levels could result from a decreased formation of this amino acid from malate (via oxaloacetate) (Fig. 1). A defect in either the transport (entrance) of malate into the mitochondria or an impaired oxidation (MDH step) of the substrate by these organelles could be the underlying mechanism. Further studies are needed to test this hypothesis.

Additional studies *(unpublished observations)* have revealed marked elevations in malate levels in postmortem brain tissues (cerebral and cerebellar cortex) from two patients of this family who came to autopsy. One of these patients was among the eight family members mentioned above. Since malate is known to be stable, its accumulation in brain tissues of patients with dominant OPCA strongly suggests that a block in the metabolism of this compound may exist in the brains of these patients. The decreased brain aspartate and glutamate levels found by Perry et al. (29; see Perry, *this volume*) in members of this family are probably directly related to defective malate metabolism. Thus a genetic defect in the metabolism of amino acid putative transmitters or Kreb's cycle substrates may be the underlying biochemical basis of the various forms of OPCA.

ACKNOWLEDGMENTS

This work was supported by NIH grants NS-16871 and NS-11631 and by the Clinical Center for Research in Parkinson's and Allied Diseases and NIH Division of Research in Parkinson's Resources grant RR-71. I thank Shirley Keel, Rochelle Cohen, and Natassa Khelemskaya for their excellent assistance and Dr. S. Berl for reading this manuscript and for his useful suggestions. I am indebted to Dr. L. J. Schut for his invaluable help in the studies on dominant OPCA.

REFERENCES

1. Bayley, P. M., and Radda, G. K. (1966): Conformational changes and the regulation of glutamate dehydrogenase activity. *Biochem. J.*, 98:105–111.
2. Berl, S. (1971): Cerebral amino acid metabolism in hepatic coma. *Exp. Biol. Med.*, 4:78–84.
3. Berl, S., Nicklas, W. J., and Clarke, D. D. (1970): Compartmentation of citric acid cycle metabolism in brain: Labeling of glutamate, glutamine, aspartate and GABA by several radioactive tracer metabolites. *J. Neurochem.*, 17:1009–1015.
4. Berl, S., Clarke, D. D., and Schneider, D., editors (1975): *Metabolic Compartmentation and Neurotransmission: Relation to Brain Structure and Function*. Plenum, New York.
5. Bodnar, R. J., Abrams, G. M., Zimmerman, E. A., Krieger, D. T., Nicholson, G., and Kizer, J. S. (1980): Neonatal monosodium glutamate. *Neuroendocrinology*, 30:280–284.
6. Chee, P. Y., Dahl, J. L., and Fahien, L. A. (1979): The purification and properties of rat brain glutamate dehydrogenase. *J. Neurochem.*, 33:53–60.
7. Chokroverty, S., Duvoisin, R. D., Khedekar, R., and Derby, B. (1983): Olivopontocerebellar atrophy (OPCA) with glutamate dehydrogenase (GDH) deficiency: A clinical-pathologic study. *Neurology (Minneap.) [Suppl. 2]*, 33:78.
8. Cooper, A. J. L., McDonald, J. M., Gelbard, A. S., Gledhill, R. F., and Duffy, T. E. (1979): The metabolic fate of ^{13}N-labelled ammonia in rat brain. *J. Biol. Chem.*, 254:4982–4992.
9. Coyle, J. T. (1982): Neurotoxic amino acids in human degenerative disorders. *Trends Neurosci.*, 5:287–288.
10. Coyle, J. T., London, E. D., Biziere, K., and Zaczek, R. (1979): Kainic acid neurotoxicity: Insights into the pathophysiology of Huntington's disease. In: *Advances in Neurology Vol. 23, Huntington's Disease*, edited by T. N. Chase, N. S. Wexler, and A. Barbeau, pp. 593–608. Raven Press, New York.
11. Curtis, D. R., and Watkins, J. C. (1963): Acidic amino acids with strong excitatory action on mammalian neurones. *J. Physiol.*, 166:1–14.
12. Desclin, J. C., and Escubi, J. (1974): Effects of 3-acetylpyridine on the central nervous system of the rat as demonstrated by silver methods. *Brain Res.*, 77:349–364.
13. Eadie, M. J. (1975): Olivo-ponto-cerebellar atrophy. In: *Handbook of Clinical Neurology, Vol. 2*, edited by P. J. Vinken and G. W. Bruyn, pp. 415–431. North-Holland, Amsterdam.
14. Engel, P. C. (1973): Evolution of enzyme regulator sites: Evidence for partial gene duplication from amino-acid sequences of bovine glutamate dehydrogenase. *Nature*, 241:118–120.
15. Gowers, W. R. (1902): Abiotrophy. *Lancet*, 1:1003–1007.

16. Hassin, G. B., and Harris, T. H. (1937): Olivopontocerebellar atrophy: Clinical and pathologic considerations. *Arch. Neurol. Psychiatry*, 37(1):1371–1382.
17. Herken, H. (1968): Functional disorders of the brain induced by synthesis of nucleotides containing 3-acetylpyridine. *Z. Klin. Chem.*, 6:357–367.
18. Lucas, D. R., and Newhouse, J. P. (1957): The toxic effect of sodium L-glutamate on the inner layers of retina. *AMA Arch. Ophthalmol.*, 58:193–204.
19. McGeer, E. G., and McGeer, P. L. (1976): Duplication of biochemical changes of Huntington's chorea by intrastriatal injections of glutamic and kainic acids. *Nature*, 263:517–519.
20. McGeer, E. G., McGeer, P. L., and Singh, K. (1978): Kainate-induced degeneration of neostriatal neurons: Dependency upon corticostriatal tract. *Brain Res.*, 139:381–383.
21. McGeer, E. G., Onley, J. W., and McGeer, P. L. (1978): *Kainic Acid as a Tool in Neurobiology.* Raven Press, New York.
22. Marrs, T. C., Salmona, M., Garattini, S., Burston, D., and Matthews, D. M. (1978): The absorption by human volunteers of glutamic acid from monosodium glutamate and from a partial enzymic hydrolysate of casein. *Toxicology*, 11:101–107.
23. Miller, A. L., Hawkins, R. A., and Veech, R. L. (1973): The mitochondrial redox state of rat brain. *J. Neurochem.*, 20:1393–1400.
24. Nelson, K. L., Povey, M. S., Hopkinson, D. A., and Harris, H. (1977): Electrophoresis of human L-glutamate dehydrogenase: Tissue distribution and preliminary population survey. *Biochem. Genet.*, 5:87–91.
25. Olney, J. W., and Sharpe, L. G. (1969): Brain lesions in an infant rhesus monkey treated with monosodium glutamate. *Science*, 166:386–388.
26. Olney, J. W., Ho, O. L., and Rhee, V. (1971): Cytotoxic effects of acidic and sulfur containing amino acids of the infant mouse central nervous system. *Exp. Brain Res.*, 14:61–76.
27. Orton, S. T. (1925): The pathology of the hereditary and familial nervous and mental disease. *Arch. Neurol. Psychiatry*, 13:96–115.
28. Perry, T. L., Currier, R. D., Hansen, S., and MacLean, J. (1977): Aspartate taurine imbalance in dominantly inherited olivopontocerebellar atrophy. *Neurology (Minneap.)*, 27:257–261.
29. Perry, T. L., Kish, S. J., Hansen, S., and Currier, R. D. (1981): Neurotransmitter amino acids in dominantly inherited cerebellar disorders. *Neurology (Minneap.)*, 31:237–242.
30. Plaitakis, A. (1982): The olivopontocerebellar atrophies. *Semin. Neurol.*, 2:334–342.
31. Plaitakis, A., Nicklas, W. J., and Desnick, R. J. (1979): Glutamate dehydrogenase deficiency in three patients with spinocerebellar ataxia. A new enzymatic defect? *Trans. Am. Neurol. Assoc.*, 104:54–57.
32. Plaitakis, A., Nicklas, W. J., and Desnick, R. J. (1980): Glutamate dehydrogenase deficiency in three patients with spinocerebellar syndrome. *Ann. Neurol.*, 7:297–303.
33. Plaitakis, A., Berl, S., Nicklas, W. J., and Yahr, M. D. (1980): Glutamate dehydrogenase deficiency in spinocerebellar degenerations: Correlation with adult-onset recessive ataxia. *Trans. Am. Neurol. Assoc.*, 105:476.
34. Plaitakis, A., Berl, S., and Yahr, M. D. (1981): Amino acids as putative transmitters: The role of aspartate and glutamate in nervous system dysfunction and degeneration. *Neurology*, 568:259–273.
35. Plaitakis, A., Berl, S., and Yahr, M. D. (1982): Abnormal glutamate metabolism in an adult-onset degenerative neurological disorder. *Science*, 216:193–196.
36. Plaitakis, A., Berl, S., Schut, L. J., and Yahr, M. D. (1982): Abnormal aspartate/malate metabolism in dominantly inherited olivopontocerebellar degeneration. *Ann. Neurol.*, 12:79.
36a. Plaitakis, A., Colon, A., Perrakis, A., Berl, S., and Clarke, D. D. (1983): Evidence for the presence of two forms of GDH in mammalian tissues. One is reduced in a neurological disorder. *Soc. Neurochem. Abstr.*, 9:1171.
37. Plaitakis, A., and Berl, S. (1983): Oral glutamate loading in disorders with spinocerebellar and extrapyramidal involvement: Effect on plasma glutamate, aspartate and taurine. *J. Neural Transm.*, 19(Suppl.):65–74.
38. Plaitakis, A., Berl, S., and Yahr, M. D. (1984): Neurological disorders associated with deficiency of glutamate dehydrogenase. *Ann. Neurol.*, 15:144–153.
38a. Pogacar, S., Amber, M, Conlin, W. J., O'Neil, W. A., and Yong Lee, H. (1978): Dominant spinopontine atrophy. Report of two additional members of family W. *Arch. Neurol.*, 35:156–162.

39. Puranen, J., and Arstila, A. (1967): Inhibition of glutamic dehydrogenase by clomiphene. *Nature*, 213:78–79.
40. Quastel, J. H. (1978): Cerebral glutamate-glutamine interrelations *in vivo* and *in vitro*. In: *Dynamic Properties of Glial Cells*, edited by E. Schoffeniels, G. Franck, D. B. Towers, and L. Hertz, pp. 153–162. Pergamon Press, Oxford.
41. Schoolwerth, A. C., Nazar, B. L., and LaNoue, K. F. (1978): Glutamate dehydrogenase activation and ammonia formation by rat kidney mitochondria. *J. Biol. Chem.*, 253:6177–6183.
42. Schut, J. W. (1980): Hereditary ataxia. Clinical study through six generations. *Arch. Neurol. Psychiatry*, 63:535–568.
43. Shy, G. M., and Drager, G. A. (1960): A neurological syndrome associated with orthostatic hypotension. *Arch. Neurol.*, 2:511–527.
44. Stanbury, J. B., Wyngarden, J. B., Fredrickson, D. S., Goldstein, J. L., and Bran M. S. (1983): *The Metabolic Basis of Inherited Disease*. McGraw-Hill, New York.
45. Van Gelder, N. M. (1982): Changed taurine glutamic acid content and altered nervous tissue cytoarchitecture. In: *Taurine in Nutrition and Neurology*, edited by R. J. Huxtable and H. Pasantes-Morales, pp. 239–256. Plenum, New York.
46. Van Gelder, N. M. (1982): Glutamic acid in nervous tissue and changes of the taurine content: Its implication in the treatment of epilepsy. In: *Amino Acid Neurotransmitters*, edited by F. V. DeFeudis and P. Mandel, pp. 115–125. Raven Press, New York.
47. Wolf, J. (1968): The effect of thyroxine on isolated dehydrogenases. II. Sedimentation changes in glutamate dehydrogenase. *J. Biol. Chem.*, 237:230–242.
48. Yielding, K. L., and Tomkins, G. M. (1962): Studies on the interaction of steroid hormones with glutamic dehydrogenase. *Recent Prog. Horm. Res.*, 18:467–489.
49. Yielding, K. L., and Tomkins, G. M. (1961): An effect of L-leucine and other essential amino acids on the structure and activity of glutamic dehydrogenase. *Proc. Natl. Acad. Sci. USA*, 47:983.
50. Yielding, K. L., and Tomkins, G. M. (1960): Structural alterations in crystalline glutamate dehydrogenase induced by steroid hormones. *Proc. Natl. Acad. Sci. USA*, 46:1483–1488.
51. Young, A. B., Oster-Granite, M. L., Herdon, R. M. and Snyder, S. H. (1974): Glutamic acid: Selective depletion by viral induced granule cell loss in hamster cerebellum. *Brain Res.*, 73:1–13.
52. Yu, A. C., Schousboe, A., and Hertz, L. (1982): Metabolic fate of ^{14}C-labeled glutamate in astrocytes. *J. Neurochem.*, 39:954–960.

The Olivopontocerebellar Atrophies, edited by R.C. Duvoisin and A. Plaitakis. Raven Press, New York © 1984.

Amino Acid Metabolism in the Central Nervous System: Role of Glutamate Dehydrogenase

William J. Nicklas

Department of Neurology, University of Medicine and Dentistry of New Jersey, Rutgers Medical School, Piscataway, New Jersey 08854

Several of the studies in this volume are concerned with the clinical ramifications of olivopontocerebellar atrophies (OPCAs) in which it is suggested that there are alterations in either the metabolism or function of the amino acid L-glutamate. It is the purpose of this chapter to render an overview of what is known (and unknown) about the metabolism and physiologic function of this amino acid in various tissues but with emphasis on the mammalian central nervous system (CNS). Since a deficiency of the enzyme glutamate dehydrogenase (GDH) has been found in a subset of these OPCAs (18,42,43,55), this chapter focuses primarily on GDH: the interesting properties of the isolated protein, its role in amino acid metabolism, and what is known of its physiologic role in several tissues.

Glutamate is a so-called "nonessential" amino acid; i.e., it is not needed in the diet but is synthesized readily in all tissues by several routes, as discussed below. However, it is far from "nonimportant." Among the numerous documented types of disturbances in amino acid metabolism that have clinical relevance, many involve glutamate. A partial list of these is as follows:

1. Pyroglutamic aciduria and glutathione synthetase deficiency
2. Glutathionuria and γ-GTP deficiency
3. Glutathione reductase deficiency
4. Glutathione peroxidase deficiency
5. γ-Glutamyl cysteine synthetase deficiency
6. Cysteinyl glycinuria
7. Type I hyperprolinemia and proline oxidase deficiency
8. Type II hyperprolinemia
9. Histidinemia
10. Homocarnosine accumulation
11. Vitamine B_6-dependent seizures and glutamate decarboxylase
12. Huntington's chorea and glutamate decarboxylase
13. Hyper-β-alaninemia and GABA aciduria
14. Hereditary protein intolerance and glutaminase

15. Carbamyl-phosphate synthetase deficiency
16. Hepatic insufficiency and encephalopathy
17. Glutamate intolerance and toxicity

Many of these disorders have peripheral and CNS features. These disturbances range from the minor problems associated with the anecdotal "Chinese-restaurant syndrome," caused by overingestion of monosodium glutamate, to life-threatening conditions, such as hepatic encephalopathy.

METABOLISM AND FUNCTION OF GLUTAMATE IN THE MAMMALIAN CNS

Metabolism

In brain, as in many other tissues, GDH forms part of a complex enzymatic machinery for transferring amino groups between α-keto acids and the corresponding α-amino acids (Fig. 1). Several transaminases (e.g., aspartate, alanine, and tyrosine aminotransferases) act to transfer amino groups between various α-keto acids and glutamate using tightly bound pyridoxal phosphate as a cofactor. These generally are freely reversible and are regulated by mass action (and, to some extent, by vitamin B_6 availability). On the other hand, GDH does not transfer a $-NH_2$ group as such; rather, it is capable of either the reductive amination of α-ketoglutarate using ammonia as a substrate or the oxidative deamination of L-glutamate to form α-ketoglutarate and ammonia. The rate and direction of reaction of GDH in the cell, therefore, is dependent on factors, such as ammonia levels and the redox potential of its metabolic surround. In fact, use has been made of the

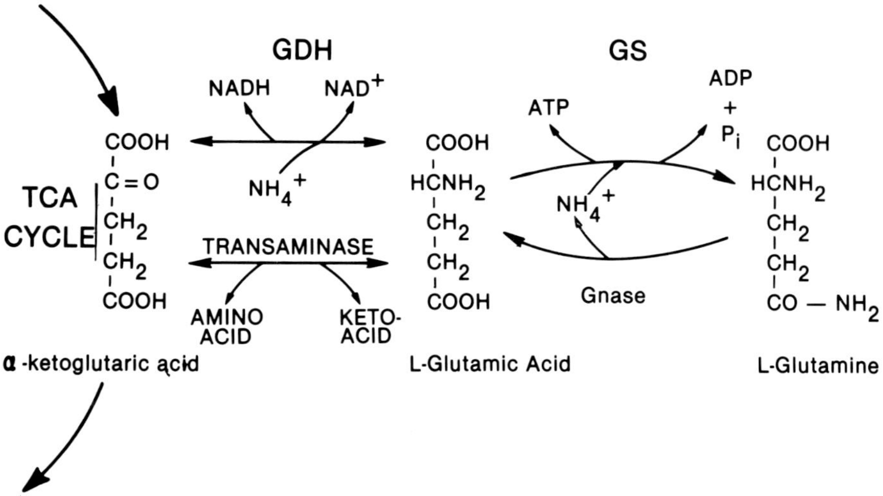

FIG. 1. Schematic of pathways of glutamate metabolism.

GDH redox couple to calculate the redox state of brain mitochondria *in situ* (23,31). Particulars of the kinetics of GDH and its allosteric regulation are detailed below.

The enzyme GDH is not the only one involved in cellular ammonia metabolism. Glutamate is amidated by the enzyme glutamine synthetase (GS) in most tissues. This enzyme is especially important in CNS since this tissue does not have a functional urea cycle for clearing ammonia. It is essentially unidirectional toward the formation of glutamine; in the process, ATP is hydrolyzed to ADP and inorganic phosphate. The regulation of the activity of the mammalian enzyme is not known beyond the obvious dependence on the energy state of the cell and ammonia availability. In terms of relative ammonia fixation potential, GS is preferred over GDH. This is because the apparent K_m for NH_4^+ of GS is about 0.4 mM, approximately 30 to 50 times lower than the apparent K_m for NH_4^+ of GDH (17,51). The reverse reaction, the deamidation of glutamine, is brought about by another enzyme, glutaminase (Gnase). This enzyme is activated by polyanionic species, such as phosphate, and allosterically inhibited by its product, glutamate; decreasing glutamate levels in the tissue initiate glutamine breakdown (9).

This metabolism by which the tricarboxylic acid cycle, ammonia fixation, and amino acid metabolism are linked is further complicated by cellular compartmentation. In all mammalian cell types studied, Gnase and GDH appear to be primarily mitochondrial enzymes; GS is cytoplasmic, but there are both mitochondrial and cytoplasmic isozymes of transaminases, such as aspartate transaminase (for discussion, see ref. 34). Thus another level of regulation is added, namely, the distribution and transport of metabolites among various cellular compartments. This means that possible regulation by substrate and product levels, as well as by allosteric activators and inhibitors, should be evaluated in terms of the presence and concentrations of these moieties in specific cellular spaces and not by whole tissue measurements alone. Needless to say, this information is often difficult or impossible to obtain.

The metabolism of glutamate in the CNS has additional complexities. Glutamate metabolism in brain has been extensively studied for the past 30 years. These investigations have been amply compiled and reviewed (2,5,7,21). The CNS is made up of heterogenous cell types—various types of neurons as well as glial cells—and this heterogeneity is also observed in the enzymes associated with glutamate metabolism (53). Central to this "compartmentation" is the astrocytic localization of GS in animal (27,36) and human (41) CNS. This localization had previously been inferred from experiments *in vivo* and *in vitro* using various labeled metabolites (53).

Computer simulation studies of the disparate distribution of amino acid-metabolizing systems led Van den Berg and Garfinkel (52) to suggest a stoichiometry of the flow of glutamine and γ-aminobutyric acid (GABA) between nerve endings and glia. In this model, GABA is released from nerve endings. After its physiologic action, some is actively taken up by the surrounding astrocytes and converted to glutamine via GS. This glutamine mixes with the extracellular glutamine and can then replenish the amino acid pools in the nerve endings via the action of Gnase.

By extrapolation, a similar "balance sheet" has been suggested for glutamate released from nerve endings as neurotransmitter (4,8,9). Direct evidence is accumulating that these neuronal-glial interactions do exist (33,35). The role of GDH in this process is not known. There has been some suggestion that GDH is a glial enzyme (6); other studies indicate it may be more active in neurons (34,45). It is probable that GDH is ubiquitously distributed among cell types, but some may have more or less enzyme. Regulation of its activity may be more important than its absolute level.

Function of Glutamate

Glutamate has many functions in cellular metabolism, and its role in nitrogen metabolism in CNS probably parallels that in other tissues. In the CNS, however, this amino acid may play a special role, that of a neurotransmitter. Several neuronal pathways in the mammalian CNS have been suggested to use glutamate (see ref. 29). This role is still somewhat in dispute, but there is no doubt that L-glutamate is a potent neuroexcitant. Since the initial demonstrations of the convulsive effects on cortex of topically applied glutamate (25) and the first experiments from Curtis' laboratory (14) on excitation of spinal neurons, numerous laboratories have demonstrated this property of glutamate and related dicarboxylic amino acids. From this work, a pharmacology of the "glutamate receptor" has been emerging (54). This has led to the recent demonstration of the possible anticonvulsive efficacy of excitatory amino acid antagonists (13). Obviously, such work may point the way to a new therapy for the treatment of epilepsy.

A corollary of the potent depolarizing action of dicarboxylic amino acids, such as glutamate, is the concomitant neurotoxicity of these substances. Glutamate, and certain structural analogs, can cause neuronal damage when administered either peripherally or directly into CNS tissue (37). In fact, the neurotoxic potency parallels the neuroexcitatory potential of these analogs, hence, the appellation "excitotoxins" (37). Because of the capacity of CNS tissue to inactivate exogenous glutamate by active uptake processes, large amounts of this amino acid are required to cause damage. In addition, the blood-brain barrier is impermeable to glutamate. Therefore, under normal circumstances, one would not expect extracellular glutamate to be neurotoxic. Under conditions where the blood-brain barrier is compromised, however, or prior to its development, peripheral glutamate can be neuropathic. For example, in neonatal animals given glutamate systemically. there is rapid degeneration of the inner layers of the retina as well as neuronal degeneration in the developing brain itself (see ref. 37). Less understood are possible problems that might occur if either the active uptake of glutamate by glial cells (see ref. 26) is somehow decreased or the ability of the tissue to neutralize the glutamate by metabolism is altered. It is known that convulsions can be caused by the potent glutamine synthetase inhibitor methionine sulfoximine (24). These are certainly areas for futuie active investigation. Again, exactly how GDH is involved in glutamate breakdown in CNS is unclear (for recent review, see ref. 12). Plaitakis et al. (43) showed that GDH-deficient patients have higher glutamate levels in plasma after a glutamate or protein bolus than do control patients. This probably reflects peripheral metabolism (liver or kidney), and its meaning for CNS events is unclear.

STUDIES ON PROPERTIES AND METABOLIC ROLE OF GDH

The structural and kinetic properties of mammalian GDH, especially of commercially available preparations from ox and rat liver, have been studied extensively (for review, see ref. 19). There are fewer published studies on the isolated protein from mammalian brain (11,28). The amino acid sequence of the protein appears to be highly conserved between species (48), and there is immunologic cross reaction between liver and brain enzymes (11). As are many other highly regulated enzymes, GDH is an oligomer; it has a single subunit of 56,000 daltons which is enzymatically inactive. The native state appears to be a hexamer of 330,000 to 360,000 daltons. In contrast to higher plants (50), there is no unequivocal evidence for isozymes of GDH from mammalian sources (32), but this possibility has not been ruled out.

The most intriguing aspect of this enzyme is the allosteric regulation of its activity by a number of physiologically relevant substances, including nucleotides (22), metal ions (38), steroids (49), branched chain amino acids, such as leucine (30), and prostaglandins (47).

The substrate NAD(P)H at high concentrations can bind to a site different from the active site, causing conformational changes which result in an inhibition of GDH activity (3). The activation of enzyme activity by ADP and its inhibition by GTP also appears to interact at this site. Sequencing of the isolated protein indicates that an evolution of this regulatory function for a second nucleotide binding site has occurred, possibly by partial gene duplication (20). Most vertebrate GDHs studied have molecular weights of about 330,000 daltons, which have a duplicated sequence of 155 residues. The corresponding enzymes from yeast, *Escherichia coli* and *Neurospora*, are not regulated by nucleotides, and their molecular weights are smaller, in the range of 250,000 daltons, and may lack the duplicated sequence (see ref. 20 for discussion). The mechanisms of the potent inhibition of GDH by steroids, such as estradiols, diethylstilbestrol, and clomiphene (44), have been less well characterized but may be of great potential significance physiologically. The recent finding of a mixed activation and deactivation of GDH by prostaglandins (47) is similarly intriguing for regulation of GDH *in situ*. In this regard, it is of interest that falsely low levels of GDH activity have been found in leukocytes from non-OPCA subjects who have been on long-term therapy with antiinflammatory agents, such as aspirin or indomethacin (R. C. Duvoisin and W. J. Nicklas, *unpublished observations*; A. Plaitakis, *personal communication*).

The activation by leucine of GDH from rat liver (30), diaphragm (40), and pancreatic islets (46) is also of possible physiologic significance. Nonmetabolizable leucine analogs, such as bis-2-aminobicyclo[2,2,1]heptane-2-carboxylic acid (BCH), also activate GDH activity (46). The latter have suggested that there is a coupling between activation of islet GDH activity by leucine and stimulation of insulin secretion. Figure 2 shows that these substances can also stimulate GDH activity in a preparation from rat brain. It should be noted that the BCH used in these experiments was a racemic mixture, and it is probable that only one of the isomers is responsible for the activity increase. For example, D-leucine does not stimulate GDH activity (46). Addition of 25μM ADP to the mixture in itself only partially activated the GDH, but it allowed the maximal activation by leucine to be attained with much lower amino acid concentrations.

Leucine added to isolated brain mitochondria can stimulate GDH activity in the direction of both glutamate synthesis (17) and glutamate oxidation (J. B. Clark, *personal communication*). The contribution to brain glutamate metabolism of its oxidative deamination by GDH is especially controversial (see ref. 15 for discussion). Thus under normal circumstances, brain, like other tissues, metabolizes

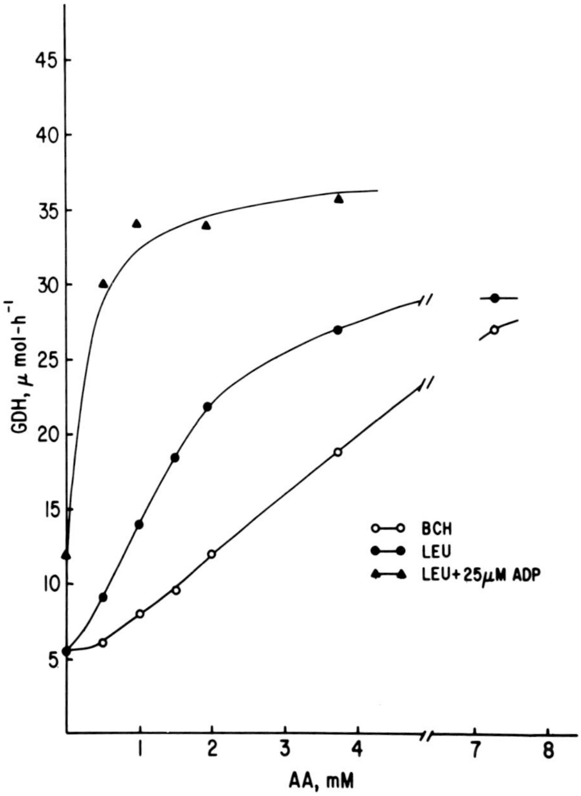

FIG. 2. Effect of adenosine diphosphate (ADP), leucine (LEU), and bis-2-aminobicyclo[2,2,1]heptane-2-carboxylic acid (BCH) on the GDH activity of a rat brain homogenate. The GDH activity was measured following the disappearance of NADH at 340 nm, as previously described (18).

glutamate primarily via aspartate aminotransferase (1,16). Under special circumstances, however, brain tissue does seem capable of forming a fair amount of ammonia from glutamate via GDH (4). The general properties of glutamate metabolism do not differ qualitatively in bulk-prepared "synaptic" and "nonsynaptic" mitochondria (16). It is possible however, that there is a small subset of mitochondria in which GDH has relatively more metabolic importance. This remains to be examined.

Each of the above substances that can potentially regulate GDH is either found normally in brain and other tissues or is of relevance to the clinical state. Studies with enzyme preparations point the way to determining the mechanisms by which GDH is regulated in the cell. It is only by studying more intact metabolic models of each tissue, however, that real understanding will come.

ACKNOWLEDGMENT

This work was supported in part by USPHS grant NS 17360.

REFERENCES

1. Balazs, R. (1965): Control of glutamate metabolism. The effect of pyruvate. *J. Neurochem.*, 12:63–76.
2. Balazs, R., and Cremer, J. E. (1973): *Metabolic Compartmentation in the Brain*. MacMillan, London.
3. Bayley, P. M., and Radda, G. M. (1966): Conformational changes and the regulation of glutamate dehydrogenase activity. *Biochem. J.*, 98:105–111.
4. Benjamin, A. M., and Quastel, J. H. (1974): Fate of L-glutamate in the brain. *J. Neurochem.*, 23:457–464.
5. Berl, S., Clarke, D. D., and Schneider, D. (1975): *Metabolic Compartmentation and Neurotransmission: Relation to Brain Structure and Function*. Plenum, New York.
6. Berl, S., Nicklas, W. J., and Clarke, D. D. (1978): Glial cells and metabolic compartmentation. In: *Dynamic Properties of Glial Cells*, edited by E. Schoffeniels, G. Franck, L. Hertz, and D. B. Tower, pp. 143–149. Pergamon Press, Oxford.
7. Bradford, H. (1982): *Neurotransmitter Interaction and Compartmentation*. Plenum, New York.
8. Bradford, H. F., and Ward, H. K. (1976): On glutaminase activity in mammalian synaptosomes. *Brain Res.*, 110:115–125.
9. Bradford, H. F., Ward, H. K., and Thomas, A. J. (1978): Glutamine as a substrate for nerve endings. *J. Neurochem.*, 30:1453–1459.
10. Bremer, H., Duran, M., Kamerling, J. P., Przyrembel, H., and Wadman, S. (1981): *Disturbances of Amino Acid Metabolism: Clinical Chemistry and Diagnosis*. Urban and Schwarzenberg, Baltimore.
11. Chee, P. Y., Dahl, J. L., and Fahien, L. A. (1979): The purification and properties of rat brain glutamate dehydrogenase. *J. Neurochem.*, 33:53–60.
12. Clark, J. B., and Nicklas, W. J. (1984): Brain mitochondria. In: *Handbook of Neurochemistry, Vol. 7*, second edition, edited by A. Lajtha. Plenum, New York.
13. Croucher, M. J., Collins, J. F., and Meldrum, B. S. (1982): Anticonvulsant action of excitatory amino acid antagonists. *Science*, 216:899–901.
14. Curtis, D. R., Phillis, J. W., and Watkins, J. C. (1959): Chemical excitation of spinal neurones. *Nature*, 183:611–612.
15. Dennis, S., and Clark, J. B. (1977): The pathway of glutamate metabolism in rat brain mitochondria. *Biochem. J.*, 168:521–527.
16. Dennis, S., Lai, J. C. K., and Clark, J. B. (1977): Comparative studies on glutamate metabolism in synaptic and non-synaptic rat brain mitochondria. *Biochem. J.*, 164:727–736.
17. Dennis, S., and Clark, J. B. (1978): The synthesis of glutamate by rat brain mitochondria. *J. Neurochem.*, 31:673–680.

18. Duvoisin, R., Chokroverty, S., Lepore, F., and Nicklas, W. (1983): Glutamate dehydrogenase deficiency in patients with olivopontocerebellar atrophy. *Neurology*, 33(10):1322–1326.
19. Eisenberg, H., Josephs, R., and Reisler, E. (1976): Glutamate dehydrogenase. *Adv. Protein Chem.*, 30:101–181.
20. Engel, P. C. (1973): Evolution of enzyme regulator sites: Evidence for partial gene duplication from amino acid sequence of bovine glutamate dehydrogenase. *Nature*, 241:118–120.
21. Fonnum, F. (1978): *Amino Acids as Chemical Transmitters*. Plenum, New York.
22. Frieden, C. (1959): Glutamic dehydrogenase. II. The effect of various nucleotides on the association-dissociation and kinetic properties. *J. Biol. Chem.*, 234:815–820.
23. Gibson, G., and Blass, J. P. (1976): A relationship between NAD/NADH potentials and glucose utilization in rat brain slices. *J. Biol. Chem.*, 251:4127–4130.
24. Gutierrez, J. A., and Norenberg, M. D. (1977): Ultrastructural study of methionine sulfoximine-induced Alzheimer Type II astrocytosis. *Am. J. Pathol.*, 86:285–294.
25. Hayashi, T., (1954): Effects of sodium glutamate on the nervous system. *Keio J. Med.*, 3:183–192.
26. Hertz, L. (1979): Functional interaction between neurons and astrocytes. I. Turnover and metabolism of putative amino acid transmitters. *Prog. Neurobiol.*, 13:277–323.
27. Martinez-Hernandez, A., Bell, K. P., and Norenberg, M. D. (1977): Glutamine synthetase: Glial localization in brain. *Science*, 195:1356–1358.
28. McCarthy, A. D., Johnson, P., and Tipton, K. F. (1981): Sedimentation properties of native and proteolysed preparations of ox glutamate dehydrogenase. *Biochem. J.*, 199:235–238.
29. McGeer, P. L., and McGeer, E. G. (1981): Amino acid neurotransmitters. In: *Basic Neurochemistry*, third edition, edited by G. Siegel, R. W. Albers, B. W. Agronoff, and R. Katzman, pp. 233–253. Little, Brown, Boston.
30. McGiven, J. D., Bradford, N. M., Crompton, M., and Chappell, J. B. (1973): Effect of L-leucine on the nitrogen metabolism of isolated rat liver mitochondria. *Biochem. J.*, 134:209–215.
31. Miller, A., Hawkins, R. A., and Veech, R. L. (1973): The mitochondrial redox state of rat brain. *J. Neurochem.*, 20:1393–1400.
32. Nelson, R. L., Povey, M. S., Hopkinson, D. A., and Harris, H. (1977): Electrophoresis of human L-glutamate dehydrogenase: Tissue distribution and preliminary population survey. *Biochem. Gen.*, 15:87–91.
33. Nicklas, W. J. (1982): Is glutamine formed in glial cells a precursor for neuronal glutamate and GABA? *Trans. Am. Soc. Neurochem.*, 13:221.
34. Nicklas, W. J., Nunez, R., Berl, S., and Duvoisin, R. (1979): Neuronal-glial contributions to transmitter amino acid metabolism: Studies with kainic-acid-induced lesions of rat striatum. *J. Neurochem.*, 33:839–844.
35. Nicklas, W. J., and Krespan, B. (1982): Studies on neuronal-glial metabolism of glutamate in cerebellar slices. In: *Neurotransmitter Interaction and Compartmentation*, edited by H. Bradford, pp. 383–394. Plenum, New York.
36. Norenberg, M. D., and Martinez-Hernandez, A. (1979): Fine structural localization of glutamine synthetase in astrocytes in brain. *Brain Res.*, 161:303–310.
37. Olney, J. W. (1978): Neurotoxicity of excitatory amino acids. In: *Kainic Acid as a Tool in Neurobiology*, edited by E. G. McGeer, J. W. Olney, and P. L. McGeer, pp. 95–121. Raven Press, New York.
38. Olson, J. A., and Anfinson, C. B. (1952): The crystallization and characterization of L-glutamic acid dehydrogenase. *J. Biol. Chem.*, 197:67–79.
40. Palaiologos, G., and Felig, P. (1978): Influence of L-leucine on glutamate dehydrogenase activity in isolated rat diaphragm. *Yale J. Biol. Med.*, 51:19–26.
41. Pilkington, G. J., and Lantos, P. L. (1982): The role of glutamine synthetase in diagnosis of cerebral tumors. *Neuropathol. Appl. Neurobiol.*, 8:227–236.
42. Plaitakis, A., Nicklas, W. J., and Desnick, R. J. (1980): Glutamate dehydrogenase deficiency in three patients with spinocerebellar syndrome. *Ann. Neurol.*, 7:297–303.
43. Plaitakis, A., Berl, S., and Yahr, M. (1982): Abnormal glutamate metabolism in adult-onset degenerative disorder. *Science*, 216:193–196.
44. Puranen, J., and Arstila, A. (1967): Inhibition of glutamic dehydrogenase by clomiphene. *Nature*, 213:78–80.
45. Quastel, J. H. (1978): Cerebral glutamate-glutamine interrelations *in vivo* and *in vitro*. In: *Dynamic*

Properties of Glial Cells, edited by E. Schofeniels, G. Franck, L. Hertz, and D. B. Tower, pp. 153–162. Pergamon Press, Oxford.
46. Sener, A., and Malaisse, W. J. (1980): L-leucine and a non-metabolized analogue activate pancreatic islet glutamate dehydrogenase. *Nature*, 288:187–189.
47. Shafer, P. T., and Fiskin, A. M. (1982): Prostaglandin and acyl chain effects on glutamate dehydrogenase activity. *Lipids*, 17:297–306.
48. Smith, E. L., Austen, B. M., Blumenthal, K. M. and Nya, J. F. (1975): Glutamate Dehydrogenase. *Enzymes*, 11:293–367.
49. Tomkins, G. M., Yielding, K. L., Talal, M., and Curran, J. E. (1963): Protein structure and biological regulation. *Cold Spring Harbor Symp. Quant. Biol.*, 28:461–471.
50. Thurman, D. A., Palin, C., and Laycock, M. V. (1965): Isoenzymatic nature of L-glutamic dehydrogenase of higher plants. *Nature*, 207:193–195.
51. Van den Berg, C. J. (1970): Glutamate and glutamine. In: *Handbook of Neurochemistry, Vol. 3*, edited by A. Lajtha, pp. 355–379. Plenum, New York.
52. Van den Berg, C. J., and Garfinkel, D. (1971): A simulation study of brain compartments: Metabolism of glutamate and related substances in mouse brain. *Biochem. J.*, 123:211–218.
53. Van den Berg, C. J., Reijinierse, A., Blockhuis, G., Ronda, G., Clarke, D. D., and Garfinkel, D. (1975): A model of glutamate metabolism in brain. In: *Metabolic Compartmentation and Neurotransmission*, edited by S. Berl, D. D. Clarke, and D. Schneider, pp. 515–543. Plenum, New York.
54. Watkins, J. C. (1981): Pharmacology of excitatory amino acid receptors. In: *Glutamate: Transmitter in the Central Nervous System*, edited by P. J. Roberts, J. Storm-Mathisen, and G. A. R. Johnston, pp. 1–24. Wiley, Chichester, England.
55. Yamaguchi, T., Hayashi, K., Murakami, H., Ota, K., and Maruyama, S. (1982): Glutamate dehydrogenase deficiency in spinocerebellar degeneration. *Neurochem. Res.*, 7:627–636.

The Olivopontocerebellar Atrophies, edited by R.C. Duvoisin and A. Plaitakis. Raven Press, New York © 1984.

Glutamate and Pyruvate Dehydrogenase Deficiency in Spinocerebellar Degeneration

*Shoichi Maruyama and **Tomoko Yamaguchi

**Department of Neurology, Neurological Institute, and **Department of Biochemistry, Tokyo Women's Medical College, Tokyo, Japan*

For several years, we have investigated cases of spinocerebellar degeneration (SCD) by neuroradiologic, neurophysiologic, endocrinologic, and biochemical methods. In these studies, cases of olivopontocerebellar atrophy (OPCA), one type of SCD, showed several characteristic features in comparison with the other types of SCD. The OPCA group (including the hereditary Menzel type) showed a significant decrease in the width of the pons and cerebellar peduncles and an increase of the width of the fourth ventricle on computerized tomography (CT) examination (14). Abnormal late components of somatosensory evoked potentials (SEP) (16), remarkable fluctuations of the baseline on plethysmography records, as in dysautonomia (15), frequently abnormal pupils with Horner's sign, poor ocular responses to vestibular caloric stimulation (17), decreased and delayed responses to thyroid-stimulating hormone (TSH) and a lower basal level and hyperresponse of prolactin in the thyrotropin releasing hormone (TRH) loading test (18) were observed. From these results, we tentatively concluded that the OPCA type of SCD, including the Menzel type, showed abnormalities referable to disorders in the brainstem (especially the pons) and the hypothalamus, as well as in the cerebellum itself. These are compatible with the neurologic features of OPCA, which include extrapyramidal and autonomic nervous system signs and with histopathologic observations in which the main locus of degenerative lesions is seen in the brainstem as well as the cerebellum (19).

Many biochemical investigations of the cerebellum have appeared recently in the literature. To elucidate biochemical changes in these ataxic disorders, several studies have been made to detect enzyme deficiencies or changes in coenzyme affinity to enzymes, such as lipoamides (28), pyridine nucleotides, or their allosteric effector (24); no decisive abnormalities have yet been demonstrated.

Kark and Rodriguez-Budelli (11) reported SCD patients deficient in lipoamide dehydrogenase complexes, such as pyruvate dehydrogenase (PDH) and α-ketoglutarate dehydrogenase, and also in Friedreich's ataxia in cultured skin fibroblasts (3). Later, deficiencies in platelet-enriched fractions were reported by Blass et al. (4). Stumpf and Parks (28) claimed that no abnormalities in the kinetics of lipoamide dehydrogenases in Friedreich's ataxia and in OPCA have been demonstrated. Plaitakis et al. (24) described glutamate dehydrogenase (GDH) deficiency in cultured skin fibroblasts and in white blood cell (WBC) specimens in three OPCA patients, including siblings.

In order to confirm the indications that enzyme deficiency might play a role in the pathogenesis of SCD, GDH in different types of SCD was measured in WBC and platelet-enriched fractions prepared from 5 ml venous blood of patients. Activity of PDH in the platelet-enriched fraction was also assayed for comparison with results obtained by previous authors (11).

Data obtained from this study are somewhat different from those reported in previous years (32). Two cases of OPCA showed no progression or definite extrapyramidal signs after several years of clinical observation; the diagnosis of SCD should be changed to late cortical cerebellar atrophy (LCCA). On the other hand, rigidity was remarkable in one female with Holmes type SCD; her diagnosis was changed from the Holmes type to the Menzel type.

MATERIALS

We studied the enzymatic activity of GDH and PDH in 23 SCD cases. These included 3 cases of OPCA, 10 cases of Menzel-type SCD, 6 cases of Holmes-type, and 4 cases of LCCA.

Among the degenerative diseases of the nervous system, SCD is particularly difficult to classify (15–19) because (a) ataxic SCD cases show similar cerebellar syndromes; and (b) even at autopsy, many cases show traditional histopathologic findings in the localization of their lesions.

The clinical diagnostic criteria used in this study for identifying each type of SCD are shown in Table 1 (7,13,21,29). The Holmes type is hereditary with onset at 30 years of age or later. Pyramidal signs, extrapyramidal signs, autonomic nerve dysfunction, or disturbances of deep sensation are all absent.

Marie-Foix-Alajouanine type of LCCA is nonhereditary, with onset at 45 to 70 years of age. Pyramidal signs may be present, but there are no extrapyramidal signs or autonomic nerve disturbances, and deep sensation is normal. The Menzel type of OPCA is hereditary, with onset at 20 to 30 years. Pyramidal and extrapyramidal signs are present, deep sensation is disturbed, and there may be autonomic dysfunction. Sporadic OPCA (Dejerine-Thomas type) is nonhereditary, with onset at 40 to 50 years of age. There may or may not be pyramidal signs, and extrapyramidal signs and autonomic nerve dysfunction usually are present. Our 33 controls included six cases of amyotropic lateral sclerosis (ALS), eight cases of cerebrovascular disease, five cases of neurologic disorders other than SCD, and 14 healthy subjects.

METHODS

We collected WBC from 5 ml heparinized venous blood to which 1 ml of 6% Dextran T-500 in phosphate-buffered saline was mixed; the sample was held

TABLE 1. *Classification of SCD*

Form	Type	Heredity	Age of onset (year)	Pyramidal signs	Extrapyramidal signs	Autonomic signs	Deep sensation
Cerebellar	Holmes	+	>30	–	–	–	–
	LCCA	–	45–70	– or +	–	–	–
Spinocerebellar	Menzel	+	20–30	+	+	±	+
	OPCA	–	40–50	– or +	+	+	–
Spinal	Friedreich	+	<20	+	–	+	+

vertically in the syringe, needle upward, for 30 min at 40° C; then the WBC in the supernatant were separated according to the method described by Christlieb et al. (5). The blood platelet-enriched fraction was prepared in the same manner, except that the syringe was kept vertical for 45 min and the platelet-enriched fraction was then collected from the supernatant by the method of Blass et al. (4). We then assayed GDH by the method of Schmidt (27), using the reaction direction forming glutamate from α-oxoglutarate, NADH, and ammonia. We assayed PDH according to Blass et al. (1) using [1-^{14}C] pyruvate sodium salt 5 mCi/mmole; (Radio Chemical Centre). The decarboxylation assay was done according to the method described by Ichiyama et al. (10) with phenethylamine as absorbant of the CO_2 evolved by the decarboxylation reaction. Protein was determined by the method of Lowry et al., modified by Daughady et al. (6). The preparations of WBC and platelet homogenates were stored at − 80° C until the enzyme assays were conducted.

RESULTS

Activity of GDH (per milligram protein) in WBC preparations from various types of SCD, other neurologic patients, and normal controls is listed in Table 2. In OPCA, the hereditary type of Menzel, and the hereditary type of LCCA (Holmes), GDH activity was lower in WBC compared with other neurologic patients, except for ALS, in which GDH activity was also somewhat decreased as compared to the control value. Those values were variable as also found by Blass et al. (4), who pointed out that WBC specimens used for detecting certain enzyme deficiencies are not reliable because of variations in number and in composition of granulocytes obtained from venous blood drawn on different occasions from the same subject. On the other hand, since blood platelets are rather stable components in individuals, and more active in energy metabolism than are WBC, rapid diagnosis may be possible by using platelet-enriched preparations rather than cultured skin-fibroblasts in detecting certain enzyme deficiencies (4). Activity of GDH obtained in platelets from patients with each type of SCD, as well as neurologic patients, are shown in Table 3.

Activity of GDH in platelet preparations is nearly twice as high as in WBC preparations on a protein basis, and standard deviations are smaller. Results ob-

TABLE 2. *GDH in WBC*

Group	Case no.	GDH (nmol/min/mg protein)	Group	Case no.	GDH (nmol/min/mg protein)
SCD			Neurologic disease		
OPCA	3	2.06 ± 1.09	ALS	6	2.34 ± 0.72
Menzel	10	2.02 ± 0.59	CVA	8	2.70 ± 0.17
LCCA	4	2.67 ± 0.38	Others[a]	5	2.51 ± 0.18
Holmes	6	2.08 ± 0.58	Control	12	2.69 ± 0.27

[a]Includes Meniere's syndrome, vertigo, Addie syndrome, and multiple neuritis.

TABLE 3. *GDH in blood platelets*

Group	Case no. determined	GDH (nmol/min/ mg protein)	Group	Case no. determined	GDH (nmol/min/ mg protein)
SCD			Neurologic disease		
OPCA	5	3.52 ± 0.35[a]	ALS	5	4.40 ± 0.64
Menzel	4	4.42 ± 0.44	CVA	2	4.40 ± 0.21
LCCA	2	3.15 ± 0.38[a]	Others[b]	3	4.13 ± 0.42
Holmes	7	4.67 ± 0.72	Control	14	4.46 ± 0.61

[a] $p < 0.001$.
[b] Includes myotonic dystrophy and Shy-Drager syndrome.

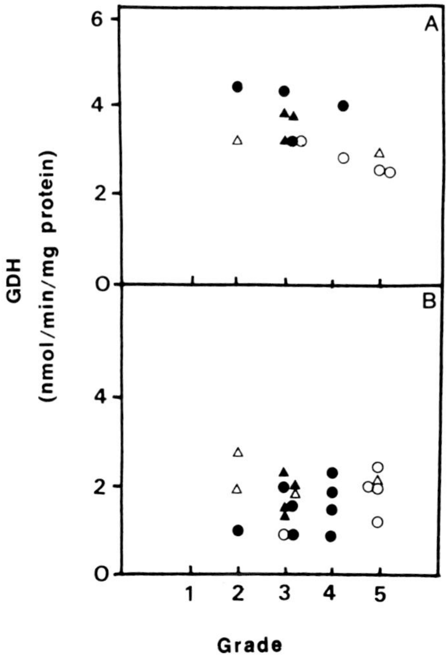

FIG. 1. GDH in SCD in relation to symptom grade in *(A)* platelet and *(B)* WBC preparations: (○) OPCA; (●) Menzel; (△) LCCA; (▲) Holmes. Clinical grades are classified as described in the text.

tained in the OPCA and LCCA groups show significantly low values of GDH activity, with a specific activity about 30% below the normal range (Table 3). Patients with OPCA whose GDH activity in WBC specimen was rather high usually had low activity of GDH on reexamination of blood platelets.

Correlation between clinically determined severity of SCD and the GDH activities in both WBC and platelet preparations are plotted in Fig. 1. The grades were expressed as the disability percentage of each patient as follows: grade 1, normal in daily activity; grade 2, 25% disturbance; grade 3, 50%; grade 4, 75%; and grade 5, 100% (bedridden).

Activities of GDH in WBC are polydisperse, regardless of the severity of clinical symptoms; with platelets, however, the grade of symptoms is somewhat proportional to the lowering of GDH activity, especially in cases of OPCA of the Menzel type. To determine whether GDH activity varies with age, GDH activities in WBC and platelets were plotted (Fig. 2). In WBC of the 30 to 60 year age group, there was a slight correlation with age but no obvious age-dependent change in SCD patients.

To assess whether GDH deficiency is specific, or if other oxidoreductive enzymes are also involved, PDH activity in platelets was assayed. As shown in Table 4, PDH activity in all five OPCA patients and in three of the four Menzel type patients was decreased to half the value of the controls. The PDH assay data are divided into two groups: high (or normal) and low PDH activity. These data are similar to those reported by Kark and Rodriguez-Budelli (11), who demonstrated low PDH activity in six of 14 patients in the platelet-enriched fraction. In our classification of SCD, if the Menzel hereditary type of OPCA is included in the OPCA group, then eight of nine OPCA patients showed low PDH activity. On the other hand, none of the LCCA cases and two of seven patients of the Holmes type showed decreased PDH activity. If the LCCA and Holmes type patients are included in the LCCA group, then only two of nine patients showed low PDH activity. The differences in PDH activity between the groups [OPCA (including Menzel) and LCCA (including Holmes)] are shown in Fig. 3.

It may be concluded from these data that PDH activity in the OPCA group is statistically lower than that in the LCCA group (Table 5; $p<0.001$). All patients

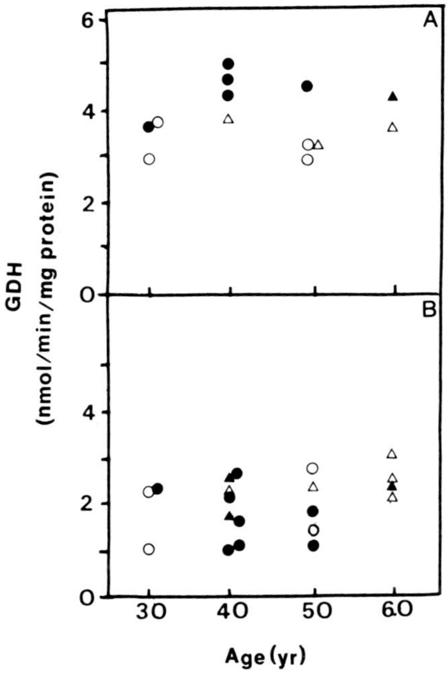

FIG. 2. GDH in SCD in relation to age group in *(A)* platelet and *(B)* WBC preparations: ○-OPCA; *solid circles*, Menzel; *open triangles*, LCCA; *solid triangles*, Holmes. Clinical grades are classified as described in the text.

TABLE 4. *PDH in blood platelets*

Group	Case no. determined	PDH (pmol/min/mg protein) Normal range	Occurrence ratio	Low range	Occurrence ratio
SCD					
OPCA	5			80.9 ± 17.5	5/5
Menzel	4	143.4	1/4	76.3 ± 16.1	3/4
LCCA	2	179.3 ± 5.9	2/2		
Holmes	7	153.2 ± 31.9	5/7	80.6 ± 12.8	2/7
Neurologic disease					
ALS	4			69.3 ± 15.5	4/6
CVA	2	152.7 ± 6.3	2/2		
Others[a]	3	164.2 ± 23.4	3/3		
Control	14	160.7 ± 25.2	14/14		

[a]Includes myotonic dystrophy and Shy-Drager syndrome.

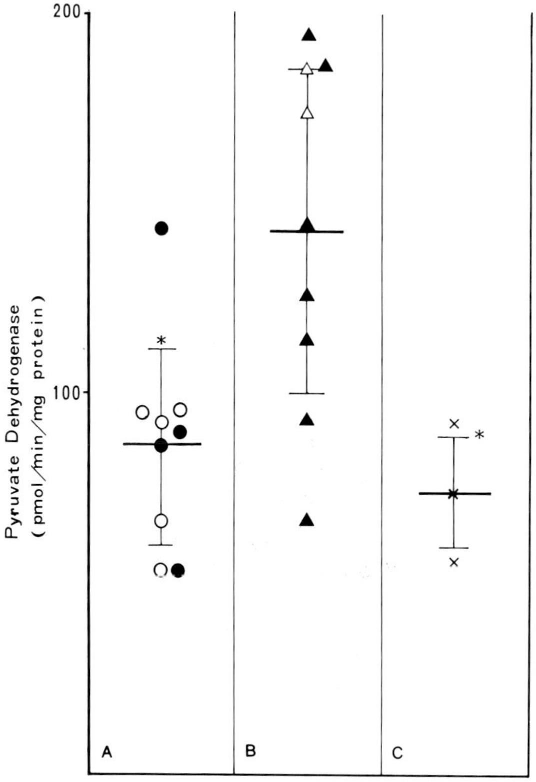

FIG. 3. Differences in PDH activity between OPCA *(A)* and LCCA *(B)* patient groups: (○) OPCA; (●) Menzel; (*) $p<0.001$; (△) LCCA; (▲) Holmes; *(C)* ALS.

TABLE 5. *PDH in blood platelets*

Group	PDH (pmol/min/mg protein)		Total no. of cases
	Normal range	Low range	
OPCA (OPCA and Menzel)	1	8[a]	9
LCCA (LCCA and Holmes)	7[a]	2	9
Total no. of cases:	8	10	18

[a]Statistically significant ($p < 0.001$).

with other neurologic diseases, except ALS, had normal PDH activity in the platelet-enriched fraction.

DISCUSSION

For the purpose of finding a possible relationship between GDH and SCD, leukocytes from patients with various neurologic diseases (Table 2) were assayed for GDH. Although a tendency toward a decreased activity of GDH in SCD other than LCCA was indicated, the differences were not statistically significant. In our study, variable data were obtained from the same patient in different preparations. This variability might be caused by different cell populations on each sampling occasion or by the rather low energy metabolism of leukocytes. On one occasion, for instance, when the patient had a remarkable leukocytosis, the activity of the enzyme was different. These facts suggest that leukocytes are improper materials for estimating enzyme activity, as stated by Blass et al. (4).

In subsequent studies, therefore, we used platelets instead of leukocytes for assay of the enzyme. Blood platelets are rather stable elements and have a higher energy metabolism than WBC. The data obtained were closer and less variable in different preparations from the same patients compared with the leukocyte data (Table 3). The specific activity of GDH was twice as high as that in leukocytes.

Activity of PDH was also measured with GDH in platelets and shown to be lower in those specimens with lower GDH activity (Table 4). Stumpf and Parks (28) have found normal enzyme kinetics for lipoamide dehydrogenase in Friedreich's ataxia patients whose PDH and α-ketoglutarate dehydrogenase levels were lowered. Kark and Rodriguez-Budelli (11) also reported low levels in some cases of OPCA. The varying results from different investigators may be due to differences in clinical diagnostic criteria, type classification, nature of the specimens from the patient, severity of symptoms, or duration of the disease. Although enzymic deficiencies can be detected in cultured skin fibroblasts, leukocytes, or blood platelets, nothing is decisive unless missing enzymes are demonstrated. For this purpose, the platelet preparation is easier than that of skin fibroblasts and more reliable than leukocyte preparations.

In our study, GDH was demonstrated to be significantly lower in platelets from OPCA and LCCA than in control subjects or the Menzel and Holmes types of SCD and was shown to be correlated with the grade of clinical manifestations. Plaitakis et al. (24) reported GDH in leukocytes and fibroblasts to be low in patients with a hereditary type of OPCA. We found reduced GDH activities in nonhereditary types of SCD, OPCA, and LCCA. These differences may reflect differences in clinical diagnostic criteria and in the materials examined. Plaitakis et al. (24) also pointed out that GDH deficiency may occur in some forms of SCD, but whether or how this enzyme defect relates to the pathogenesis of the clinical syndrome is not clear. Little is known about the role of GDH and the consequence of its inhibition in nervous tissue function.

From our data, it may be postulated that reduced GDH activities are related not only to genetic factors but also to the clinical type of SCD or the severity of the clinical manifestations.

The second part of this study is concerned with PDH activity in SCD. In platelets, PDH is significantly lower in the OPCA group (OPCA and Menzel type) than in the LCCA group (LCCA and Holmes type). Reduced PDH activity is also related to heredity and to some types of SCD with extrapyramidal features or dysfunction of the autonomic nervous system. Reynolds and Blass (25) postulate a possible mechanism for selective cerebellar damage in partial pyruvate dehydrogenase deficiency. In their opinion, because the brain is biochemically and anatomically heterogenous, it is reasonable to expect that reduced activity of an enzyme could affect the metabolic pathway in certain parts of the brain before other parts. Their data show that the cerebellum has low PDH activity and is high in oxygen consumption. These characteristics are especially remarkable in the anterior cerebellar vermis. If these measurements reflect relative activities *in vivo*, then the flux of pyruvate to acetyl coenzyme A might be impaired in the anterior cerebellar vermis by deficiencies of PDH too mild to affect flux in other areas.

In animal experiment, McCandless and Schenker (20) and Dreyfus and Hauser (8) found that homogenates of whole rat cerebellum oxidized pyruvate more slowly than did homogenates of other regions of the brain. The authors also reported that the oxidation of pyruvate was more sensitive to thiamine deficiency in homogenates of rat cerebellum than in other regions. The anterior cerebellum is frequently damaged in the brain of thiamine-deficient human alcoholics (31). Patients with mild deficiency of PDH show cerebellar ataxia in the lower limbs as the earliest clinical sign. This is compatible with dysfunction in the anterior vermis (2,31).

In our study, we observed low activity of PDH not only in hereditary OPCA but also in nonhereditary cases. The initial symptom in nearly all these cases was gait disturbance or ataxia in the lower extremities. The speculation of Reynolds and Blass (25) and Dreyfus and Hauser (8) may also apply to our cases.

From the results of the present study, it may be concluded that in some cases, the decreased enzyme activities of oxidoreductive processes may cause cerebellar dysfunction, resulting in clinical manifestations of some types of ataxia, including OPCA and LCCA. In our study, PDH activity in platelets was lower in ALS patients than in controls. Although this finding could not be understood exactly, it may offer a possibility of correlating the localization of a degenerative lesion, of which the main focus would be in the pyramidal system, and the clinical course or a general reduction of energy metabolism. The enzyme PDH is more indicative of cellular energy metabolism controlling the tricarboxylic acid cycle, and more universal changes were observed in some types of SCD and in ALS. Some changes may be quite specific, however, such as low GDH activity for OPCA and LCCA.

As reported by Plaitakis et al. (24), reduced GDH activity was observed in hereditary OPCA in our study. However, platelet GDH activity was low in both OPCA and LCCA, a nonhereditary type of SCD, while PDH was low in both sporadic and hereditary OPCA (Menzel), in which the main pathologic lesions are thought to be in the brainstem. From these results, it may be postulated that abnormal GDH activity may have particular effects on some area of the central nervous system, just as PDH abnormality may correspond to specific damage in some site of the brain that is sensitive to PDH enzyme disturbance. In our study, GDH activity in ALS, a pyramidal system degeneration was normal. The GDH abnormality may have some relationship to degeneration of systems other than the pyramidal tract.

A low glutamate content in the cerebellum was observed in ataxic mutant mice (9,12,22,26). Low GDH activity in OPCA and LCCA may indicate reduced activity in glutaminergic neurons in this type of disorder. Although we do not yet know the significance of these enzymes in cerebellar function, the biochemical basis of enzymatic deficiencies in cerebellar ataxia will be clarified in the near future, and a biochemical approach may be one of the most promising ways to reveal the etiology of SCD.

REFERENCES

1. Blass, J. P., Avignan, J., and Uhlendorf, B. W. (1970): A defect in pyruvate decarboxylase in a child with an intermittent movement disorder. *J. Clin. Invest.*, 49:423–432.
2. Blass, J. P., Kark, R. A. P., and Engel, W. K. (1971): Clinical studies of a patient with pyruvate-decarboxylase deficiency. *Arch. Neurol.*, 25:449–460.
3. Blass, J. P., Kark, R. A. P., and Menon, N. K. (1976): Low activities of the pyruvate and oxoglutarate dehydrogenase complexes in five patients with Friedreich's ataxia. *N. Engl. J. Med.*, 205:62–67.
4. Blass, J. P., Cederbaum, S. D., and Kark, R. A. P. (1977): Rapid diagnosis of pyruvate and ketoglutarate dehydrogenases deficiencies in platelet enriched preparations from blood. *Clin. Clim. Acta*, 75:21–30.
5. Christlieb, A. R., Sbarra, A. J., and Bardawil, W. A. (1962): Isolation of highly purified, viable leukocytes from blood. *Am. J. Clin. Pathol.*, 37:257–262.
6. Daughady, W. H., Lowry, O. H., Rosenbrough, N. J., and Fields, W. S. (1952): Determination of cerebrospinal fluid protein with the Folin phenol reagent. *J. Lab. Clin. Med.*, 39:663–665.
7. Dejerine, J., and Thomas, A. (1900): Latrophie olivo-ponto-cerebelleuse. *Nouv. Iconogr. Salpet.*, 13:330–370.
8. Dreyfus, P. M., and Hauser, G. (1965): The effect of thiamine deficiency on the pyruvate decarboxylase system of the central nervous system. *Biochim. Biophys. Acta*, 104:78–84.
9. Holmes, G. (1907): A form of familial degeneration of cerebellum. *Brain*, 30:446.
10. Ichiyama, A., Nakamura, S., Nishizuka, Y., and Hayaishi, O. (1970): Enzymic studies on the biosynthesis of serotonin in mammalian brain. *J. Biol. Chem.*, 245:1699–1709.
11. Kark, R. A. P., and Rodriguez-Budelli, M. (1979): Pyruvate dehydrogenase deficiency in spinocerebellar degenerations. *Neurology*, 29:121–131.
12. Macbride, W. J., Aprison, M. H., and Kusano, K. (1976): Contents of several amino acids in the cerebellum, brain stem and cerebrum of "staggerer," "weaver" and "nervous" neurologically mutant mice. *J. Neurochem.*, 26:867–870.

13. Marie, P., Foix, C. H., and Alajouanine, T. H. (1922): De latrophie cerebelleuse tardive a predominance corticale. *Rev. Neurol.*, 29:849–1082.
14. Maruyama, S., Okayama, K., Aikawa, T., Kobayashi, N., and Saito, Y. (1977): Analysis of spinocerebellar degenerations by CT-scan. In: *1976 Annual Report of the Ministry of Health and Welfare, Spinocerebellar Degenerations Research Committee, Japan*, pp. 119–129.
15. Maruyama, S., Takemiya, T., Yamaguchi, S., and Sakaguchi, J., (1977): Plethysmography in OPCA and LCCA. In: *1976 Annual Report of the Ministry of Health and Welfare, Spinocerebellar Degenerations Research Committee, Japan*, pp. 138–143.
16. Maruyama, S., and Okayama, K. (1978): Somatosensory evoked potentials of spinocerebellar degenerations. In: *1977 Annual Report of the Ministry of Health and Welfare, Spinocerebellar Degenerations Research Committee, Japan*. pp. 151–154.
17. Maruyama, S., Aikawa, T., Uemura, T., and Shimazaki, C. (1980): Abnormal eye movement in patient with spinocerebellar degeneration. In: *1979 Annual Report of the Ministry of Health and Welfare, Spinocerebellar Degenerations Research Committee*, Japan, pp. 182–187.
18. Maruyama, S., and Okayama, K. (1980): The responses of thyrotropin releasing hormone (TPH) test in patients with spinocerebellar degeneration (SCD). In: *1979 Annual Report of Ministry of Health and Welfare,* The Research Committee of Therapeutic Agents for SCD, the Ministry of 1979, pp. 229–232.
19. Maruyama, S., Takemiya, T., Miura, A., Okayama, K., and Aikawa, T. (1980): Clinical study of spinocerebellar degeneration—Type diagnosis by clinical examination methods. *Jpn. Med.*, 19(4)375.
20. McCandless, D. W., and Schenker, S. (1968): Encephalopathy of thiamine deficiency: Studies of intracerebral mechanisms. *J. Clin. Invest.*, 47:2268–2280.
21. Menzel, P. (1891): Beitrag zur Kenntnia der hereditaren Ataxie und Kleinhirnatrophie. *Arch. Psychiatr.*, 22:160.
22. Mikoshiba, K., Teichberg, I.V., and Changeux, J. P. (1977): Biochemical studies on the cerebellum of neurological mutant of mice: Role of glutamic acid and cholinergic system. *Proc. Intern. Soc. Neurochem.*, 6:286.
23. Mikoshiba, K., Takamatsu, K., Akagawa, K., Kohsaka, S., and Tsukada, Y. (1981): Immunohistochemical and neurochemical studies on the cerebellar hypoplasia in the Gunn rat with hereditary hyperbilirubinemia. *1980 Annual Report of the Ministry of Health and Welfare, Spinocerebellar Degenerations Research Committee, Japan*, pp. 181–188.
24. Plaitakis, A., Nicklas, J., and Desnick, R. J. (1980): Glutamate dehydrogenase deficiency in three patients with spinocerebellar syndromes. *Ann. Neurol.*, 7:297–303.
25. Reynolds, S. F., and Blass, J. P. (1976): A possible mechanism for selective cerebellar damage in partial pyruvate dehydrogenase deficiency. *Neurology*, 26:625–628.
26. Roffler-Tarlov, S., and Sidman, R. L. (1978): Concentration of glutamic acid in cerebellar cortex and deep nuclei of normal mice and weaver, staggerer, and nervous mutants. *Brain Res.*, 142:269–283.
27. Schmidt, E. (1974): Glutamate dehydrogenase. In: *Methods in Enzymatic Analysis, Vol. 2*. edited by H. U. Bergmeyer, pp. 650–656. Academic Press, New York.
28. Stumpf, D. A., and Parks, J. K. (1979): Friedreich ataxia. II. Normal kinetics of lipoamide dehydrogenases. *Neurology*, 29:820–826.
29. Victor, M. (1978): Spinocerebellar degeneration—Cerebellar and brainstem forms. In: *Spinocerebellar Degenerations*, edited by Jpn. Med. Foundation, pp. 53–66. Univ. of Tokyo Press, Tokyo.
30. Victor, M., Adams, R. D., and Mancall, E. L. (1959): A restricted form of cerebellar cortical degeneration occurring in alcoholic patients. *Arch. Neurol.*, 1:579–588.
31. Victor, M., Adams, R. D., and Collins, G. H. (1972): *The Wernicke-Korsakoff Syndrome*. F. A. Davis, Philadelphia.
32. Yamaguchi, T., Hayashi, K., Murakami, H., Ota, K., and Maruyama, S. (1982): Glutamate dehydrogenase deficiency in spinocerebellar degenerations. *Neurochem. Res.*, 7:627–636.

The Olivopontocerebellar Atrophies, edited by
R. C. Duvoisin and A. Plaitakis. Raven Press,
New York © 1984.

Clinical Expression of Glutamate Dehydrogenase Deficiency

Roger C. Duvoisin and Sudhansu Chokroverty

Department of Neurology, University of Medicine and Dentistry of New Jersey, Rutgers Medical School, Academic Health Science Center, New Brunswick, New Jersey 08903

With the aim of defining the clinical expression of glutamate dehydrogenase (GDH) deficiency, we have routinely assayed this enzyme in patients with Parkinson's disease, atypical parkinsonism, chronic progressive ataxia, spastic paraplegia of undetermined cause, progressive supranuclear palsy, the Shy-Drager syndrome, and unclassified progressive extrapyramidal syndromes, as well as in patients diagnosed on clinical grounds as having olivopontocerebellar atrophy (OPCA). Over a period of 3 years we have tested a total of 220 such patients; 10 (4.5%) had values for GDH activity less than 50% of our normal control values. Low values were confirmed by repeat assays on additional blood samples drawn on other occasions. We present here a summary of the clinical features of these patients. We also tested all their available siblings and offspring to gain some notion of the inheritance of GDH deficiency and of the degree of clinical expression of neurological disorder in GDH-deficient individuals.

Early in the course of this work a number of patients with low, usually borderline depression of GDH activity on an initial sample were found to have normal values on repeat testing in a drug-free state. It was found in this way that spurious depression of leukocyte GDH could be caused by a variety of drugs, notably salicylates in antiarthritic doses, indomethacin and related nonsteroidal anti-inflammatory agents, and dietary supplements with linoleic and folic acids. Accordingly, we have been careful to have the patients discontinue all drugs, so far as possible, at least 3 days prior to obtaining a blood sample. Carbidopa, levodopa, amantadine, the anticholinergic antiparkinsonian drugs, diuretics, and cardiac glycosides were not found to interfere with the assay, and these agents were not routinely discontinued in all parkinsonian patients.

GDH ASSAY

The activity of the enzyme was quantitated as previously described (7). Briefly, blood was collected by routine venipuncture in a heparinized syringe and mixed with a 6% solution of dextran in physiological saline. The syringe was allowed to stand inverted for 1 hr. The supernatant plasma was then removed and centrifuged.

The resulting leukocyte pellet was washed in cold isotonic saline, quick-frozen, and stored at − 20°C.

Assays were performed when a sufficient number of samples had been collected. On the day of assay, the leukocytes were disrupted by several freeze/thaw cycles then homogenized in triethanolamine buffer with Triton X-100. GDH activity was initiated by adding sodium oxoglutarate and measured by following the oxidation of NAD(P)H fluorometrically. The results were expressed in micromoles per hour per milligram protein of glutamate formed. All assays were done at least in duplicate; most were done in triplicate.

The values for GDH activity ranged from 227 to 494 μmoles/hr/mg protein (mean 343 + 49.9 SE) in the 10 deficient patients (Table 1). In contrast, the mean value in 20 normal controls was 828 μmoles/hr/mg protein + 151.1 SE. There was no overlap between the normals and the GDH-deficient patients. The latter represented a distinct group.

CLINICAL FEATURES

The history and clinical findings in the 10 patients found to be GDH deficient were those of a chronic, slowly progressive degenerative disease affecting principally the central nervous system and culminating ultimately in severe invalidism in 5 to 20 years. The salient clinical features are summarized in Table 2. The age at diagnosis varied from 48 to 82 years (mean 63.7); the duration of the disease at the time GDH deficiency was established also varied considerably: from 2 to 23 years. The sexual distribution was 7 men and 3 women. One patient died during the period of observation after 26 years of illness, another after only 8 years.

Despite some individual variation, certain features were consistently noted. These included an ataxic gait and impaired coordination of limb movements consistent with cerebellar system disease, extrapyramidal features resembling parkinsonism, a dysarthria progressing in some cases to anarthria, a supranuclear disturbance of eye movement, and a mild peripheral neuropathy. Unsteadiness when walking was the most frequent initial symptom and was always prominent early in the course of the disorder. In one patient, difficulty swallowing was the initial symptom;

TABLE 1. *Glutamate dehydrogenase activity in 10 deficient patients[a] and in 20 normal controls[b]*

Patient	GDH activity (μmol/hr/mg protein)	Patient	GDH activity (μmol/hr/mg protein)
1	342	6	372
2	227	7	297
3	375	8	365
4	315	9	359
5	285	10	494

[a]Mean, 343 + 49.9 SE, GDH activity (μmol/hr/mg protein).
[b]828 + 151.1 SE, GDH activity (μmol/hr/mg protein).

TABLE 2. *Clinical data on 10 symptomatic patients with GDH deficiency*

Patient	Age (yr)	Sex	Duration (yr)	Initial manifestation
1	76	M	4	Bradykinesia, shuffling gait, stooped posture
2	48	M	28	Limb and gait ataxia
3	61	F	4	Unsteady gait, bradykinesia
4	69	M	20	Unsteady gait, bradykinesia
5	70	M	7	Bradykinesia, dysarthria
6	78	M	5	Diplopia, dysphagia, dysarthria
7	76	M	6	Bradykinesia, tremor, rigidity, abnormal gait
8	77	F	12	Right hemiparkinsonism
9	82	F	3	Unsteady gait, bradykinesia
10	61	F	2	Tremor of head and right hand

in another, tremor of the head. In yet another, the clinical picture was primarily cerebellar with truncal and limb ataxia and intention tremor. The gait was slow, short-stepped, shuffling, and festinating in character resembling that of Parkinson's disease. There was loss of associated movements and the patients turned *en bloc*. The patients also displayed features of cerebellar dysfunction; they walked on a broad base, had difficulty performing tandem walking, and were unsteady on turns. However, the lurching and staggering of the typical cerebellar gait was not observed, apparently being obscured or masked by the parkinsonian features. Bradykinesia developed early in the course of the illness in all our patients and was often the most prominent feature. By the time they came to medical attention, a primarily bradykinetic parkinsonism dominated the clinical picture and a diagnosis of Parkinson's disease or parkinsonism was entertained in 9 of our 10 patients. Facial hypomimia was particularly striking, but there was a generalized slowness of all bodily movement, a paucity of spontaneous movement, and a loss both of associated movements and of the automatic movements of postural adjustment.

The plastic resistance to passive movement characteristic of extrapyramidal hypertonicity was found, in some degree, in all patients. Cogwheel rigidity was found in 9 patients. A resting tremor with alternating pronation and supination of the hand and a "pill-rolling" movement of the fingers was seen in several patients, at least on some occasions. Tremor, however, was never a prominent feature and, in most patients, was quite minimal. The remainder had an intention or action tremor. A postural tremor of the arms and a nodding tremor of the head suggestive of essential tremor was present in one patient. The speech was soft and monotone. In this respect, it was reminiscent of that of Parkinson's disease, but it was also slow, slurred, and scanning in quality. Tachyphemia was not noted. In nearly half our patients, dysarthria and dysphagia ultimately became extremely severe. In several patients there was great difficulty eating and 3 patients with long-standing disease were anarthric and aphonic. Nasogastric tube feedings or a feeding gastrotomy were necessary to maintain nutrition, and communication required the use of an alphabet board or electronic communicator. Tongue movements were slow and the gag reflex was diminished or absent, but there was no atrophy of the tongue and no fasciculations were observed.

The jaw jerk was normal. Released oral reflexes were not seen. However, 2 patients had episodes of involuntary laughter and 1 had involuntary weeping. Some impairment of ocular motility was detected in all our patients. Hyperactive vestibuloocular reflexes and fixation instability were the most common abnormalities. Slow saccades were seen in 9 cases. Limitation of vertical and horizontal movements were seen in 5 patients; in 2 of these, there was severe ophthalmoplegia, yet oculocephalic maneuvers elicited a full range of excursions. Minimal gaze-evoked nystagmus was found in several patients. There was no evidence of optic nerve atrophy on funduscopic examination.

Hyperactive reflexes in both the upper and lower extremities and extensor plantar responses were noted in approximately half our patients. These signs of corticospinal tract involvement tended to appear after the disease had progressed for several years. In later stages, the Achilles tendon reflexes were diminished or absent and the patellar reflexes also tended to become less brisk, whereas the plantar responses became more prominent.

Diminished appreciation of vibration distally in the lower extremities was a common finding. Slight impairment of position sense in the toes and a reduction of two-point discrimination in the toes and fingers were found in several patients. Other sensory modalities were not affected on clinical examination. Urinary urgency and incontinence occurred late in the course of the illness in several patients. Orthostatic arterial hypotension was not found in any patient. Pupillary reflexes were preserved. There was no indication of any decrease or loss of sweating.

Formal psychometric testing was not attempted in our patients. Clinical evaluation of mental status was limited in one patient who was also a chronic schizophrenic and in the severely dysarthric or anarthric patients. However, mental faculties appeared to be generally well preserved in the remainder of the group. Even the anarthric patients appeared to be able to communicate intelligently.

Electrophysiological Studies

The clinical findings consistent with a mild peripheral, primarily sensory neuropathy were substantiated on studies of peripheral nerve conduction. Evidence of peripheral nerve dysfunction was detected in all patients tested. Sural nerve sensory potentials were reduced or absent in all 8 patients tested. Median and ulnar nerve sensory potentials were altered in 5 patients. Motor conduction velocities were slowed in the peroneal and tibial nerves in 4 patients. Thus the neuropathy was greater in the lower than in the upper limbs, was distal, and preferentially affected sensory function. Comparable evidence of peripheral neuropathy was not found in other patients classified as having OPCA on clinical grounds with CT scan confirmation of cerebellar atrophy.

Pattern-reversal visual evoked responses were studied in 5 patients. The latency of the major positive wave (P100) was mildly prolonged in 2 patients and was normal in the remainder. Brainstem auditory evoked responses were also studied in these patients. Components I, II, III, and V were prolonged in 3 patients, but the interpeak latencies were all normal. These findings are consistent with a peripheral auditory nerve dysfunction and suggest a parallel involvement of spiral and dorsal root ganglion cells.

Electroencephalography was either normal or showed minimal diffuse slowing and disorganization. Polygraphic studies of sleep revealed episodes of sleep apnea in 2 of 4 patients so studied.

Brain CT Scans

The varied spectrum of atrophic changes seen on CT scanning in our patients was generally consistent with the clinical features. In order to obtain good visualization of the posterior fossa and brainstem, 3 to 5 mm sections were done through the posterior fossa up to the foramina of Munro without contrast. In all but one case, the third and fourth ventricles were enlarged. The widening of the third ventricle, which assumed a tear drop shape, was quite striking in some cases (Fig. 1A). Mild to moderate atrophy of the lateral ventricles was present in some cases. In several cases, the shape of the cerebral peduncle was altered; its normally rounded contour was replaced by an angular appearance and the interpeduncular cistern was widened (Fig. 1B) to suggest atrophy of the corticospinal and corticobulbar tracts. The mesencephalon appeared diminished in size, with the surrounding subarachnoid spaces enlarged. Cerebellar atrophy was very prominent in some cases (Fig. 2), especially in patients with the most striking cerebellar manifestations, but was minimal in other cases.

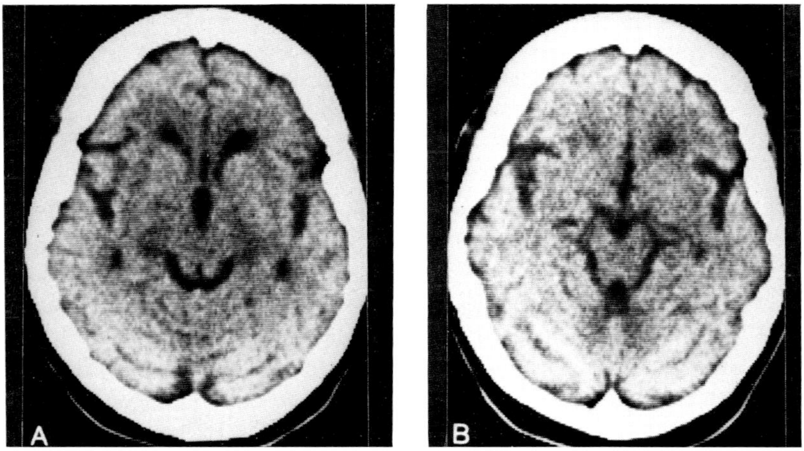

FIG. 1. CT scan of a patient with GDH-deficient OPCA showing atrophy of the mesencephalon and cerebellum with enlargement of the third and fourth ventricles. Note tear drop shape of third ventricle and large ambient cistern **(A)** and atrophied peduncles with wide interpeduncular fossa **(B)**.

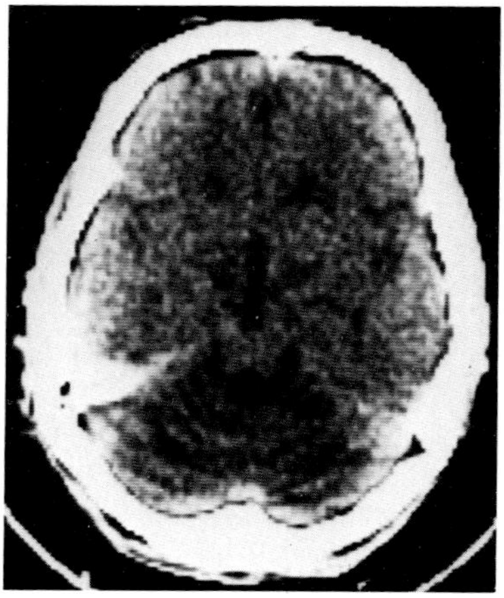

FIG. 2. CT scan of a patient with GDH-deficient OPCA showing particularly severe cerebellar atrophy. Note prominent cerebellar folia.

Genetic Aspects

A positive family history was obtained in 5 of our patients. One may have had a similarly affected parent; another had a granduncle and a maternal grandfather who may have been affected; a third had a sibling who died some years previously with a disorder manifesting ataxia; a fourth proband reported a sibling said to have had multiple sclerosis; another proband had a monozygotic twin who was clinically normal but also GDH deficient. One of the twin's children was clinically affected but unfortunately could not be tested for GDH deficiency. Since many members of this family, the "R" family, were examined and tested, a more detailed account may be of interest.

The proband of the R family was a housewife and former textile mill worker who was noted at age 65 to walk with her arm carried stiffly at her side flexed at the elbow and to drag her right foot. Her handwriting became cramped and small. A diagnosis of Parkinson's disease was made and treatment with trihexyphenidyl prescribed. There was some initial benefit, but her symptoms gradually worsened. At age 70 she had a stooped posture and an expressionless face with infrequent eye blink; she spoke slowly and softly. Her physicians noted cogwheel rigidity more evident on the right side and general bradykinesia. There was no tremor or dysmetria, but alternating movements were performed slowly and awkwardly. She walked on a broad base with short shuffling steps. The tendon reflexes were normally active and the plantar reflexes were flexor. The diagnosis of Parkinson's disease was confirmed by a consulting neurologist. Treatment with trihexyphenidyl was continued. Later, amantadine and levodopa were given, but these yielded little or no benefit. A second consultant described the patient's condition as an atypical form of parkinsonism.

On examination at age 77 the patient was severely bradykinetic with marked facial hypomimia; a soft, slurred scanning speech; and plastic rigidity greater in the right limbs. Eye movements were slow with jerky pursuit and fixation instability.

Alternating movements were performed very slowly. The patient required assistance to arise from her chair and stood in a moderately stooped posture. She walked very slowly on a broad base with short shuffling steps using a walker for support. Her feet frequently seemed glued to the floor. Left standing alone she fell backwards spontaneously, without retropulsion. The tendon reflexes were normally active. The left plantar reflex was extensor; the right was flexor. Vibration sense was decreased at the iliac crests and knee, and absent at the ankles. Mental function appeared grossly normal. A CT brain scan showed moderate ventricular enlargement, especially of the third and fourth ventricles.

When seen again at age 79, the patient was confined to bed and chair, profoundly bradykinetic, and unable to walk even with assistance. There was very little voluntary eye movement, but a full range of movements could be elicited on oculocephalic maneuvers. She could neither maintain eye contact on conversation nor look down at her plate in attempting to eat. Owing to severe dysarthria she could only eat soft foods. Her voice was barely audible and her speech extremely slow and slurred. The patellar reflexes were less active and the ankle jerks were markedly depressed. The plantar reflexes were now both extensor.

A genealogical table of this patient's family is shown in Fig. 3. The patient had two offspring aged 48 and 49 years. Both were clinically normal, but one was GDH deficient. She had 6 siblings including an identical twin. A brother had died of heart disease at age 64. One sister in addition to her twin sister was GDH deficient. Both were asymptomatic. The patient's twin proved to be monozygotic on genotyping performed at the clinical center at the National Institutes of Health, as previously described by Ward et al. (16). She had 6 offspring; 5 were tested and found to be GDH deficient but clinically normal. The sixth was not tested but was affected with a chronic neurological disease characterized by his physicians as postencephalitic parkinsonism. On examination this 57-year-old man was confined

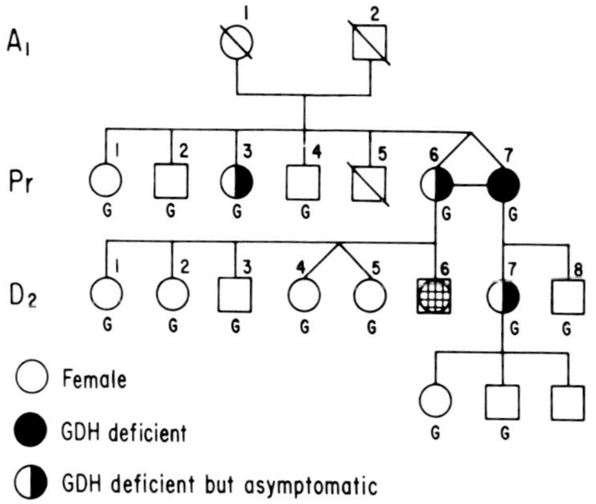

FIG. 3. Genealogical table of the "R" family. The proband is Pr-7. Her monozygotic twin Pr-6, another sister Pr-3, and her daughter DI-7 are GDH deficient but asymptomatic; her nephew DI-7 is clinically affected, but his GDH activity was not measured. Family members tested for GDH deficiency are indicated by "G".

to bed and chair, noticeably bradykinetic with severe generalized rigidity. His speech was severely dysarthric and barely intelligible. Dysphagia, constant drooling, and episodes of involuntary crying were observed. Alternating movements of the hands and feet were performed poorly and very slowly. He was able to stand up only with assistance and stood with the trunk flexed. He was, however, able to walk with a cane, very slowly on a broad base with short shuffling steps. Retropulsion was easily elicited. The tendon reflexes were hyperactive with wrist and ankle clonus. The plantar reflexes were bilaterally extensor. Although a GDH assay could not be obtained, it appears reasonable to conclude that he had the same illness as the proband, discussed above.

At present, excluding the monozygotic twin from consideration, GDH had been assayed for in 25 first-degree relatives (8 siblings and 17 children) and found deficient in 4 of these relatives, comprising 2 women and 2 men. If we assume that both the affected son of the monozygotic twin of our proband in the R family and the ataxic deceased sibling mentioned above had GDH deficiency disease, then 6 of 27 proband relatives had the enzyme defect. These data suggest an autosomal dominant pattern of inheritance with incomplete penetrance.

The data also indicate that GDH deficiency is clinically silent in a large proportion of affected individuals, most likely because the first-degree relatives tested were younger than the mean age of onset of the symptoms in the clinically affected family members. It seems likely that at least some of the asymptomatic GDH-deficient individuals will develop neurological manifestations. (On the other hand, it also seems clear that some individuals deficient in the enzyme will not experience any neurological disease.) Thus, patients with GDH-deficient disease having no clinically affected relatives, may appear to represent, albeit falsely, a sporadic disorder. It would be impossible to understand the genetic basis of the clinical disorder in these cases without knowledge of the underlying enzyme defect.

It is tempting to speculate that GDH deficiency may represent a Mendelian homozygous state, but there are problems in this formulation. First, the enzyme appears to be only partially deficient, not totally absent. Second, one would expect to find that one-half the first-degree relatives, being heterozygous, would have a minor decrease in the activity of the enzyme.

The first point might be explained by the existence of two forms or moeities of the enzyme under different genetic control. The suggestion of Plaitakis et al. (13) that there are two isoenzymes is thus of great interest. Possibly, also, the deficient activity of the enzyme may reflect a defect elsewhere in the cascade of control mechanisms regulating GDH.

With regard to the second point, our data do not indicate a bimodal distribution of values for GDH activity among the first-degree relatives, as would be expected if there were a heterozygous population. However, the variability in the enzyme assay from one run to another is such that the data may not be adequate to fairly exclude this possibility. Further research is needed to resolve these issues and clarify the nature of the enzyme deficiency in this disorder.

PATHOGENESIS

The pathogenesis of the neurological disorder associated with GDH deficiency remains to be defined. It appears plausible to suggest, however, that the enzyme deficiency is more than a mere diagnostic marker, useful as that may be. Abnormal regulation of GDH could permit the accumulation of toxic levels of glutamic acid in synaptic compartments where it could then induce neuronal degeneration in accordance with the concept of neuroexcitotoxic action proposed by Olney (11). However, that not all GDH-deficient individuals are clinically affected indicates that some additional factor plays a role.

Anecdotal data in several of our patients suggest that dietary factors may precipitate the clinical disorder. Because the branched-chain amino acids, and especially L-leucine, activate the enzyme, treatment with a high leucine diet or with a dietary supplementation with mixtures of amino acids has been attempted to arrest the progression of the neurological disorder. The results have been encouraging. Plaitakis et al. (13) reported arrest of the disorder in 4 patients treated with amino acid supplements. It is possible to provide approximately 10 g daily of L-leucine by means of a high protein diet. One of our patients has shown no progression of his disease after 3 years on such a diet, with an improvement in peripheral nerve conduction velocities in the lower extremities. This patient had eaten such a diet most of his adult life, but had adopted a low protein diet to diminish the risk of arteriosclerosis shortly before the onset of his first symptoms. Another patient had a postgastrectomy dumping syndrome which severely impaired his nutrition and resulted in substantial weight loss before the onset of his neurological symptoms. A third had a diaphragmatic hiatal hernia resulting in considerable discomfort, poor nutrition, and weight loss prior to the development of her neurological disorder. A fourth patient was placed on a severe reducing diet to combat obesity and diabetes mellitus. Possibly, a loss of an adequate protein intake may have resulted in decompensation in the regulation of glutamate metabolism in these individuals. These observations can, at present, only support speculation, but they do suggest that careful evaluation of dietary factors in both the genesis of the neurological disorder and its treatment is warranted.

Nosology of GDH Deficiency

In the combination of cerebellar, extrapyramidal, and pyramidal manifestations; supranuclear oculomotor dysfunction; bulbar palsy and peripheral neuropathy; the clinical features of GDH deficiency resemble those of the apparently sporadic type of olivopontocerebellar atrophy (OPCA) first described by Dejerine and Thomas (6). Eadie's comprehensive and detailed review of 35 cases studied postmortem (9) depicts a chronic, slowly progressive disorder usually beginning in late adult life with gait ataxia, general bradykinesia, rigidity, tremor, and dysarthria. Some of these cases had been thought to have Parkinson's disease until OPCA was discovered on postmortem study. Parkinsonism was present in 55% of 63 previously published cases of OPCA recently reviewed by Berciano (1).

Although they received little attention until recently, oculomotor abnormalities other than nystagmus have been noted by various authors in "sporadic" forms of OPCA. Indeed, Dejerine and Thomas (6) described peculiarities of eye movement in their 2 cases. Elevation of the eyes occurred in several steps and rapid eye movements were "uncertain" in their first case. Their second case experienced diplopia. Oculomotor defects were also present in the sporadic case reported by Thomas (15) and in the case of Maas and Scherer (10). "Instability" of the eyes was described in one patient with OPCA reviewed at the clinical pathology conference of the Massachusetts General Hospital (3); and in another, reviewed more recently (4), there was "saccadic breakdown of pursuit eye movements"; lateral eye movements were slow and upward gaze was impaired. It is now well recognized that complex abnormalities of eye movement occur regularly in both the dominant and sporadic forms of OPCA (F. Lepore, *this volume*).

Peripheral neuropathy has not been recorded in the apparently sporadic forms of OPCA. Eadie (9) specifically stated that "no abnormalities of sensation" had been found on "adequate examination" in typical cases of sporadic OPCA even though the lateral and posterior columns of the spinal cord showed degenerative changes post mortem. However this may reflect the lack of electrophysiological techniques for measuring peripheral nerve function at the time those cases were studied. In any case, the peripheral neuropathy in our cases was often minimal and might readily have been overlooked on clinical examination alone or considered normal in elderly subjects. Similar evidence of peripheral neuropathy was noted by Plaitakis et al. (14) in 2 of their cases of GDH-deficient OPCA.

Thus the differences between our GDH-deficient patients and the Dejerine–Thomas type of OPCA described in the literature appear to reflect recent improvements in clinical neurology, notably an increased interest in eye movements and the development of clinical neurophysiology rather than significant differences in clinical phenomenology. It appears likely that GDH deficiency accounts for an important subset of the patients currently classified as sporadic OPCA.

Only 1 case has so far been followed to postmortem examination (5). We are hesitant to draw firm conclusions from a single case, but the findings in the patient are of sufficient interest to warrant mentioning here. Grossly, there was atrophy of the olive, pons, and cerebellum with involvement of the middle cerebellar peduncle confirming the CT scan and the clinical diagnosis of OPCA. Microscopically, there was loss of the Purkinje cells and the granule cells of the cerebellum. There was also degeneration of the posterior columns, particularly the fasciculus gracilis, and some loss of anterior horn cells in the spinal cord. An unexpected finding was a marked accumulation of lipofuscin pigment which frequently distended the nerve cell bodies and displaced the nuclei to one side. The pigment was found widely distributed throughout the nervous system and was also present in the dorsal root ganglia (Fig. 4) and in the myenteric plexus. A somewhat similar case with widespread neuronal lipofuscinosis was reported some years ago by Fine et al. (8). These authors referred to similar cases in the literature. A number of separate disorders have been associated with neuronal lipofuscinosis including the Ramsay-

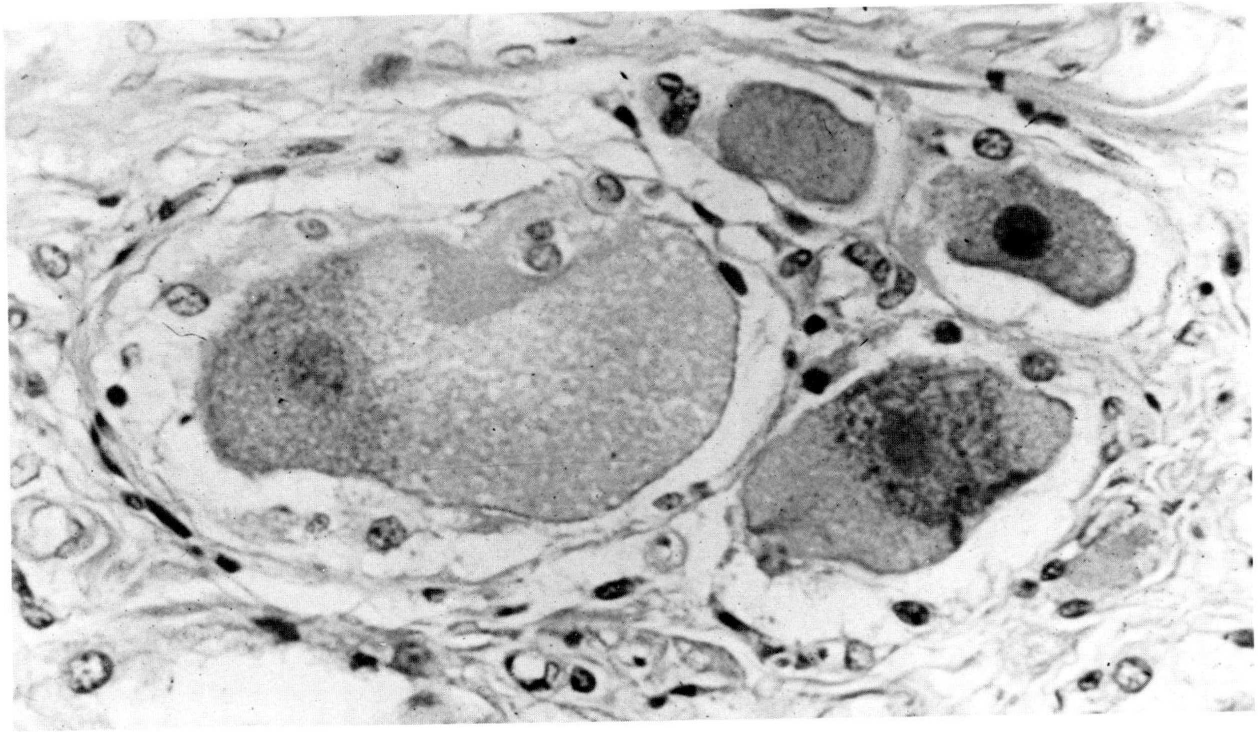

FIG. 4. Neurons distended with lipofuscin pigment in a lumbar dorsal root ganglion of a patient with GDH-deficient OPCA studied post mortem, H & E $\times$ 1,160. (From Chokroverty et al., ref. 5, with permission.)

Huint syndrome (12), Kufs' disease (16), and a distinct, dominantly inherited disorder which has also been reported as a form of Kufs' disease (2). Apparently, we may now add GDH-deficient OPCA to the list of disorders associated with neuronal lipofuscinosis.

Differential Diagnosis

The differentiation of GDH deficiency from other neuronal system degenerations involving the basal ganglia and cerebellum may be quite difficult on clinical grounds alone. Most of our patients were initially considered by their physicians to have parkinsonism. However, as the disease progressed, it became apparent that the parkinsonism was atypical for Parkinson's disease. The development of supranuclear oculomotor impairment caused some difficulty, in several cases, in distinguishing the disorder from progressive supranuclear palsy. None of our patients developed dystonic hyperextension of the neck. The consistent absence of orthostatic hypotension appears to sharply distinguish the GDH-deficiency disease from the Shy-Drager syndrome. Patients presenting a primarily bradykinetic syndrome with minimal cerebellar features would be very difficult to distinguish from those with striatonigral degeneration.

In these circumstances, the recognition of GDH deficiency must depend on appropriate assay of the enzyme. Accordingly, routine screening of all newly diagnosed cases of parkinsonism, and especially those with atypical features, now seems indicated. The diagnostic recognition of GDH deficiency may be of practical value, especially if dietary management proves effective. It will also be of value in improving our understanding of the large heterogenous group of neurodegenerative disorders primarily affecting the basal ganglia and cerebellum.

REFERENCES

1. Berciano, J. (1982): Olivoponto-cerebellar atrophy—A review of 117 cases. *J. Neurol. Sci.*, 53:253–272.
2. Boehme, D. H., Cottrell, J. C., Leonberg, S. C., and Zeman, W. (1971): A dominant form of neuronal ceroid lipofuscinosis. *Brain*, 94:745–760.
3. Case Records of the Massachusetts General Hospital (1981): Case 39–1980. *N. Engl. J. Med.*, 303:803–809.
4. Case Records of the Massachusetts General Hospital (1983): Case 23–1983. *N. Engl. J. Med.*, 308:1406–1414.
5. Chokroverty, S., Khedaker, B., Derby, B., Sachdeo, C., Yook, C., Lepore, F., Nicklas, W., and Duvoisin, R. C. (1984): Olivopontocerebellar atrophy with glutatmate dehydrogenase deficiency: A clinical-pathological study. *Neurology*, 34*(in press)*.
6. Dejerine, J., and Thomas, A. (1900): L'atrophie olivo-ponto-cerebelleuse. *Nouv. Iconogr. Salpet.*, 13:330–370.
7. Duvoisin, R. C., Chokroverty, S., Lepore, F., and Nicklas, W. (1983): Glutamate dehydrogenase deficiency in patients with olivopontocerebellar atrophy. *Neurology*, 33:1322–1326.
8. Fine, D. I. M., Barron, K. D., and Hirano, A. (1960): Central nervous system lipidosis in an adult with atrophy of the cerebellar granular layer. *J. Neuropathol. Exp. Neurol.*, 19:355–369.
9. Eadie, M. J. (1975): Olivoponto-cerebellar atrophy (Dejerine-Thomas type). In: *Handbook of Clinical Neurology*, Vol. 21, edited by P. J. Vinken and G. W. Bruyn, pp. 415–431. Elsevier-North Holland, Amsterdam.

10. Maas, O., and Scherer, H. J. (1933): Zur klinik und anatomie einiger seltener kleinhirnerkrangungen. *Z. Gesamte Neurol. Psychiatr.*, 145:420–444.
11. Olney, J. W. (1978): Neurotoxicity of excitatory amino acids. In: *Kainic Acid as a Tool in Neurobiology*, edited by E. G. McGeer, J. W. Olney, and P. L. McGeer, pp. 95–122. Raven Press, New York.
12. Pallis, C. A., Duckett, S., and Pearse, A. G. E. (1967): Diffuse lipofuscinosis of the central nervous system. *Neurology*, 17:381–394.
13. Plaitakis, A., Berl, S., Yahr, M. D. (1983): The treatment of GDH-deficient olivopontocerebellar atrophy with branched chain amino acids. *Neurology*, 33(Suppl 2):78 (abstr.).
14. Plaitakis, A., Nicklas, W., and Desnick, R. J. (1980): Glutamate dehydrogenase deficiency in three patients with spinocerebellar syndrome. *Ann. Neurol.*, 7:297–303.
15. Thomas, A. (1903): Atrophie du cervelet et sclerose en plaques. *Rev. Neurol.*, 1:121–131.
16. Ward, C. D., Duvoisin, R. C., Ince, S., Nutt, J. D. F., Eldridge, R., and Calne, D. (1983): Parkinson's disease in 65 pairs of twins and in a set of quadruplets. *Neurology* 33:815–824.
17. Zeman, W. (1976): The neuronal ceroid-lipofuscinosis. In: *Progress in Neuropathology*, Vol. 3, edited by H. M. Zimmerman, pp. 203–223. Grune & Stratton, New York.

Subject Index